The Eight
Immortal Healers

The Eight Immortal Healers

Taoist Wisdom for Radiant Health

Mantak Chia and
Johnathon Dao, M.D. (A.M.), L.Ac.

Destiny Books
Rochester, Vermont • Toronto, Canada

Destiny Books
One Park Street
Rochester, Vermont 05767
www.DestinyBooks.com

Destiny Books is a division of Inner Traditions International

Library of Congress Cataloging-in-Publication Data
Names: Chia, Mantak, 1944– author. | Dao, Johnathon, author.
Title: The eight immortal healers : taoist wisdom for radiant health / Mantak Chia, Johnathon Dao, M.D. (AM).
Description: Rochester, Vermont : Destiny Books, [2017] | Includes index. | Description based on print version record and CIP data provided by publisher; resource not viewed.
Identifiers: LCCN 2016057823 (print) | LCCN 2017013644 (e-book) | ISBN 9781620556504 (paperback) | ISBN 9781620556511 (e-book)
Subjects: LCSH: Qi gong. | Qi gong—Therapeutic use. | Mind and body therapies. | Health—Popular works. | BISAC: HEALTH & FITNESS / Alternative Therapies. | BODY, MIND & SPIRIT / Healing / Energy (Chi Kung, Reiki, Polarity). | PHILOSOPHY / Taoist.
Classification: LCC RA781.8 C46925 2017 (print) | LCC RA781.8 (e-book) | DDC 613.7/1489—dc23
LC record available at https://lccn.loc.gov/2016057823

Printed and bound in the United States

10   9   8   7   6   5   4   3   2

Text design by Priscilla H. Baker and layout by Virginia Scott Bowman
This book was typeset in Garamond Premier Pro and Futura with Present and Futura used as display typefaces

Photographs by Sopitnapa Promnon
Illustrations by Udon Jandee

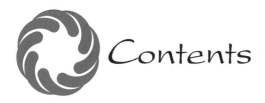 Contents

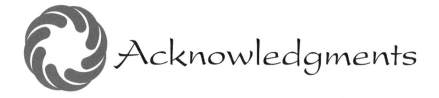

Acknowledgments

The authors and Universal Healing Tao Publications staff involved in the preparation and production of *The Eight Immortal Healers* extend our gratitude to the many generations of Taoist masters who have passed on their special lineage in the form of an unbroken oral transmission over thousands of years. We thank Taoist master Yi Eng (One Cloud Hermit) for his openness in transmitting the formulas of Taoist Inner Alchemy.

We offer eternal gratitude to our parents and teachers for their many gifts to us. Remembering them brings joy and satisfaction to our continued efforts in presenting the Universal Healing Tao system. For their gifts, we offer our eternal gratitude and love. As always, their contribution has been crucial in presenting the concepts and techniques of the Universal Healing Tao.

We wish to thank the thousands of unknown men and women of the Chinese healing arts who developed many of the methods and ideas presented in this book. We offer gratitude to Bob Zuraw for sharing his kindness, healing techniques, and Taoist understandings.

We thank the many contributors essential to this book's final form: the editorial and production staff at Inner Traditions/Destiny Books for their efforts to clarify the text and produce a handsome new edition of the book, and Margaret Jones for her line edit of the new edition.

We wish to thank the following people for their assistance in producing the earlier edition of this book: Colin Drown for his editorial work and writing contributions, as well as his ideas for the cover.

And special thanks goes to our Thai production team: Hirunyathorn Punsan, Sopitnapa Promnon, Udon Jandee, and Suthisa Chaisarn.

• • •

Johnathon Dao would love to offer his personal gratitude to Diana and Peter Smith, Dr. Tony Holt, Jessa O'My Heart, Theme Rains, Maree Thomas, Liz and Jill Henry, Emma and Alex Grant, Neal Hoptman, Jacqueline and Marco Vasquez. Also big thanks to Francisco, Audrey and Luke Oliveira, Etta Win, Jenni Stott, Jenni Saukonen, Patrick Riddall, Arthur Lane, Gillian Miller, Dr G Sofi, Eric Freymond, Glen Pelham-Mather, Owen Formosa, Dr. Brad Jones, Carey O'Sullivan, Jennifer Kelly, Ian and Jenny Curnow at Tweed Coast Chiropractic, and all dear friends who guide and help me so much. And he wishes to thank Eden Health Retreat, Australia's most successful health retreat, and Oliver's Real Food Restaurants, the first all-organic restaurant chain.

Thanks also to senseis Masakazu Ikeda, Edward Obaidey, and Alan Jansson, who have taught me traditional Japanese acupuncture and Chinese medicine. To Lama Gyurme for Buddhist teachings and to Master Mantak Chia for teaching me the wisdom of the Tao.

Master Chia and Johnathon Dao are both so grateful to share the Eight Immortals with the world to assist in their radiant health transformation.

Putting the Taoist Immortal Principles into Practice

The information presented in this book is based on the authors' personal experience and knowledge of the Eight Immortals, the legendary Taoist healers of Chinese mythology. Some of the practices described in this book have been used successfully for thousands of years by Taoists trained through personal instruction from a lineage of masters. Readers should not undertake these Taoist practices without receiving personal transmission and training from a certified instructor of the Universal Healing Tao, since some of these practices, if done improperly, may cause injury or result in health problems. This book is intended to supplement individual training by the Universal Healing Tao and to serve as a reference guide for these practices. As well, many other practices described herein stem from various traditions and sources, including modern naturopathic medicine, traditional Chinese medicine, yoga, ayurveda, and modern Western medicine practices. Anyone who undertakes these practices on the basis of this book alone does so entirely at his or her own risk.

The meditations, practices and techniques described in this book are not intended to be used as an alternative or substitute for professional medical treatment and care. If any readers are suffering from illnesses based on physical, mental, or emotional disorders, an appropriate professional health care practitioner or therapist should be consulted. Such problems should be corrected before you start Universal Healing Tao training.

Neither the Universal Healing Tao nor its staff and instructors are responsible for the consequences of any practice or misuse of the information contained in this book. If the reader undertakes any exercise without strictly following the instructions, notes, and warnings, the responsibility lies solely with the reader.

This book does not attempt to give any medical diagnosis, treatment, prescription, or remedial recommendation in relation to any human disease, ailment, suffering, or physical condition whatsoever.

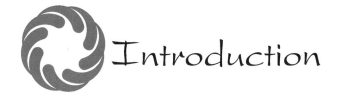 # Introduction

You can fool some of the people all of the time, and all of the people some of the time, but you cannot fool all the people all the time.

ATTRIBUTED TO ABRAHAM LINCOLN

Be careful about reading health books. You may die of a misprint.

MARK TWAIN

In his 1996 book *The Electric Universe,* David Elliott says, "Never before has there been so much talk about health. Never before have people been so unhealthy." Today, the sicker we are as a society, the more money the medical industry makes, including the doctors, hospitals, and drug companies that compose this system. To put it plainly, our health care system gains wealth and power from sickness rather than from health. This has caused the health care system to spin out of control, allowing the system's "authorities" to keep us in the dark on the real causes of disease and how to prevent them or effectively cure them.

We now live in a world of human-made diseases. During the early part of the past century the four main causes of death were all infectious diseases such as pneumonia and tuberculosis. Due to technological advancements in diagnosing and as a result of more advanced scientific understanding of how disease microorganisms spread, there has been a decrease in the number of people perishing from infectious disease. So today, although we are living longer, we are also getting sick and dying of degenerative "lifestyle diseases" and various environmental factors, and this includes children as well as adults. The American Cancer Society reports that in the United States in 2007, approximately 10,400 children under the age of fifteen were diagnosed with cancer, and about 1,545 children will die from this disease, making cancer the leading cause of disease-caused death among U.S. children between the ages of one and fourteen.

While modern medicine takes credit for its amazing discoveries of viruses and bacteria and its invention of antibiotics and vaccines (more about those later in this book), it seems to be doing little to protect and teach the general population about the true causes of chronic degenerative diseases and how to effectively prevent them. Most people living in developed countries today do not die at the hands of a virus, but rather by their own hands, and they haven't even a clue as to how this happens. Heart disease, cancer, stroke, and diabetes are the major killers in the developed world today. These diseases didn't even rank in the top ten causes of death a hundred years ago. So what happened? What about the mountains of scientific studies on prevention through diet, nutrition, exercise, meditation, and other lifestyle factors? After all, the true causes of these human-made degenerative diseases are well known and can actually be prevented provided there is correct education. So why are we not doing this effectively in our schools or in the media?

Some scholars say that today's medical institutions are no longer run by honest people and have become more like giant corporations, moving away from finding cures to spend most of their time and money creating expensive symptomatic treatments that rely on costly pharmaceutical drugs (that many people can't even afford). It seems that when you cure the patient, you lose the patient, and therefore the profits. When a medical system is based on profiting from sickness rather than from health, it becomes a "disease-care industry" rather than a true health care system.

Make no mistake: modern medicine is not without its many successes, one being the increase in life span. The place where allopathic medicine excels over natural medicine is in emergency situations, where patients can be stabilized by means of powerful drugs, surgery, and other technological interventions. Allopathic medicine also succeeds in treating serious injuries from motor-vehicle accidents and gunshot wounds, and in reconstructive surgery, general trauma diagnostics, organ transplants, scanning technology, and certain kinds of blood tests. What we are questioning is its inability to treat and prevent illness and promote true health and wellness through fostering harmony within and without.

As a result of our improved standards of living in the developed world we are exposed to less contagious diseases, but this is all beginning to change. Antibiotic usage in the last decades has led to super-resistant infectious diseases, and it's getting out of control. We regularly read about stronger and more mutated pathogens that threaten to become another plague for humanity, and immunizations supposedly designed to address this have not really saved us at all. In fact, widespread antibiotic use has made our immune systems weaker than ever before. So modern medicine has not really succeeded in keeping us healthy over the long term, but it has made a "quick buck" that could spell big trouble for humanity in the near future.

There is no room for greed and politics to exist in our system of medicine, but it does. There is no room for corruption to exist where human life is concerned, but it does. There is no room for the public to be ignorant as to what is going on all around us, pretending this is not happening, but by and large they are. So now it is time to take back our power and reeducate ourselves on the immense possibilities that other forms of medicine and health care can provide in these extremely challenging times.

In this book we refer to modern mainstream medicine as *allopathic medicine* or *allopathy*. We refer to natural medical practices such as traditional Chinese medicine (TCM), ayurvedic medicine, naturopathy, and other modalities as *natural medicine* (rather than *alternative medicine*) because in many cases these forms of medicine are beneficial as primary treatment methods rather than as some New Age alternative.

The Different Approaches of Allopathic and Natural Medicine

Having a thorough understanding of the differences between allopathic medicine and natural medicine can allow you to make a clearer and more educated choice about your health care.

Basic Premise of Health Care

Allopathic Medicine: Invade, attack, dissect, remove, or destroy diseased tissue and organs by surgically cutting or dissecting the malfunctioned parts, removing them altogether or replacing them with another person's organs or artificial mechanical parts; treat symptoms with drugs that have toxic side effects.

Natural Medicine: Eliminate the cause of the disease, whether it be chemical, nutritional, environmental, mental, or spiritual; educate the person in how to maintain lifestyle habits, diet, and mental/emotional health that promotes self-healing; integrate a combination of different and complementary natural therapies addressing all levels of body, mind, and spirit.

Medications Used

Allopathic Medicine: Man-made, inorganic, synthetic drugs derived from petrochemicals, coal tar, animal products, and other substances that suppress or stimulate the body's chemical processes, causing symptomatic relief only rather than curing, and may cause dependence; radiation and chemotherapy result in cell death, with severe side effects.

Natural Medicine: Organic substances derived from Mother Nature, including foods and herbs that detoxify, cleanse, nourish, and promote the body's innate self-healing processes, with little or no side effects when used correctly; additional, complementary techniques may be physical, energetic, or spiritual healing therapies such as loving touch and gentle manipulation of the physical body to remove blockages in the physical, emotional, and spiritual levels.

Role of Patient

Allopathic Medicine: Person is a passive recipient of treatment by medical authority figure and is regarded as a victim of external circumstances and therefore of disease that "attacks" the person.

Natural Medicine: Person is actively involved in healing process and encouraged by practitioner to take full responsibility for his/her own health and well-being by understanding the underlying causes, be they physical, mental, emotional, or spiritual.

The number-one cause of disease and premature death in today's world is not really cancer or heart disease; it's ignorance—ignorance about the true nature of what constitutes physical, emotional, and spiritual health. Yet this is changing. We are constantly astounded by the amount of health information clients seem to have when they come to our clinics and health retreats for the first time. People are beginning to do more research and take an open stand on their natural health care. Many don't buy into the allopathic medical establishment's fearmongering anymore, but also be careful about becoming an armchair expert. People nowadays are taking the initiative to become informed, and that is good as Taoists have always encouraged us to learn as much as we can about our bodies and cultivate our wisdom, but self-help, health, and diet books are being pumped out almost faster than cola bottles. Books on natural healing have become a staple item, in turn making many readers instant experts. These days, if you read a book on herbs, you're suddenly an herb expert, or if you do a weekend Reiki workshop and get a Reiki master certificate, you're suddenly a master healer, but Taoist wisdom has taught us that it is not that easy!

We openly encourage you to research and question everything we offer you in this book; don't just accept it on blind faith. We need to trust health professionals, but we must also take responsibility for our own health and acknowledge that *we* are the ones responsible for our state of health. Strive to be an ardent listener and learn from your practitioner, and participate in your own healing process each day. Of course, feel free to express your doubts and concerns to your natural medicine practitioner (and to your allopathic doctor especially), but understand that they are doing their job to the best of their knowledge and experience, and they are not the godlike figures we so often have come to expect doctors to be. We recommend that you use this book to educate yourself and learn what to look for. Work with a trusted practitioner, whether of allopathic or natural medicine, who is willing to communicate and work with you for your benefit.

THE NEXUS OF NATURAL AND ALLOPATHIC MEDICINE

All truth passes through three stages: first it is ridiculed, second it is violently opposed, and third it is accepted as self-evident.

ARTHUR SCHOPENHAUER,
NINETEENTH-CENTURY PHILOSOPHER

When we look at traditional systems of medicine, we often find the use of certain symbols as a means of demonstrating the importance of addressing the body-mind-spirit connection. Tai Chi, which translates as "Supreme Ultimate," is commonly depicted as the yin-yang symbol that almost everyone is familiar with. The Tai Chi symbol is used to represent Taoist teachings and traditional Chinese medicine (TCM), as well as many other oriental art forms that demonstrate the philosophy of the laws of complementary opposites and the laws of nature.

The yin-yang symbol has two aspects or sides; however, there are in reality three aspects to this symbol. Yin is said to be feminine, like the moon and nighttime, while yang is masculine and is represented by the sun and daytime. The third aspect is the connection between them that allows both to exist together in harmony, just like a normal day, where the sun goes down in the evening and the moon comes up. This third aspect is known as the spirit-soul, or *shen*. This aspect connects the two, for without spirit (shen) and body (yin), the mind (yang) would cease to exist. The spirit could be likened to space in this example, as it allows the sun and moon to exist and live together in harmony. Without space, neither the sun nor the moon would exist; similarly, we need shen, and not only a body and mind, to exist. Just like the yin-yang symbol, our health also reflects this same principle.

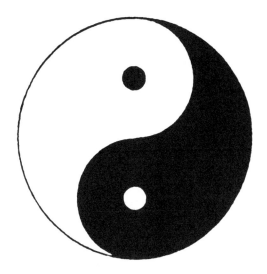

The yin-yang symbol

The yin-yang symbol originates in the ancient sages' study of the seasons and elements of nature and how they affect us and our health, and not all that New Age stuff it's often associated with. You see, the ancient Chinese understood that we are connected in some way to nature and the elements, and this means that we must be connected to the seasons that create them. When observing the cycle of the sun, ancient Chinese Taoist scholars simply used a pole about eight feet long and posted it at right angles to the ground to record the position of the shadows. From this they discovered that the length of a year is approximately 365.25 days. They evenly divided the year's cycle into twenty-four parts using the sunrise and Dipper positions to delineate the vernal equinox, the autumnal equinox, the summer solstice, and the winter solstice. They then used six concentric circles to mark the twenty-four segment points and divided the circles into twenty-four sectors and recorded the length of the shadow each day. The shortest shadow is found on the summer solstice, while the longest, of course, is found on the winter solstice. After connecting all the lines and dimming the yin part from summer solstice to winter solstice, the sun chart looks like it does in the figure on page 8. The ecliptic angle of 23.26.19 degrees of Earth can be seen in this diagram.

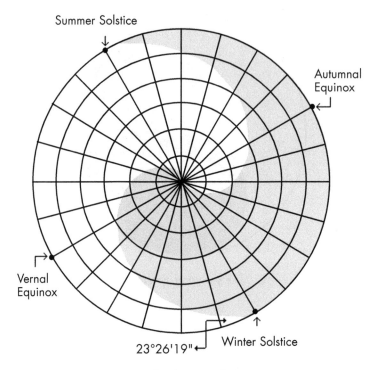

Seasonal solstice and equinox

In ancient China, Taoist doctors were known to be superior clinicians. One reason for this is that they did not have the advanced technology that we rely on so heavily today to measure bodily functions. Instead they intuitively evolved other forms of diagnosing illness, such as pulse, tongue, and meridian diagnosis. Medicine at that time had an entirely different approach and attitude compared to what exists in allopathy today. Prevention was regarded as the ultimate cure, so much so that the practice of seeing illness before it actually manifested physically was a highly respected skill in traditional medicine. Taoist doctors were employed by villages to keep people healthy rather than to just medicate their ills; in fact, in most cases they were paid only when their patients got well. Consequently, Chinese medicine was forced to develop a strong understanding of the true causes of diseases, and in turn they had to educate people on how to prevent them. As medicine at that time based its success on people's health and not their sicknesses, it had an entirely different approach. It was common knowledge that sick people gave no rewards and offered no financial gain to doctors, whereas healthy people in a community brought more respect to doctors and therefore financial success.

The preamble to the constitution of the World Health Organization as adopted by the International Health Conference in 1946 defines health as "a state of complete physical, mental and social well-being and not merely the absence of disease or infirmity." Today, most forms of natural medicine are termed "alternative" or "New Age"; however, most of these forms of medicine are not New Age, nor are they alternative. By combining the more modern discoveries of anatomy, physiology, chemistry, and pathology with the ancient ways of treating the *cause* rather than the *symptoms* of illness, both allopathic and natural medicine can come together to form something special, delivering effective solutions to today's so-called incurable diseases. So while treating symptoms is important when someone is in severe pain or needs surgery, eliminating the cause of the problem must be the first step in bringing about any possible cure.

Many traditional forms of healing have had long and successful histories, including ancient Egyptian, ayurvedic, and traditional Chinese medicine (TCM). What all these systems have in common is that they understand that the human being is more than just a physical body; it is a subtle-energy body made of many elements that make us whole. Disease can manifest as a result of poor diet, environmental factors, genetic weakness, and even the emotions. The study of the connection between the mind and the emotions and its relationship to specific health problems is sometimes called *metaphysics*. This advanced subject is not taught, nor is it even mentioned, in allopathic medical institutions today, and if mentioned at all, it's laughed at. What allopathic medicine does state is that stress can aggravate health conditions and sometimes cause them, while the finer details of this complex subject are not properly understood. A truly holistic system of medicine must effectively address *all* levels of imbalance, educating the patient on the true causes of a disease while effectively treating it, and incorporating educational steps on how to prevent it in the future. Understanding the different elements of the human body, mind, and spirit, and how they are interrelated, is the key to having true health, the truest of all wealth. To do this we must first understand the basic laws of health before complete healing can occur. As an Egyptian proverb states, "Disregarding the absurd or unorthodox may mean a lost chance to understand the universal laws."

Sixteenth-century Swiss-German philosopher and physician Paracelsus believed that physical health relied on the harmony of man (microcosm) with nature (macrocosm), an idea that was considered heretical at the time, although this view had been commonly accepted in Asia for thousands of years. Now, even after massive advancements in modern medical technology, many of us are returning the views of Paracelsus.

THE EIGHT FORCES OF NATURE

When I (Johnathon Dao) first began studying natural medicine I was confused about one particular aspect: unlike allopathic medicine, which is organized into innumerable specialties and subspecialties, natural medicine did not seem to be arranged in any logical order in terms of core foundational protocols. Therefore, if you wanted to give it a try, your understanding as to which particular form of natural medicine would best work for your particular problem or disease could be problematic, with the results sometimes even dangerous. It seems that all the various natural medicine practitioners do not understand enough about one another's area of specialty either. For example, osteopaths sometimes do not have a clue as to what an herbalist or acupuncturist does, and they do not refer patients or communicate regularly with other types of natural-medicine practitioners to understand what they are doing. Frequently, the homeopath only understands homeopathy and hasn't a clue as to what the naturopath, who may be practicing in the room next door, is doing. Even conventional allopathic medical doctors of different specialities get together and have their seminars and discuss the latest pharmaceutical drugs and diseases and are required to have the same basic formal training, as in the case of the M.D. or M.B.B.S. (Bachelor of Medicine, Bachelor of Surgery) degrees.

What sort of so-called holistic medicine is this, I thought, when practitioners are not educated in the basics of one another's disciplines and lack the same basic formal training across all these disciplines? It often seems to me to be more like a hodgepodge than a complete, integrated system of holistic medicine, as each form of therapy, from homeopathy to crystal healing, claims to cure you of this or that. For a layperson deciding to skip the symptomatic approach and often dangerous treatment that uses drugs or surgery and give natural medicine a try, it can seem very confusing as to where to start and whom to trust. The majority of people using natural medicine just try this or try that, as no standard protocol currently exists for the many different natural medicine practitioners to follow, nor are there a standard set of guidelines for patients. There had to be some organizing principle in this profusion, so I made it my life's work to find it.

Around this time I was blessed to happen upon a rare bookshop, where I found a book by Master Mantak Chia. There I discovered that traditional Taoist wisdom organizes all the different types of natural medicine into the eight forces of nature. As I began learning more and more about the different natural medicine disciplines, I began placing each of them into categories determined by these eight forces, thus aligning them with the *pakua* (or *bagua*), the eight trigrams used in Taoist cosmology to represent the fundamental principles of reality, seen as a range of eight interrelated concepts. This ancient Chinese model for understanding the interrelated system of the body was there all along; its principles are easy to follow and understand, and the protocols involved in this model can help us maintain our physical, mental, and spiritual health in these demanding and stressful times.

The eight forces of nature are as follows:

Kan/Water: the gathering yin power, connected with the kidneys, ears, and sexual organs; therapies connected with water hydration

Li/Fire: the prospering power, connected with the heart; therapies connected with internal exercises

Chen/Thunder: the gathering power; wood element, connected with the liver and eyes; therapies involving electrical medicine

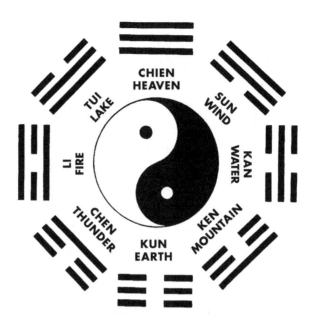

The pakua: the eight trigrams of the eight forces

Tui/Lake: contracting power, connected with the lungs and nose, the metal element; therapies that address chemical poisons

Kun/Earth: the stabilizing power of harmony, connected with the stomach and mouth, spleen and pancreas; therapies that involve cleansing and purification

Ken/Mountain: stability and strength, connected with the bladder, right sexual organs, and back of skull; therapies involving nutritional healing

Sun/Wind: connected with the gallbladder and the base of the skull; therapies involving oxygenation

Chien/Heaven: expanding yang energy, connected with left sexual organs, large intestine, and forehead bone; therapies that involve emotional and spiritual healing

Each of these eight forces of nature is also associated with a geographical direction, season, color, planet, animal, organ of the body, and so forth. So when one fully understands and practices all eight elements of the pakua, only then does true healing take place. If any aspect of the eight forces is neglected, the body cannot do what it is designed to do implicitly, which is to heal itself.

Note that the number 8 holds special significance for Taoists. Aside from being a Fibonacci number, it is the only positive Fibonacci number, aside from 1, that is a perfect cube. It also represents the eight solar terms of the year and maps with the yin-yang symbol. Notably, the importance of the number 8 to Chinese culture came to the attention of the Western world when the Beijing Olympics commenced at exactly 8:08 p.m. on the eighth day of the eighth month of the year 2008.

THE FIVE ELEMENTS

In addition to the eight forces of nature, the principle of the five elements comes into play in Taoist medicine, as each of the eight forces represents one of the five elements. Through careful observation of their surroundings, traditional doctors who lived thousands of years ago began to understand the importance of being in harmony with the five universal elements and cosmic energies. This fundamental understanding of the universe was considered a good basis for understanding health as being determined by all five of the elements at work in our bodies, those both seen and unseen—and five-element theory was born.

Five-element medicine classifies imbalances in the body according to the five different natural elements present in our bodies, in the environment, and in the universe at large: water, wood, fire, earth, and metal. Such diverse things as compass direction, taste, human organs, sounds, food groups, emotions, animals, and stages of growth can all be classified according to the five elements.

According to traditional Chinese medicine, when the body is in disharmony with the environment, a stage of unease or "dis-ease" enters it through one or more of five elements, in turn affecting all the other elements. Some in the health profession are under the assumption that the emotions are the prime cause of all our ailments. The reason our emotions and beliefs have such a profound effect on our physical body is primarily because the emotional and mental bodies are less dense than the physical body, allowing them to have the power to greatly affect it on an energetic level. You can see as well as feel when your physical body is sick; just look in the mirror. On the other hand, if your emotions are sick you can suppress them, sweeping them under the rug until they creep up on you and attack your organs and physical structures. The emotions, which stem from the egoic mind, have the power to override chemical processes inside the organs and tissues, so in most cases they must be treated alongside the physical body when there is a health problem.

FIVE-ELEMENT TABLE OF CORRESPONDENCES

ELEMENT	WATER	WOOD (ETHER)	FIRE	EARTH	METAL (AIR)
Season	Winter	Spring	Summer	Indian summer	Autumn
Climate	Cold	Wind	Heat	Damp	Dryness
Yang organs	Bladder	Gallbladder	Small Intestine	Stomach	Large Intestine
Yin organs	Kidneys	Liver	Heart	Spleen	Lungs
Sense	Ears	Eyes	Tongue	Mouth	Nose
Tissue	Bone	Tendons	Vessels	Muscles	Skin
Emotions	Fear	Anger	Anxiety	Worry	Sadness
	Gentle	Kindness	Patience	Grounded	Courage
Color	Blue	Green	Red	Yellow	White
Taste	Salty	Sour	Bitter	Sweet	Spicy

The five elements are demonstrated in the form of a nourishing cycle, which explains how harmony occurs in the body through mutual promotion:

• Water promotes wood (nourishing it to grow)
• Wood promotes fire (burning medium)
• Fire promotes earth (by creating ash)
• Earth promotes metal (minerals formed)
• Metal promotes water (through condensation)

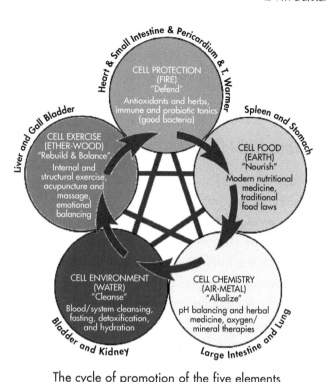

The cycle of promotion of the five elements

On the other hand, when illness occurs in the body, the five elements take on a completely different flow. This is called the *control cycle,* where the elements, instead of nourishing one another, which leads to good health, begin to control one another:

- Metal controls wood (chopping it down)
- Fire controls metal (melting it)
- Water controls fire (putting it out)
- Earth controls water (damming it)
- Wood controls earth (covering it)

Five-element theory is based on careful observation between humans and their relationship to their environment. This practical framework for understanding and determining energetic and physical imbalances within the body's organs has proved effective for more than three thousand years. Only relatively recently has it begun to receive attention in the West because many people have come to realize that the prevailing medical paradigm, based largely on the use of drugs and surgery, has failed to cure disease and has done long-term damage to our environment.

THE EIGHT IMMORTAL HEALERS

Each of the eight forces of nature is represented by one of the Eight Immortal Healers, a group of eight Taoist yogis from Chinese history, each of whom is briefly introduced in each of the following chapters. That said, it is not the purpose of this book to focus on the history or mythology of these legendary Taoist sages. Here we use them simply as guides or organizing principles for the eight healing forces of nature that each represents. All the different forms of natural medicine can be categorized according to these Eight Immortals, because as keepers of Taoist wisdom they contain the secrets of the eight forces of nature and the eight parts, or trigrams, of the pakua. Each Immortal is a symbol of an aspect of health and spiritual wealth and a keeper of wisdom who helps to enlighten seekers on the way of the Tao.

The Eight Immortals and their associated forces of nature as delineated in the pakua are:

> Han Hsien-Ku: Sun/Wind
> Chang Kuo-Lao: Kan/Water
> Tsao Kuo-Chiu: Ken/Mountain
> Ho Hsien-Ku: Kun/Earth
> Lu Tung-Pin: Tui/Lake
> Li Tieh-Kuai: Li/Fire
> Chuan Chung-Li: Chen/Thunder
> Lan Tsai-Ho: Chien/Heaven

These Eight Immortal Healers are called "immortal" because they have always been and always will be *universal* laws for the health of humankind. Each of the Eight Immortals has many aspects, and no individual Immortal is more important than any other. In fact, it is by the loving assistance provided by all eight of these healers combined that the body is able to self-heal.

Again, please remember that all eight of these healers need to be respected for their importance in affecting the totality of the body, mind, and spirit-soul. I have come to understand that there is only one disease: sick cells. And there are only two causes of sick cells: too much of something (excess) or not enough of something (deficiency). Maintaining a balance that is free from deficiency or excess and learning the Eight Immortal Healers is the key to Taoist wisdom and radiant health, and the subject of this book.

Today, allopathy says that many conditions, from obesity to autoimmune diseases, are genetic, but it has been proven that while most of us hold the genes for these diseases, we don't necessarily suffer from them. What really happens is that these genes are "ignited" when we do not adhere to the principles underlying the Eight Immortal Healers. I am not saying that everything can be healed; some things we are born with as a result of our genetics. But many times by using the principles of the Eight Immortals, these kinds of factors, often considered beyond our control, can be managed.

The idea behind this book when I first began compiling information for it was to create a personal resource for understanding the profusion of natural medicine protocols while assembling a valuable healing checklist for my clients. With more than twenty years of clinical practice under my belt now, combined with Master Chia's many decades of practice and teaching, we have begun to realize the purpose of accumulating these vital protocols, which is to simplify the healing process.

We have been reminded time and time again that information is useless unless acted on, and it's not so important how much we know, but what we do with the little we do know. When you begin applying the simple health habits outlined in this book, you may be amazed at how effective and powerful they can be. Knowledge is power, so take back your innate healing power and discover the simplicity of healing your body, mind, and spirit with the Eight Immortal Healers. Here in these writings you will learn that medicine is about to undergo a paradigm shift (with your participation), and that prevention is truly the ultimate cure. And as with ancient physicians like Hippocrates, the doctors of the future will treat the whole person—body, mind, and spirit—seeing these three aspects as inseparable and interrelated, totally dependent on one another for true health to occur. This is the foundation of the teachings of the Taoist sages.

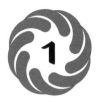

First Immortal Healer—Han Hsien-Ku

Oxygen Is the Body's Prime Nutrient

Oxygen to a healthy cell is like an electrically charged screen door to flies: a virus, like a fly, cannot penetrate these defenses.

DR. OTTO WARBURG

The healing that relates to wind concerns oxygenation, specifically, our vital breath; it is symbolized by Immortal Han Hsien-Ku. This sage was born in the eighth century CE and was a nephew of the great Tang poet and scholar Han Yu. While still a teenager Han Hsien-Ku was initiated into the secrets of Taoism by his fellow Immortal Lu Tung-Pin, and he quickly became absorbed in the practice of internal alchemy, eschewing all worldly distractions. He probed the mysteries of heaven and mastered the five phases (i.e., elements) of energy. He is often depicted carrying a magical flute on which he plays the Six Healing Sounds, and he rides a buffalo, symbol of the Hsi Wang Mu, the shamanic Queen Mother or Great Goddess of China who controls the cosmic forces, ordains life and death and disease and healing, and determines the life spans of all living beings.

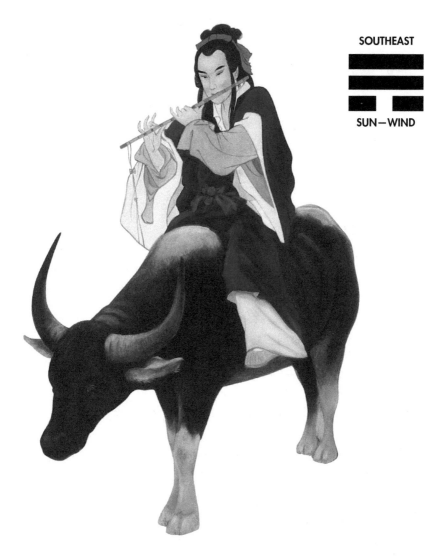

SOUTHEAST

SUN—WIND

Han Hsien-Ku (Han Xiang Zi)

THE COMPOSITION OF THE HUMAN BODY

The human body is anywhere from 50 to 75 percent water (actually, salt water), while the brain is almost 90 percent water. When we break it down into precise chemical content, this is what it looks like: 96.2 percent of your body composition is made up of organic elements present in many different forms. These elements combine to form substances akin to DNA, RNA, proteins, fats, and sugars. And so the 96.2 percent looks like this:

Oxygen: 65 percent
Carbon: 18.5 percent
Hydrogen: 9.5 percent
Nitrogen: 3.2 percent

Most of the carbon listed here is in the form of CO_2 (carbon dioxide), which is the by-product of oxygen usage by our bodies. This means that approximately 90 percent of our body is made up of gas. Basically, you are made of hot air! The rest of the body is composed of inorganic elements and trace elements, of which 3.8 percent is in the form of salts. Most of the calcium in your bones is in the form of salts. Although these levels are small compared to that of the above elements, the correct balance of minerals is vital for health and proper biological functioning within every cell of the body, or as Leonardo da Vinci said, "Vitality and beauty are gifts given to those who live according to its laws."

The 3.8 percent of salts in the body breaks down as follows:

Calcium: 1.5 percent
Phosphorous: 1 percent
Potassium: 0.4 percent
Sulphur: 0.3 percent
Sodium: 0.2 percent
Chlorine: 0.2 percent
Magnesium: 0.1 percent
Iodine: 0.1 percent
Iron: 0.1 percent

Trace elements make up less than 0.5 percent of your body, yet they are called *essential elements* because they are regarded as all-important for the myriad chemical reactions that take place inside your cells, such as manufacturing hormones, synthesizing vitamins, DNA protection, and other vital chemicals necessary to create homeostasis (balance). Some of the trace elements we know about are chromium, cobalt, copper, fluorine, manganese, molybdenum, selenium, tin, vanadium, and zinc. There are an estimated eighty macro, micro, and trace elements present in the body, most in very small amounts. The mineral content of the sea (excluding the higher sodium content), which contains all these seventy-plus minerals, is almost identical to healthy human blood, excluding the higher sodium content. This may be why many ancient cultures regarded unprocessed sea salt as sacred and traded it at a higher price than gold.

All these trace minerals have specific functions at the cellular level. Nutritional scientists are now researching the functions of these trace elements and how they work. What is important to understand is that your body needs all of them to stay in balance and function correctly. When you are missing just one, things go wrong at a chemical level. That's why when you are ill, trace mineral supplementation is critical.

Oxygen and water are the body's prime nutrients. We know that we can do without food for weeks, but without water we quickly dehydrate and die within days, and without oxygen we die within minutes. Therefore, when disease or ill health appears in the body's cells, it is only common sense to first look at one's basic nutritional requirements and deficiencies of water and oxygen. Then look at mineral salts and trace elements. It seems ridiculous that modern allopathic medicine tells us that the first place to go to when you are sick is to pharmaceutical drugs, which only suppress symptoms and hide the real cause of an illness. Humans seem to have become so carried away with medical technology that they seek extremely complicated cures for even more complicated sicknesses. Simple cures for complex ills do not sell well. Drug companies know this full well, but the average person today is just beginning to discover this truth.

THE ROLE OF OXYGEN
IN THE HUMAN BODY

In his *Textbook of Medical Physiology,* Arthur C. Guyton, M.D., says, "All chronic pain, suffering and diseases are caused by a lack of oxygen at the cell level." As most of us know, trees, plants, and even algae produce oxygen in a process called *photosynthesis*. This process involves plants taking in the CO_2 (carbon dioxide) and converting it into oxygen with the help of sunlight. Our body uses oxygen to give life to cells. The human body is aerobic—it needs oxygen—and harmful bacteria and viruses are anaerobic and rob the body of oxygen. A lack of oxygen in any of the body's tissues creates a breeding ground for viruses and other diseases; thus, for example, cancer cannot and does not survive or thrive in well-oxygenated tissue. Of all the elements needed by the body, only oxygen is in constant demand, so much so that its absence brings death within minutes. Our bodies are composed mostly of water, which is eight-ninths oxygen. Unfortunately, in the last few decades nutritional studies have tended to get caught up in the minor details of biochemistry, overlooking our most abundant and essential element, along with the fundamental role its depletion plays in creating disease.

Generally, the brighter the color red your blood is, the more oxygen it carries; conversely, the darker its red color, the less oxygen it carries. Arterial blood is generally a much brighter red color because it has just passed through the lungs, while the venous blood is generally a darker red because it has passed through the tiny capillaries where oxygen is transferred from these vessels to the surrounding tissues. Your body runs on a fuel called *adenosine triphosphate,* commonly known as ATP. This ATP is created by all your cells, for energy. The chemical manufacturing process of ATP is called *oxidation phosphorylation* and is totally dependent on oxygen. All healthy cells require an alkaline, oxygen-rich environment to produce enough ATP for the body to function optimally and to avoid the proliferation of cancerous cells. Unlike healthy cells, cancerous cells, which are oxygen depleted, manufacture ATP by fermenting glucose (sugars), which requires a combination of low oxygen and an acidic environment to flourish. Yet if you ask people in the street if they know what the cause of cancer is, they will tell you that doctors still don't know. The sincere ignorance of the public to investigate what the modern medical industry would like us to believe is astounding, yet proves that we seem to just believe what we are told. In fact, two-time Nobel Prize winner Linus Pauling (1901–1994) declared that "everyone should know that the 'war on cancer' is largely a fraud."

Probably the simplest reason our bodies lack the level of oxygen needed for optimal health is due to poor breathing, pollution, and cigarette smoking (primary or secondhand). Even though cities have poorer-quality air, there is still plenty to go around, yet most people suffer from illness of one sort or another because of a lack of cellular oxygen. In traditional Chinese medicine, patients are taught to increase their oxygen level by learning breathing techniques through Chi Kung exercises. These are taught as part of medical Chi Kung, and they are useful for physical rehabilitation and to enhance strength in martial arts. In some hospitals in China today, before one can be treated by a doctor one must first attend a specified number of Chi Kung classes. This is done because the hospitals find that in most cases after Chi Kung training the illness has been cured. In fact, China has discovered many simple cures to complex illnesses due to its overpopulation, pollution, and shortage of drugs and doctors. Teaching a person to heal his or her own disease is much cheaper and more effective in the long term.

A lack of aerobic exercise, which activates and strengthens oxygen-carrying blood cells, is another reason many people suffer from oxygen deficiencies. Smoking and pollution, of course, minimize oxygen absorption in the lungs and make breathing shallower, but one does not have to be a smoker to suffer from oxygen starvation; shallow breathing is common in nonsmokers as well. It is noteworthy that scientists have discovered that several thousand years ago air contained approximately 40 percent more oxygen. Rainforest destruction, pollution, and massive overpopulation over just the past few centuries may have something to do with these findings. Whatever the cause, it is a sure sign that increasing your oxygen level is necessary.

Cancer and Viruses Linked to Low Oxygen Levels

German biochemist and two-time Nobel Prize winner Dr. Otto Warburg (1883–1970), who devoted his entire life to the study of the cause of cancer, proved that cancer cells can only begin to proliferate in the human body when the cells are oxygen deficient, and he further asserted that when the body has ample oxygen, cancer cells cannot proliferate. "Deprive a cell of 35 percent of its oxygen for forty-eight hours," he said, "and it may become cancerous." Dr. Warburg maintained that oxygen deficiency leads to an acidic state in the body that promotes cancer, whereas cancer cells cannot live in a sufficiently alkaline environment. He claimed that the difference between normal cells and cancerous cells is so great that one can scarcely picture a greater difference. Oxygen, a gas, the provider of energy in plants and animals, is replaced within cancerous cells by an energy-producing reaction of the lowest form, the fermentation of sugar, which has been dubbed "the Warburg effect." In other words, instead of fully respiring in the presence of adequate oxygen, cancer cells ferment.

This groundbreaking information unveiled by Dr. Warburg and other scientists who aided in this discovery led to the development of research into the use of therapeutic ozone and oxygen as treatments for many health problems, especially cancer, with great success. Of course, cancer can have countless secondary causes, such as exposure to chemical carcinogens, which must be eliminated by the body; but here as well, oxygen and ozone treatment appears to help in terms of increasing the detoxification process.

So to summarize: the prime cause of cancer is the replacement of the respiration of oxygen in normal body cells by the fermentation of sugar. All of the body's cells obtain their energy needs through the respiration of oxygen, whereas cancerous cells meet their energy needs mainly by fermentation. All normal body cells are thus obligate aerobes, whereas all cancerous cells are partial anaerobes. Oxygen, which is a gas and the donor of energy in plants and animals, is dethroned in cancerous cells and replaced by an energy-yielding reaction of the lowest form, the fermentation of glucose. If it is true that the replacement of oxygen respiration by fermentation is the prime cause of cancer, then all cancerous tissue without exception must ferment, and no normal, healthy tissue could exist within fermentation.

In a lecture titled "The Prime Cause and Prevention of Cancer,"

Dr. Warburg cited an experiment performed by American researchers Malmgren and Flanigan:

> If one injects tetanus spores, which can germinate only at very low oxygen pressures, into the blood of healthy mice, the mice do not sicken with tetanus, because the spores find no place in the normal body where the oxygen pressure is sufficiently low. Likewise, pregnant mice do not sicken when injected with the tetanus spores, because also in the growing embryo no region exists where the oxygen pressure is sufficiently low to permit spore germination. However, if one injects tetanus spores into the blood of tumor-bearing mice, the mice sicken with tetanus, because the oxygen pressure in the tumors can be so low that the spores can germinate. These experiments demonstrate in a unique way the anaerobiosis of cancer cells and the non-anaerobiosis of normal cells, in particular the non-anaerobiosis of growing embryos.*

For many years cancer investigators searched for a cancer that did not ferment. When finally a nonfermenting tumor appeared to have been found in slow-growing Morris tumors, it was shown to only be the result of a methodological error. Due to low cell-oxygen levels, toxins build up rapidly, and the growth of anaerobic microbes such as bacteria, viruses, fungi, and other pathogens dwell inside us. Basically, anaerobes and toxicity overloads us until we break down. This is a primary cause of most human, animal, and plant health problems, including a long list of supposedly incurable diseases.

HYDROGEN PEROXIDE, A MEDICAL REMEDY

In his book *Oxygen, Oxygen, Oxygen,* Kurt Donsbach, D.C., N.D., Ph.D., says, "I have been so impressed with the results of the use of hydrogen peroxide that every cancer patient receives infusions of the 35% food grade hydrogen peroxide/DMSO mixture throughout their

---

*Found at http://healingtools.tripod.com/primecause1.html.

entire stay. . . . This is the only substance I use in every cancer patient."

Hydrogen peroxide was first discovered by French chemist Louis-Jacques Thénard in 1818, who appropriately named it *eau oxygenée,* "oxygen water." In Spanish, hydrogen peroxide is known as *agua oxigenada,* and in Italian, *acqua ossigenata.* If you mention to someone that you are consuming hydrogen peroxide, many people are bewildered or even shocked; but if you were to say that you're supplementing with oxygen water, they will probably say, "That sounds good."

Hydrogen peroxide is produced by our own immune cells on a daily basis, and in quite substantial amounts—yes, your own cells produce hydrogen peroxide. This is how our white blood cells disable bacteria, viruses, and other anaerobic microbes in the body—by suffocating them with oxygen. Mother's milk also contains substantial amounts to boost the baby's immune system. Hydrogen peroxide in its chemical form is H_2O, water, plus one extra oxygen atom, O_1, which is released to destroy pathogens and foreign invaders. This healing chemical is also created in the atmosphere when ultraviolet light strikes oxygen in the presence of moisture. As well, it occurs naturally in rain and snow, from atmospheric ozone, and in mountain streams where rushing water is continuously aerated. When common hydrogen peroxide comes into contact with water, an extra atom of oxygen splits off, or water (H_2O) combines with an extra atom (O_1) of oxygen, thus becoming hydrogen peroxide (H_2O_2).

In his book *Hydrogen Peroxide: Medical Miracle,* William Campbell Douglass, M.D., says:

> There are over 6,100 articles in the scientific literature dating from 1920 on the scientific applications of hydrogen peroxide. It seems inconceivable that the astounding medical cures reported in science journals over the past 75 years could have been ignored. . . . Tumor cells, bacteria, and other unwanted foreign elements in the blood could usually be destroyed with hydrogen peroxide treatment. Peroxide has a definite destructive effect on tumors, and, in fact, cancer therapy may prove to be the most dramatic and useful place for peroxide therapy.

There are various forms of hydrogen peroxide:

3–3.5 percent hydrogen peroxide (drug/grocery store variety): usually made from 50 percent super D peroxide and diluted; therefore can contain stabilizers such as phenol, acetanilide, sodium stannate, tetrasodium, and phosphate

6 percent hydrogen peroxide: used by beauticians for coloring hair, comes in a strength labeled "20 volume"; must have activators added to it to be used as bleach

30 percent reagent hydrogen peroxide: used in medical research; also contains stabilizers

30–32 percent electronic-grade hydrogen peroxide: mainly used for washing transistors and integrated chip parts before assembly

35 percent technical-grade hydrogen peroxide: contains a small amount of phosphorus to neutralize any chlorine in the water it is combined with

35–50 percent food-grade hydrogen peroxide: used in food products like cheese, eggs, whey products, and to spray the inside of foil-lined containers for food storage and as an antiseptic packaging system

90 percent hydrogen peroxide: used as a military source of oxygen and also as a form of rocket fuel

Safest Form of H_2O_2

The easiest method for taking hydrogen peroxide is to purchase 35 percent food-grade hydrogen peroxide, which can be diluted in pure water at a ratio of 10:1, making 3.5 percent, which is safe for handling and storage, or 3 percent food grade is also available. This type of hydrogen peroxide is the best available for internal use and can be purchased from some compounding pharmacies or online. Most health-food stores do not sell food-grade hydrogen peroxide anymore; they instead offer stabilized oxygen supplements mentioned also in this chapter, which are beneficial but not as strong.

In his 1988 book *O₂xygen Therapies,* Ed McCabe says, "In 1920, intravenous hydrogen peroxide cut the death rate from pneumonia in half." Walter Grotz, president of Educational Concerns for H_2O_2, in *The Truth about Food Grade Hydrogen Peroxide,* says, "I drink food grade hydrogen peroxide every day and my ingesting of hydrogen peroxide didn't poison me at all. It cured my arthritis and it did so for a total of $6. If this is con artistry, it's the cheapest rip-off in history."

The use of hydrogen peroxide can also extend to purifying water on a large scale. Today there are many pools and spas turning to hydrogen peroxide as an alternative to using chemical chlorine in swimming pools, which is a well-known health hazard. To start using hydrogen peroxide in a chlorinated pool, you don't have to drain the water. Rather "shock" the water by adding 35 percent concentrated food-grade hydrogen peroxide at a ratio of one cup to 250 gallons of water in your pool. Run the pump to circulate the solution and then shut off the pump to allow the peroxide to work for twenty-four hours before swimming. After this, test your pool weekly to ensure an adequate concentration of hydrogen peroxide, typically 30 to 50 parts per million for residential pools, or up to 100 ppm for higher-volume pools. This concentration is approximately one cup of hydrogen peroxide for 500 gallons of pool volume. Peroxide testing strips are available at pool supply stores, and be sure to check online for more information regarding concerns about pool hardware reacting with peroxide. Many people are unaware that you can absorb more chlorine from one hot shower than in one day of drinking the same water.

Many natural medicine doctors prescribe food-grade (35 percent) hydrogen peroxide in many different ways to add oxygen to the body:

- Add one cup of 35 percent H_2O_2 to a half-filled bathtub for bathing (makes the bathwater less than 1 percent H_2O_2.
- Spray diluted 3 percent H_2O_2 solution on your body, especially the armpits or groin area, to kill bacteria, cure infections, and neutralize odors.
- Gargle with 3 percent H_2O_2 for throat infections.
- Brush teeth with 3 percent H_2O_2 for shiny, white teeth or to cure gingivitis or bad breath caused by gum infections.
- Add three drops of 3 percent H_2O_2 to ears three times daily

for infection or during times of cold/flu or for ear problems.

- Inhale 3 percent H_2O_2 (not through the nose) by spraying it into your mouth using a spritzer spray bottle; simply spray while taking a normal breath in; do three sprays two to three times daily for lung or respiratory diseases.
- Half fill a standard kitchen sink with water, add one tablespoon of 35 percent H_2O_2, and let your fruits or vegetables soak for a few minutes to kill bacteria and neutralize chemical pesticides.
- Some doctors inject dilute solutions (0.04 percent) into their patients using an IV.

Hydrogen Peroxide Dosages and Remedies

If you are using food-grade hydrogen peroxide (35 percent) internally, it is recommended you start with two to four drops in each glass of water you drink, so if you drink ten glasses of water daily, that makes a total of twenty to forty drops daily. Alternately, some natural medicine doctors recommend eight drops of 35 percent hydrogen peroxide in a glass of water three times daily, for a total of twenty-four drops. Oxygen can cause temporary feelings of nausea, so using the "little and often dosage" (three drops many times daily) may be better for those with sensitive stomachs. Holding the solution in the mouth and gargling before swallowing can help you avoid possible stomach upset that is sometimes associated with hydrogen peroxide therapy. If you are using diluted 35 percent food-grade hydrogen peroxide at 10:1 with water, making it 3.5 percent, simply adjust the dosage accordingly, such as twenty drops in each glass of water. We do not recommend H_2O_2 all the time; rather, only when needed.

Warning: Never use hydrogen peroxide near the eyes at any strength. Although 3 to 6 percent is very safe on the skin and even ears, 35 percent must be handled with extreme care and always diluted heavily, and kept completely away from children, as it can burn if placed directly on the skin or taken internally.

OXYGEN-BOOSTING TECHNOLOGY

There are an increasing number of oxygen boosters available today, including oxygen supplements that are readily available at health-food stores and on the Internet. These supplements contain stabilized oxygen (sometimes referred to as *vitamin O*) and are often combined with trace minerals and amino acids. Manufacturers claim these supplements reach starved oxygen cells faster than hydrogen peroxide can. They are presently being used by many Olympic athletes with great success, having been shown to increase stamina, reduce fatigue and lactic acid build-up, charge the immune system, and provide extra oxygen to the brain, thereby reducing fatigue and speeding up recovery time from injuries.

You don't need to be an Olympic athlete to benefit from these medical breakthroughs, though, as oxygen supplementation can benefit anyone. As we get older, the arteries begin to fill with plaque, leading to heart attack and stroke. Oxygen helps cleanse the arteries, reducing the risk of stroke and heart attack. The mechanical action of oxygen-rich blood flowing through the arteries acts to "scrub" the arteries clean naturally.

Oxygenated Water

Besides hydrogen-peroxide therapy, another great way to oxygenate the body is through ozone therapy. Ozone therapy dates back some time in mainstream medicine; it was used successfully in the 1930s until drugs began to take the place of simpler, less profitable treatments, and ozone is still used successfully to treat serious illnesses in Germany, Mexico, and some Asian countries. But you do not have to travel halfway around the world to get the amazing healing benefits of ozone, as ozone generators are very affordable for the average person, allowing you to treat yourself at home with oxygen-rich water.

Although ozone is very harmful when produced from air alone or when breathed directly into the lungs, if produced from pure oxygen and pumped though water it changes from O_3 to O_2 and then O—oxygen-rich water. Portable mini ozone generators for making ozonized water or ozonized oils can be purchased online for a few hundred dollars. We at Tao Garden own one that is made by Sota Instruments and is designed by Dr. Bob Beck (described in chapter 7); we use this for making ozonized drinking water and for making ozonized oils for external applications.

In 1983, at the World Ozone Conference, medical doctors from around the world listed thirty-three major diseases that had been successfully treated with ozone therapy, including AIDS, cancer, multiple sclerosis, Alzheimer's disease, and Parkinson's disease. An exhaustive survey of 644 medical doctors and ozone therapists conducted in Germany found that of the 384,775 patients receiving 5,579,238 ozone treatments, only thirty-nine incidents of any side effects occurred, giving ozone therapy a side-effect rate of 0.0007 percent per 5.5 million doses. When they do occur, ozone side effects are typically minor irritations of only short duration—nothing like the side effects of pharmaceutical drugs used today.

Ozone and oxygen therapies are safe when used correctly. Nevertheless, the U.S. Food and Drug Administration has concluded that "ozone is a toxic gas with no known medical use"—a judgment that flies in the face of evidence to the contrary and has more to do with financial interests and the influence that drug companies have on the FDA and the medical industry.

Chi Machine Increases Oxygen

I have seen some pretty amazing technology come out that benefits overall health, but none more simple and effective than the Chi Machine, also known as the Swing Machine. This simple device was first created by Japanese engineer Keiichi Ohashi in 1988 and is said to be the brainchild of Dr. Shizuo Inoue, chairman of Japan's Oxygen Health Association. It is designed to increase oxygen and circulation to the spine, organs, and limbs.

The Chi Machine rocks your body from side to side while you lie on your back. It is actually the exact same movement a fish uses to move itself through water. Traditionally, this method was called *pulsing* and was performed manually by health practitioners in Asia. Practitioners would hold your ankles and rock your legs in a wavelike motion, like a fish, from side to side. The ancient Chinese believed that this simple movement creates a wave of energy up your spine and out to the muscles, meridians, and nerves, increasing oxygen supply to the cells, oxygen metabolism, general energy (chi), circulation, blood supply, and lymph drainage. The Chi Machine does just that.

Laboratory tests show that approximately fifteen minutes on a Chi Machine is equivalent to 4.5 km of aerobic (oxygen-giving) exercise. The great thing about this technology is that you can use it without increasing your pain that might result from whatever your present ailment is. It provides the benefits of aerobic exercise to bedridden patients or the elderly and is great for spinal health and spinal-injury rehabilitation, releasing tension between vertebrae, especially the sacrum and sciatic nerves, thereby alleviating the pain associated with spinal and back problems. However, in general, any health-conscious person can benefit from the Chi Machine, as it increases oxygen and the flow of energy (chi) through the body, increasing our own natural healing abilities.

Deep Breathing

Deep-breathing exercises are probably the easiest and most natural way to increase oxygen and negative ions in the body, but only if you are breathing fresh, clean air. The way in which you breathe is also very important. For instance, shallow, spasmodic breathing accounts for many respiratory conditions, including asthma, and in turn can be a cofactor in many other ailments, as the body's needs are based on the availability of oxygen. Traditional holistic medicine encourages educating the person on correct breathing, as it promotes health recovery. In modern-day China, some hospitals insist that patients attend a certain number of medical Chi Kung breathing classes before medicine is administered; in many cases it has been found that patients are cured before the prescribed number of classes are completed.

Traditional Chinese medicine and ayurveda not only stress the importance of oxygen, they also emphasize the importance of negative ions that are taken into the body while breathing fresh air. For this reason the best places to practice breathing exercises are in parks, mountains, or wherever trees or water are present—the places where negative ions are at their maximum concentration.

Chapter 6, on internal exercises, describes some yogic forms of breath work, called pranayama, as well as other internal exercises that require the person to breathe correctly.

Second Immortal Healer—Chang Kuo-Lao

Your Body Is Water

All around us we see the bridges of life collapsing, those capillaries which create all organic life. This dreadful disintegration has been caused by the mindless and mechanical work of man, who has wrenched the living soul from the Earth's blood—water.

VIKTOR SCHAUBERGER, AUSTRIAN FOREST CARETAKER, NATURALIST, AND PHILOSOPHER

The healing that relates to the element water (Kan) is represented by Immortal Chang Kuo-Lao, an occultist-alchemist who was born in the eighth century CE. He claimed to have been a grand minister to the legendary enlightened emperor Yao (2357–2255 BCE) in a previous lifetime, and by the time the emperor Wu Zetian came to power in the eighth century, Chang claimed he was already several hundred years old (the epithet Lao added at the end of his name means "old").

Chang had a love of wine and winemaking and was known to make liquor from herbs and shrubs. The other members of the Eight Immortals drank his wine, which they believed to have healing properties. He was a master of Chi Kung and could go without food for days,

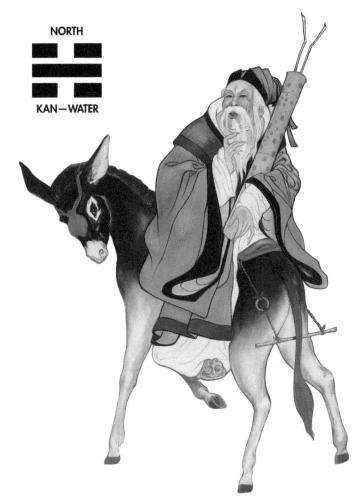

Fig. 2.1. Chang Kuo-Lao (Zang Guo Lao)

surviving on only a few sips of his medicinal wine. Many of the Tang emperors invited him to court, but he usually declined their invitations, preferring his solitary existence as a hermit on Zhongtiao Mountain. Nevertheless, he entertained one emperor by making himself invisible and by drinking poisons. Thereafter the emperor bestowed on him the title "Master of Understanding the Mystery" and offered him a high position and his daughter in marriage. Chang Kuo-Lao declined both offers, and then he received the imperial summons to accept the emperor's offer, so he lay down and died. He was buried in a coffin, but later when Chang's disciples opened it, it was found to be empty. After this he was frequently seen alive. This Immortal Taoist sage's epithet is "Original Vapor," a reference to water, our primary physical element.

THE BODY'S WATER CONTENT

Water is life. Life cannot exist without water. We must constantly recycle fresh water through our body daily to keep it properly hydrated and internally cleansed. Clean water is probably the second most important thing after clean air for our bodies to survive. It is difficult for the body to get water from any other source than water itself. Soft drinks, coffee, and alcohol steal tremendous amounts of water from the body, while other beverages such as milk and juice require water from the body to be properly metabolized.

In his book *Your Body's Many Cries for Water,* Dr. F. Batmanghelidj applies his some twenty years of clinical and scientific research into the role of water in the body to explain that chronic dehydration produces stress, chronic pain, and many other degenerative diseases and conditions such as asthma, allergies, heartburn, back pain, arthritis, colitis, and migraine headaches and contributes to premature aging. Dr. Batmanghelidj asserts that the opinion, published in the *American Journal of Physiology* in 2002, that there is no scientific merit in drinking eight eight-ounce glasses of water a day "is the very foundation of all that is wrong with modern medicine, which is costing this nation [the United States] $1.7 trillion a year, rising at the rate of 12 percent every year."

Dr. Batmanghelidj cites the following facts:

- More than half of the world's population is chronically dehydrated.
- The thirst mechanism is so weak that it is often mistaken for hunger.
- Even mild dehydration will slow down one's metabolism.
- One glass of water shuts down midnight hunger pangs for almost 100 percent of dieters.
- Lack of water is the number-one trigger of daytime fatigue.

- Preliminary research indicates that eight to ten glasses of water a day could significantly ease back and joint pain for up to 80 percent of sufferers.
- A mere 2 percent drop in body water can trigger fuzzy short-term memory, trouble with basic math, and difficulty focusing on the computer screen or on a printed page.
- Drinking at least five glasses of water daily decreases the risk of breast cancer by 79 percent, and one is 50 percent less likely to develop bladder cancer.
- The body's water content is approximately 45 liters for the average adult, meaning our daily consumption of water needs to be approximately 2.4 liters (.63 gallons).

Your Body Is Salt Water

Though science consistently states that the human body is made up of up to 70 percent water, this water is actually salt water. Your tears are salty, your sweat is salty, your blood is salty, and you are even made in salt water—embryonic fluid—inside your mother's womb. Every chemical reaction in your body depends on the correct amount of both water and cell salts. Minor dehydration in any tissues of the body results in disease. Water assists the body in cleansing wastes and removing toxins. Yes, the body is approximately 70 percent saline water, while the brain is approximately 90 percent salt water. Your body produces neither water nor these mineral salts and is constantly losing them on a daily basis through urination, perspiration, and respiration; hence the need for constant replenishment.

Sadly, in modern medical schools it is taught that water is only a sort of packing material or means of transport, having no metabolic function of its own and no direct role in any of the body's physiological functions. However, water not only acts to hydrate the body's cells, it also acts as a solvent to clean the cells, as well as a medium in which all the body's chemical reactions occur. The body produces many chemicals, from hormones to pain-killing endorphins, for healthy function. Without sufficient water, these chemical reactions become impaired and actually slow down, opening the door for virtually any disease to take root, from hormonal imbalance to memory loss. Many kinds of muscle and joint pain can also be attributed to dehydration. We know as well that our DNA can be affected as a result of a deficiency of water. The amino acid tryptophan, which is involved in DNA printouts during cell renewal, is impeded with dehydration. Tryptophan is also vital in the prevention of cancer cell development during cell renewal.

PERCENTAGE OF WATER IN THE HUMAN BODY

Blood plasma	(main body component)	approximately 92 percent water
Fetus	(our growing physical vehicle)	approximately 90 percent water
Blood	(nutrient conveyor)	up to 90 percent water
Brain cells	(intellect, creativity, and behavior)	approximately 85 percent water
Kidneys	(fluid processors and purifiers)	approximately 82 percent water
Muscles	(prime movers of the body)	average 75 percent water
Body	(our abode on Earth)	approximately 71 percent water
Liver	(metabolism and detoxification)	approximately 69 percent water
Bones	(structural support system)	approximately 22 percent water
Cells	(complete basis of growth and survival)	mostly water

Water plays a vital role in nearly every bodily function and is essential for proper digestion, nutrient absorption, chemical reactions, proper circulation, and the flexibility of the blood vessels, as well as helping to remove toxins (acidic waste) from the body, in particular from the digestive tract. Water regulates your body's temperature; imagine a car running without water in the radiator. Consistent failure to drink enough water can lead to chronic cellular dehydration, which can occur at any time of the year, and not only during the summer months when it is hot. In fact, during winter we often forget to drink enough, so we can dehydrate quicker than when it's hot. The other cause of dehydration in winter is due to central heating and the resulting dry atmosphere in most homes.

General Water Rule

Take half your body weight (in pounds) and translate that to ounces of water daily to provide your body with its minimum water replacement requirements. You can start by sipping water and gradually build up to your full requirement to prevent adverse cleansing reactions and sudden detoxification, while also training your bladder to hold water so as to reduce frequent urination, which increased water consumption obviously brings. You need to understand that a dry mouth is one of the *last* signs of dehydration, and not the first, as many people mistakenly think. As Dr. Batmanghelidj says, "Waiting to get thirsty is to die prematurely and very painfully."

Our Bodies Lack Sufficient Water

Our body is constantly using and losing water. We lose water constantly, through urination, defecation, perspiration, and respiration; therefore, its constant supply is vital. The amount of water we need to drink is hugely misunderstood. Although different ages at different times need different amounts, the average adult needs to drink a daily minimum of approximately two liters, or eight standard glasses of water. This does not include beverages such as tea, coffee, alcohol, soda, or even juices, as many of these beverages actually dehydrate the body of its vital water supplies. Most of us drink insufficient amounts of water; we also drink a lot of dehydrating beverages. Another reason most of us do not drink enough water is that the signs we look for when evaluating dehydration are vastly misinterpreted. Many gauge a dry mouth and the sensation of thirst as one of the first signs of needing to drink water, when in fact it is one of the last. There are many other signs of chronic dehydration that may present even before we feel thirsty:

- Headache
- Body aches and pains
- Gastric reflux
- Stomach upset
- Morning sickness in pregnant women
- Constipation and dry stools
- High blood pressure and high cholesterol

With age, and as illness gradually appears, we tend to overlook the correlation with insufficient water intake. Most medical doctors are vastly uneducated about the intricacies of the important role of water in the nervous and endocrine systems. Instead, drugs are prescribed to nullify the effects or imbalances that come from chronic dehydration, instead of simply addressing the underlying cause—not enough water consumption.

The Best Water to Drink

There are four types of commercially available bottled water: spring water, mineral water, drinking water, and distilled water.

Spring water is collected directly from natural springs, where it rises up from underground and must therefore be bottled at the source. Mineral water is rainwater that flows through the ground before it's collected. As a result, mineral water has a higher content of various minerals (not ionic), which are picked up as it flows over rocks. It also can contain urine from animals that live along its banks, which most of the time gets filtered out before bottling. Drinking water is merely tap water that has been filtered by reverse osmosis filters and ultraviolet light, and then bottled. Pure distilled water we will discuss shortly.

In my experience, most bottled water contains large amounts of solvents and various bacteria. Studies done on popular commercial-brand bottled water found all of them to be quite unhealthy for drinking and no better than ordinary, clean tap water. The taste of bottled water is usually better, as chemicals such as chlorine are reduced, but even if one could afford to only drink this type of water you would be no healthier. The most sensible and affordable way to consume good, clean water is to use correct home-filtering techniques and reenergize your water, which I will explain how to do shortly.

Water contamination seems to be quite prevalent today due to over-population combined with the lack of education in safe and effective ways of purifying water. If you suspect your tap water is contaminated (most are), get your own home testing kit and test your water, or take it to a private lab and post the findings on your local supermarket bulletin board to educate your fellow citizens that they need to filter their water of chemical pollutants and do something about their local environment. Most of our public drinking water has been tampered with, and many chemicals are added to purify it, but these kinds of efforts more often than not are poisoning us. The water boards in many communities use hundreds of chemicals to eliminate harmful bacteria and heavy metals; unfortunately, these methods do not remove all contaminants, so you need to do further purification in your home. Buying purified bottled water is expensive and really unwarranted, as you can make your own at home for less than a few cents a gallon with a suitable filtration system.

Remembering that the body is ionic and not metallic, a special conversion process must be done by the body to utilize any metallic minerals common in bottled mineral waters. If our bodies were designed to digest large amounts of metallic minerals as found in popular bottled mineral waters, we could simply live on eating dirt, as it contains the minerals the body needs, but in metallic form. But if we did this we would not live very long. The reason we live on plants and not dirt is because plants suck up metallic minerals from the earth and do this reconverting process for us, converting them into water-soluble minerals that the body can easily process.

Taking the Confusion Out of Buying a Water Filter

After having an analysis of our tap water, which greatly shocked us, we began to search for the most effective and affordable filtration system for my clients and myself. Filters come in all different shapes and sizes and different ways of filtering water. There was no doubt that water distillers do the best job in terms of taking out everything, including all the inorganic minerals in the water. Despite all the claims that drinking distilled water leaches minerals from the body, we have seen no clinical evidence to support this claim, which we believe originated from companies selling water-filtration systems.

Many cultures, such as the various Pacific South Sea island cultures, drink distilled water in the form of rainwater and display incredible levels of health. Many people don't realize that rainwater is actually distilled water, pure H_2O, just like snow. From our own clinical experience we have found that drinking rainwater can have a different effect on the body compared to commercial distilled water, even though structurally they are identical. This fact may be due to the emergence of living water technology and the angles of the degrees in which the water molecules are positioned. This is why after you distill your water it's good to reenergize it with life-giving plant minerals and a healing frequency.

For detoxification purposes distilled water is very useful, as it seems to have a very cleansing action in the body. It is very energy consuming to manufacture distilled water all the time, so we recommend that it be taken during fasting and on other cleansing regimens only. On the same note, there is strong evidence that our bodies cannot properly assimilate the inorganic minerals found in most mineral or tap waters. The best source of minerals needed by the body comes from plant minerals through foods.

Another type of water filtration is reverse osmosis, which usually uses a double-carbon filtration system, wherein water is fed through the system at a high pressure. These are excellent systems but can be costly, and they usually waste water. Ultraviolet light is often needed in combination with reverse osmosis, as it kills large amounts of bacteria that build up in these types of units. This process is also expensive because of filter replacement cost, and it still does not completely eliminate all heavy metals, unlike steam-distilled water. But reverse osmosis is very beneficial and the best bet if you live in an area where the water contains bacteria.

The most economical method if you have disease-free tap water is to use a simple activated carbon filtration system of 1 or 0.5 microns. This kind of system works on standard water pressure and does not waste water. The small-micron filter size filters out the most harmful organisms and heavy metals. Unfortunately, most of the jug or container filters sold in supermarkets and department stores have a filter core size of approximately 30 microns, which does not do as well as the countertop or under-sink filters that attach to the tap itself. Remember to ask for the filter core size, and make sure it is 1 micron or less.

We have been extremely impressed with water ionizers, which were first developed in Asia. They are a brilliant addition to any healthy home. They filter water thoroughly, oxygenate, alkalize, and reenergize the water into microclusters, giving it the same health-bestowing properties of the purest mountain or spring water. To this day, ionizers and distillers are the best units you can invest in for your health. Where normal water acts to hydrate the body, these waters can be highly medicinal. Until their recent exposure to Western lifestyles, the Hunza people of North Pakistan commonly lived to one hundred years of age, with men in their seventies still very fertile. The key to such longevity is the quality of glacial water the Hunza drink, which has a microcluster size that penetrates deeper into the tissues, cleansing acidic wastes that age the body while simultaneously energizing the immune system to neutralize free radicals.

There is a "new wave" of affordable filters on the market now that filter, energize, and add molecular hydrogen (H_2) to the water. Some examples are the Naturopaths Choice MinWell+ and the UltraStream units. Both these units were inspired by studies done through the Molecular Hydrogen Foundation (MHF), a nonprofit scientific organization that is the foremost authority on the science of molecular hydrogen. Molecular hydrogen appears to be an excellent and selective antioxidant and anti-inflammatory that specifically targets the hydroxyl free radical and boosts the body's natural antioxidant molecules. Compared with other antioxidants it is extremely small in size and penetrates deep into the tissues.

Revitalizing Water

Research has shown that when we attempt to completely filter unclean water using every process available, it still remains at its previous vibration and unstable molecular structure. Water does in fact contain a memory and is a living substance. It appears that when we clean water and filter it of chemicals and other impurities, somehow the memory or imprint of those impurities remains in the water at a molecular level, limiting its health-giving benefits. To understand this fully we must understand a little bit about biophotons, known in the scientific field as *somatids*. Biophotons are the tiniest energy bodies found in all living things, especially fluids. Many researchers now believe that photons are the solidification of pure light and, in turn, all life.

We have known for some time now that all life and matter is made up of atoms; but we are now learning that all atoms are made of a form of light called *biophotons*. Microscopic observations of these biophotons under a snap-freezing experiment by Japanese scientist Dr. Masaru Emoto have shown that molecular clusters change dramatically when water is subjected to sound, music, and even personal thought vibrations. Incredibly, this means that water is a living organism in its own right, just like plants. *Aqua vivens,* "living water," is a term that seems to be greatly misunderstood in modern Western medicine. Many people today, especially allopathic medical practitioners, tend to think of water as a lifeless chemical composition; namely, H_2O. That much of any given city's drinking water is recycled and treated with chlorine and fluoridation, not to mention the barrage of agricultural pesticides that find their way into water supplies via land runoff, means that our water supplies are in a state of coma.

Water does contain life force, and pioneers in the field of living water have proved this fact. Austrian naturalist Viktor Schauberger (1885–1958) was probably the first modern pioneer in the study of living water. Schauberger, through the encouragement of his father and grandfather, discovered that water shaded in mountain areas produced richer plants. He also discovered that vegetation and fields irrigated by water transported at night yielded greater harvests than neighboring meadows and fields. From his research he was able to explain the significance of water's properties, and he devised various methods for promoting and maintaining water at its optimum level of purity and vitality. This was all because he understood water as a living energy. He began to perceive water as the lifeblood of the earth and surmised that it must be allowed to follow its own course to keep its energy at a maximum level. Schauberger witnessed that a natural water course is shaped by winding curves and shaded banks, which protects it from direct sunlight, and that its low temperature and natural flow are the conditions necessary for water to preserve its supportive and carrying strength; namely, its "energy." His main discoveries regarded water as a living energy. Unfortunately, much of the water consumed in today's world is no longer what it used to be during Schauberger's lifetime because it has been damaged by chemicals while sitting in pipes or water-treatment stations.

Schauberger did not have access to today's high-tech cameras to show that light photons exist, but he understood it somehow at an intuitive level. His amazing observations led him to become a prolific writer and inventor, patenting many amazing subtle-energy devices, such as a "vortex implosion energizer machine" for restoring the life force back into water. There are many people today who continue the research of Viktor Schauberger, such as Johann Grander, a fellow Austrian, with his company Grander Technology. Grander has developed a way of revitalizing water back into its most organic form.

Because even filtered water still contains the memory of former contaminants and impurities, the process of revitalizing water is as important as filtering it. The vortex shape that most water revitalization units use to reenergize water can be seen everywhere in nature, from seashells to plant surfaces. It is always the natural path of least resistance that free-flowing water takes to keep itself healthy and full of light. Many energy healers say that this vortex is also the same motion by which energy flows into the chakras and pranic tubes of the human body; two such examples are tornados and the bathwater drain.

What we now realize is that water as a living entity records everything as an imprint, acting almost like a liquid tape recorder, storing the frequencies and magnetic influences of anything it comes into contact with into its subatomic structure. By the time it reaches our water faucet, although it may be relatively clean in some cases, it's still loaded with inharmonious vibrations from the chemicals and pollutants that have been previously removed from it. Just as nature cleans water through natural rock formations or internal pressure deep inside Earth's crust, water revitalization units can also do this to your drinking water. If you cannot afford these units, there are basic ways to filter water for only a hundred dollars a year by using standard carbon block/sediment filters. After filtering you can energize your water by stirring it vigorously, forming a funnel or vortex effect for several seconds. You can also energize the water by adding a bit of lemon juice and stirring the water vigorously. Doing so adds minerals such as hydrogen, citric acid, and charged anions, which help to detoxify the liver and increase uric acid waste removal.

Third Immortal Healer—Tsao Kuo-Chiu

The Laws of Nutrition

*The one who takes the medicine yet neglects the diet
wastes the experience of the physician.*

CHINESE PROVERB

The healing of nutrition is symbolized by Immortal Tsao Kuo-Chiu. Tsao was one of two royal brothers whose sister was a Song Dynasty empress during the eleventh century CE. He hated all the corruption that was going on at court and was so ashamed of his brother, a murderer and a hedonist, that he gave away all his wealth to the poor and went to the mountains to meditate. There he clothed his body with wild plants and lived as a hermit. While in his mountain hermitage he was visited by Immortals Lu Tung-Pin and Chuan Chung-Li, who taught him the techniques for attaining perfection. Thereafter he harmonized his mind, body, and spirit and attained immortality.

Tsao Kuo-Chiu is portrayed wearing an official's court dress and holding castanets along with an imperial jade tablet that indicates his rank, gives him access to palace audiences, and also has the power to purify the environment. He is the patron of the theater and of actors.

Tsao, it is said, had a fierce demeanor, making him one of the less popular of the Immortals, though he lived an exemplary life.

This Immortal represents the earth element as signified by the mountain (Ken), the solid foundation of the Immortals and our storage of vital chi, as well as the maker of clouds and water streams. Life force streams from this storehouse—the nutrients from the ground that nourish us and give us our vital chi from food, which is symbolized by Tsao's clothing himself in wild plants.

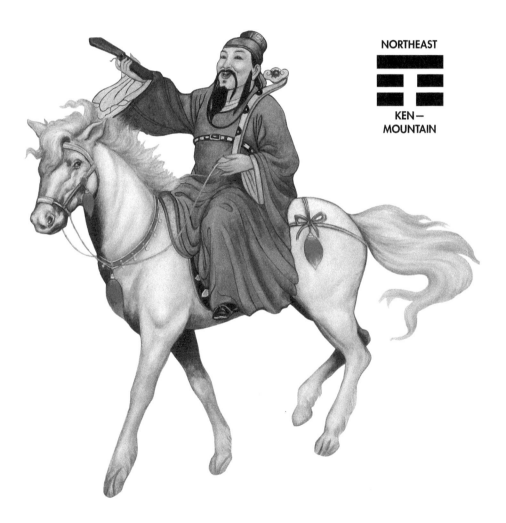

NORTHEAST

KEN—
MOUNTAIN

Fig. 3.1. Tsao Kuo-Chiu (Cao Guo Jio)

THE "MOUNTAIN" OF NOURISHING FOOD

Nutrition is the foundation—the mountain—that composes the framework of our physical body, the "we are what we eat" component of our health. Unfortunately, most of the food we eat today does not give us what we need. In various studies it was found that people who consumed the recommended daily allowances of the ten essential nutrients still do not get what the body needs for optimal health and proper functioning. This proves that not only are our modern diets lacking in nutrients, but so is the soil in which our food is grown.

At the turn of the last century there was no doubt that food was highly nutritious. Prior to the widespread use of chemical pesticides, food was, of course, 100 percent organic, grown in rich, fertile soil. GMOs did not exist, so there wasn't even a need to advertise food as "organic" because everything was, including the food eaten by livestock. But agriculture today has become big business, and big business has no time to wait for natural fertilizers to enrich the soil. True, synthetic chemical fertilizers produce food faster and bigger, but to the disadvantage of human health and the ecology of the earth. Pesticide use is commonplace in the breadbasket of the United States because of the poor quality of the soil; plants are less resistant to disease and pests as a result of these practices, so stronger and stronger pesticides must be used. Nutritional experts agree that using chemicals in the production of food is causing a downward spiral, with the result being more health problems for both humans and animals, and pollution of the environment.

Chemical fertilizers were first introduced early in the last century by petrochemical companies that realized that the by-products of the petroleum industry could be used to kill pests. Farmers at that time were totally unaware of the dangers of these chemicals and the long-term effects that cause plants' immune systems and the quality of their health to be poor. Even with all the proof of the harm of chemically grown food and GMOs, it is still not compulsory for food manufacturers to declare what's really in our food, which amounts to a chemical feast. These chemicals are then stored in human body fat, where they then affect our health.

The Depletion of Our Soil

In his book *Rare Earths: Forbidden Cures,* about the connection between minerals and disease and longevity, Joel Wallach writes, "Before written history it took one hundred thousand years to double the world's population. After the dawn of agriculture (approx. seven thousand years ago) it took only seven hundred years. Today it takes only thirty-five years to double the world's population. This has forced growers to increase production of crops unnaturally, using techniques that decrease vitamin and mineral content to NPK, nitrogen, potassium, and phosphorous, hardly enough to grow healthy human cells [and] combat disease and pollution."

Agricultural scientists now estimate that approximately 80 percent of the mineral content of our soils has been depleted in just the last hundred years. This chronic soil degradation is due to overfarming practices combined with the use of chemical fertilizers to increase crop yields each year. Organic farming, on the other hand, uses no harmful chemicals, but even organic farming, if not practiced wisely, according to soil nutrient levels, can still result in food that lacks essential nutrients. A diet of fresh fruit and vegetables may have delivered all the essential nutrients for the body to achieve optimal health in the 1920s, but in the twenty-first century it seems to be far from doing so. According to many nutritional experts, vitamin, mineral, and other nutrient deficiencies are in epidemic proportions not only in the Third World, but also in developed nations. In the United States, for example, the population's generally poor health is a result of being overfed and undernourished. Since many diseases are caused by overeating nutritionally deficient foods, malnutrition (but with obesity) is rampant here. As Linus Pauling said, "You can trace every sickness, every disease, and every ailment to a mineral deficiency."

The Necessity of Food Supplements

In his 1981 best-selling book *The Airola Diet and Cookbook,* nutritionist, naturopathic physician, and educator Paavo Airola says, "Those who advocate eating natural foods as the only source of vitamins and minerals live in a dream world of yesterday. What was yesterday's law is today's folly. It doesn't really matter how well you balance your meals, or if you're a meat-eater, vegetarian, or a raw foodist, you still run the risk of malnutrition if you try to get all your vitamins and minerals exclusively from the food you eat."

As late as the 1970s, the allopathic medical establishment was still denying the fact that we needed to supplement our diet to obtain all the necessary nutrients for health, passing off nutritional supplements as just a form of expensive urine to their patients. Today, doctors are singing a different tune, saying what naturopathic doctors were already asserting back in the 1970s: we all need to supplement our diet, particularly during times of growth and development like pregnancy, adolescence, and menopause. The evidence is now irrefutable—the normal, even healthy diet must be supplemented. Today medical journals are packed with clinical trials and studies on the amazing effects of nutritional supplementation, so much so that even naturalists have no leg to stand on when they attempt to prove that we can obtain optimal health from our food alone. Food supplements are vital in today's world to achieve optimal health; the facts are out there for all those who are willing to open their eyes to the truth of the modern world.

Nobel Prize–winning physician and biochemist Hans Krebs (1900–1981) said, "In the entire history of medical science there has not been one metabolic disease that was ever cured or prevented by drugs, surgery, or mechanical manipulation of the body. In every case the ultimate solution was found only in relation to adequate nutrition." There is strong evidence that the sudden increase in degenerative diseases such as cancer, diabetes, and heart disease, today's leading killers, are at least in part the result of soil degradation that has led to mineral deficiencies in the food we consume and therefore in the body. It's hard to believe that we have done so much damage to soil health in such a short time, but with the last century's burst in population, along with massive and unnatural changes in how we raise our food, there is really no doubt anymore as to why we get sick.

The Best Way to Supplement Your Diet

Apart from the obvious fact that we should eat a whole-foods, unprocessed diet of fresh, organic fruits, vegetables, herbs, nuts, seeds, and whole grains, we need to supplement our diet. When you visit a health-food store you will undoubtedly be bombarded with all the latest in vitamins and told that you should purchase practically the whole shop or you will be missing something. As a result, it is extremely confusing for the average person to figure out what supplements you need. You can do the old "pick and mix," choosing different bottles of this or that, but the latest studies regarding vitamin and mineral ratios prove that synergy is vital for good absorption and balance within the cells. Chances are you are making a dangerous cocktail that is not going to work, doing yourself more harm than good.

A landmark study published in 1999 by the *Journal of the American Nutraceutical Association* found that over 97 percent of store-bought nutritional products, randomly selected, were toxic or labeled untruthfully. When visiting your health-food store you need to be educated when choosing supplements, and even then most supplements have been clinically found to be useless in curbing serious health problems. Therefore, it is best to get recommendations from a qualified professional nutritionist who is educated in recent scientific findings. Unfortunately, many nutritionists and certainly many doctors are still quoting old research texts that we now know to be untrue and misleading.

When looking for complete and balanced supplements it is not only vital to get the right synergy, but also the correct amounts. For example, current studies show that the optimal daily amount of vitamin E for prevention of most cancers is 400 I.U., and most multivitamins usually provide less than 100 I.U., not nearly enough to prevent serious disease, so you end up having to buy many separate bottles of this single vitamin, playing a dangerous game of pick and mix. Nutritionists say that it takes five times more nutrition to repair and rebuild the body as it does to maintain it. This means that high-potency supplements are vital when using nutrition to reverse serious health problems. If you take multivitamin/mineral supplements in larger amounts than the bottle recommends, it can be risky because of sloppy formulations, poor synergistic ratios, and toxic excipients. That is why it is important to get a supplement that is tested on human cells and that has excellent formulation and safety. If you are taking a man-made vitamin/mineral tablet, find out if it has a potency guarantee on the bottle.

Why Vitamins and Herbs Don't Work (and How to Get Ones That Do)

Nearly 75 percent of the world's population takes some type of herbal/mineral supplement every day, and there are literally thousands of brands and millions of products to choose from. Is there really a difference between them? Well, check this out: A landmark study published in the *Journal of the American Nutraceutical Association* 2, no. 1 (1999) found that over 97 percent of nutritional products randomly selected from health-food stores were found to be toxic or labeled untruthfully.

We have been telling our clients and students to be very careful when purchasing supplements in health-food stores and to question the quality of these supplements with what we have taught them. Unfortunately, many of the supplements you buy today at stores or online are not only of poor quality in general, they also contain a lot of questionable fillers, binders, bulking agents, and stearates. Without getting myself into too much trouble here and at the same time shocking the socks off you, just think about these findings. A study at East Carolina University School of Medicine in Greenville, North Carolina, demonstrated that toxic excipients such as magnesium stearate and stearic acid found in 90 percent of health-food store supplements actually cause a collapse of T-cell membrane function and cell death, therefore suppressing the immune system (*Journal of Immunology*, July 1990).

When using herbs to detoxify and purify or to stimulate the healing of the body's internal organs or tissues you need to initially understand three main points that aren't even taught today in herb school. These important factors are the main reasons behind what established herbal medicine in the first place, so it's vital to go back to our roots and understand them well. Understanding these three main factors will make you realize why so many people say "herbs do not work," and why they are probably right.

1. Potency (dosage): Not all health supplements are created equal. Most supermarkets and many health-food store varieties of supplements are diluted or full of fillers or bulking agents. They do not contain enough of the biochemical substance that is the magic that does the job and brings about the desired healing effect. You end up having to take three to four times what the bottle recommends, and then you still need to take some more before you start to see anything happen. This can be dangerous because of point 2 below, purity. Companies today aren't providing optimal dosage levels on labels for fear of being prosecuted by consumers who overdose or have side effects as a result of mixing supplements with allopathic medicines and then blaming the herbal product. These low-dosage recommendations mean you do not get cured, which also means you have to keep coming back for more. Also, life today on the planet is totally different from what life was like in the past century and the century before that. Today, many people do not eat organic food, and at the same time we live in a much more polluted environment than ever before. This means that dosages that worked three centuries ago for a healthy-eating, hardworking organic farmer would not work for an obese, fast-food-eating couch potato today.

2. Purity (organic or wild sourced): Once upon a time before global pharmaceuticals were the norm, when herbal medicine was the only medicine available and cancer, heart disease, and diabetes were not as common, all herbs were organically grown in the wild and harvested at the correct times for potency and purity. Everyone knows (or should we say we think they know) that wild-harvested organic herbs contain several times more medicinal properties than the spray-riddled, farmed variety. On top of this, all herb barrels were filled to the top and no cheapskating occurred; this means that all that was in the final product was the strong, potent herb itself and nothing else—no additives, fillers, or binders as in most of today's so-called natural supplements.

3. Formulation (synergy): Most of today's nutritional and herbal formulas are created by what we call "armchair herbalists" or from theory-based nutritional information derived from herb books written by other armchair herbalists. Today, most supplement manufacturers have never operated a successful herb clinic, nor have they tested the formulas extensively on themselves or their clients (because they probably don't have any; they're in the herb "business"). Perhaps they just got out of herb school after studying with other armchair herbalists. When we look at a nutritional product today to determine its quality we need to look deeper, starting with who is producing it and why. Make sure the formulator is (or recently was) a successful health care practitioner. Did they really heal anybody from any serious health ailments? Did they ever run a clinic or have clients? Herbs work in synergy with one another and complement one another, creating a greater sum together than the sum of their individual parts. Different herbs can counteract one another and cause a poor electrical synergy, which in turn causes poor absorption of the nutrients. Even though there may be a fancy list of famous herbs on the bottle in the formula you are taking, it may not be synergistic. This is why I prefer to use products created by experienced master herbalists.

Most of us do not blink an eyelid when it comes to spending a lot of money on a car each year, for insurance, road tax, and getting it serviced every three to six months. Unlike your car, if your body blows up you cannot just buy another one; it's the only one you've got. Your body deserves the best supplements you can get, not some vitamins from your local health-food store of questionable provenance. Look at it this way: everyone knows the importance of cleansing your outer body each day; otherwise it smells bad. Your internal organs get dirty, too. This is why both correct nutrition and internal cleansing on a regular basis (as described in chapter 4) is the key to curing your health ailments and preventing illness.

SUPERFOODS

As Hippocrates famously said, "Let your food be your medicine and your medicine be your food." However, do not be fooled by the boom in overpriced "superfoods" that claim all kinds of medicinal benefits. There is a lot of hype out there and plenty of money to be made. Many common spices like turmeric, oregano, and cinnamon have double the ORAC (oxygen radical absorbance capacity, a method of measuring antioxidant capacities in biological sample) over expensive exotic fruits like the currently trendy acai fruit. In fact, *superfood* is just a new name that's been given to ancient foods that have always been known throughout history to be jam-packed with important nutrients or that contain high ORAC levels.

Most countries are well known for having several superfoods that grow locally and are common. One such food is alfalfa. The word *alfalfa* comes from Arabic, meaning "Father of all foods." This plant (not the sprout) has a large root system and has been known for centuries to increase the power of the immune system and clean the blood. It's little wonder what this powerhouse of a plant can do for your health when you look into how it grows, with roots reaching down twenty feet or more, far beyond the topsoil, pulling up valuable trace minerals and other nutrients. Alfalfa is also high in chlorophyll, which is the green pigment in leafy green vegetables and grasses that has a blood-cleaning action.

There are many such superfoods that we recommend because of their high levels of organic nutrients. These include maca, ground flax meal, barley grass, wheat grass, chlorella, marine phytoplankton, hemp seeds, molasses, miso, kombucha, green tea, aloe vera, and spirulina. There are also superfoods you probably have in your kitchen now that you likely don't know about, things like oregano and sumac (used in Middle Eastern cooking), which have some of the highest ORAC antioxidant values in the world. Pumpkin seeds are another superfood, rich in zinc for wound healing and immunity, and great for the prostate gland. Then there is, of course, broccoli, which is packed with anticancer compounds and antioxidants like superoxide dismutase, which stimulates the production of glutathione, the mother of all antioxidants.

We do not believe that taking only one of these superfoods can deliver all the vitamins, minerals, amino acids, and essential fatty acids we need; therefore, it is imperative to combine different superfoods for optimum nutritional synergy, which is called a *superfood formula.* It's like a cocktail of nature's most nutritionally dense foods all in one jar. There are a number of new products coming on the market that contain virtually all the major superfoods, and these make an excellent natural vitamin/mineral supplement that is an alternative to standard commercial synthetic supplements. To make your superfoods formula even more digestible and absorbable you can now purchase fermented superfood blends from companies such as NuFerm, which are higher in enzymes and probiotics due to the fermentation process. I personally have used these types of fermented superfood formulas with great success for healing gut diseases along with following the Eight Immortal Healers' guidelines.

CHLOROPHYLL, THE "BLOOD" OF PLANTS

Richard Willstätter, a German organic chemist whose study of the structure of plant pigments, chlorophyll included, won him the 1915 Nobel Prize for chemistry, observed that the chlorophyll molecule bears a striking resemblance to hemoglobin, the red pigment in human blood. So if you could say that plants have blood, chlorophyll would be it. Chlorophyll is the green pigment in plants that makes them green. It even performs functions similar to what human blood does, such as growth and respiration and delivering oxygen to cells. What's even more interesting is that a chemical molecule of human blood is almost identical to that of chlorophyll, the only difference being that chlorophyll's central atom is magnesium, whereas human blood maintains iron as its central atom.

Chlorophyll has been shown to have a blood-purifying action on the body, assisting the liver and kidneys and lowering acid wastes in the body's tissues, which can have a positive effect on any illness. Liquid chlorophyll is like detergent for our cells, cleaning and scrubbing them. Chlorophyll assists in naturally bonding to heavy metals like mercury and toxins in the blood, detoxifying them from the body. It also has an alkalizing effect along with its many nutritional benefits, while also performing as an antioxidant, mopping up free radicals. There is a valid reason behind why Grandma said, "Eat your greens." Green leafy vegetables contain high levels of chlorophyll, but even higher amounts are found in alfalfa, chlorella, spirulina, kelp, wheatgrass, and barley grass. Common household sources are green leafy vegetables, and one in particular is cilantro (coriander leaves).

Composition of Half a Kilo of Wheatgrass (7–10" tall)*

Nutrients per pound: 453.59 g

Chlorophyll: 5,000 mg

Choline: 4,000 mg

Vitamin C (ascorbic acid): 2,000 mg

Vitamin A (carotene): 360 mg

Vitamin E: 120 mg

Vitamin F: 120 mg

Vitamin K: 120 mg

Niacin (B group vitamin): 120 mg

Vitamin B_2 (riboflavin): 24 mg

Vitamin B_1 (thiamine): 12 mg

Pantothenic acid (B_5): 8 mg

Vitamin B_6: 4 mg

Although the above levels of B vitamins are lower than some other plants, these levels are more in line with recent research on recommended B vitamin levels. As you can see, grasses like wheatgrass contain almost all the nutrients to sustain life.

---

*Report to the American Chemical Society by Dr. C. F. Schnabel. See www
.grainmills.com.au/wheatgrass-juice.

Scientists have done considerable research on the healing nutrients that chlorophyll contains and have found it also acts as a liver tonic, protecting DNA breakdown due to its high enzyme content. It also has been shown to minimize the effects of radiation, especially when people undergo chemotherapy. Do not wait to get a serious disease. Start eating more greens or take liquid chlorophyll, green food concentrates, or wheatgrass juice daily. Chlorophyll is nontoxic, alkalizing, and nutritious, and when mixed with mint leaves it becomes an excellent beverage to flavor your drinking water.

Note: Wheat allergies are due to the gluten found in the wheat grain. Wheatgrass is cut before the plant forms any grain, and therefore it contains no gluten.

THE HEALING POWER OF ORGANIC SULFUR

In their book *The Miracle of MSM: The Natural Solution for Pain,* doctors Stanley W. Jacob and Ronald M. Lawrence and health writer Martin Zucker attest to the power of organic sulfur, better known as MSM: "Here is an essential nutrient that no one sees as being that! We don't learn anything about sulfur in medical school. Sulfur has been the most understudied and overlooked nutrient."

Methylsulfonylmethane (MSM) is the scientific term for the naturally occurring organic element sulfur, which is found in every living cell of our bodies. MSM is not a drug, medicine, herb, or synthetic substance, but rather an organic nutrient that plays a key role in forming the structure of every human cell. Organic sulfur has a governing effect on hormonal production and balance, enzyme activity, and immunity. Unlike calcium and magnesium, sulfur is quite abundant in a variety of foods, but at the same time is much more easily destroyed by heating, drying, or any other cooking method for that matter. So unless your diet consists of a large percentage of raw food on a daily basis, you are likely lacking in organic sulfur. MSM's richest sources are in raw vegetables such as cabbage, peppers, asparagus, brussels sprouts, garlic, onions, and grasses such as wheat and barley. Some key signs that arise when your body becomes sulfur-deficient are pain and inflammation in the form of arthritis, as well as other autoimmune conditions like asthma; fatigue; unhealthy skin, hair, nails; and memory loss.

It is important not to be confused about the difference between organic sulfur (MSM) and sulfur-based drugs. While MSM is organic and needed by the body, sulfite drugs are synthetic versions that don't occur naturally except as waste products produced by our bodies. Although sulfur drugs were invented more than a century ago by European chemists prior to the advent of antibiotics, many people do not tolerate sulfur drugs even in small doses, as in the case of sulfur dioxide, which is used as a preservative in many foods and beverages, especially dried fruits and wine. As MSM is organic and vital for the body, there is no allergic reaction as in some sulfur drugs, but instead the opposite occurs.

Organic Sulfur (MSM) May Help with Common Ailments

- Improves the quality of the skin by increasing connective tissue
- Aids in forming proteins that strengthen hair and nails
- Decreases the effects of allergens
- Prevents the buildup of bad bacteria and parasites in the abdomen
- Relieves migraines
- Alleviates snoring
- Improves tooth whitening
- Helps correct
  - Constipation
  - Candida
  - Cramps and spasms
  - Arthritis
  - Blood-sugar problems

Sulfur is referred to in the Bible as "brimstone," and its medicinal use goes back thousands of years, to the Trojan Wars, when soldiers healed their wounds in the sulfur baths of Agamemnon. Even today sulfur baths (hot springs) are renowned for treating a variety of joint and other ailments. Sulfur is commonly regarded as the fourth most important mineral in the body after calcium, phosphorous, and potassium, accounting for just under 0.5 percent of your body weight.

DMSO

As we know, most of us are deficient in organic sulfur, not only because we do not eat enough greens (the case for many of us), but because cooking and processing destroys it. Here we introduce you to another form of sulfur like MSM that can greatly assist in many health ailments; this type is not intended for internal use, rather for applying to the skin, to be absorbed by muscles and associated structures for many purposes. It is particularly useful when doing any kind of exercise or as a complement to internal exercises.

DMSO is the naturally occurring organic sulfur that binds the cells of trees together. It is extracted as a by-product while making pulp and was previously discarded as a waste by-product of the wood pulp industry. It was first researched by Stanley Jacob, M.D., the codiscoverer of MSM. DMSO (dimethyl sulfide), just like MSM (dimethyl sulfone, also known as methylsulfonylmethane), is an organic sulfur nutrient.* DMSO and MSM are natural forms of sulfur compounds that have been used for many years and are safe and nontoxic. DMSO, like MSM, has very much the same healing properties, but with a few added ones. DMSO is not intended for internal use (for this, MSM is preferred) because it can cause some side effects, such as garlic breath, intestinal gas, and allergic reactions (although none of these side effects is life-threatening). However, one property of DMSO

---

*Both these forms of organic sulfur are not to be confused with sulfur-based drugs, which are inorganic and synthetic. These inferior inorganic forms are used as antibiotics, which many people have allergic reactions to.

when applied externally that MSM does not have is its ability to act as a powerful carrier for other substances through the skin. DMSO literally acts as an organic solvent, carrying other substances that are mixed with it into the body through the skin and mucous membranes. DMSO can also be added in small amounts (5 to 10 percent) to internal solutions of MSM to assist in better absorption of the MSM into the body. It also becomes a powerful supercarrier of nutrients and essential oils—whatever it is combined with—into the local tissues it is applied to. Nutritional supplements can be dissolved in DMSO solution and then applied to the skin for fast absorption into the bloodstream if digestive function is poor and one is not able to absorb nutrients correctly, as with the elderly. DMSO is antibacterial and antiviral, so it does not necessarily cause surface bacteria or infections on the surface skin to absorb further; instead it can be applied successfully to open herpes sores (on the mouth or genitals), assisting in their healing. For this purpose and in most cases for external use it is best diluted in a 50:50 solution with aloe vera to decrease possible irritation, itchiness, or a slight burning sensation, while also working with the aloe vera, which is a powerful skin-healing substance.

DMSO has also shown remarkable effects on joint pain and spinal problems such as disc inflammation and nerve pain and even in paralysis, and it is currently being researched by spinal centers for the treatment of nerve paralysis. James A. Howenstine, author of *A Physician's Guide to Natural Health Products That Work,* says:

> Diseases of the nervous system, brain injury and spinal cord injury physicians around the world have found DMSO to be invaluable in treating head injuries and injury to the spinal cord. Use of DMSO within a few hours of brain injuries and within one hour of injury to the spinal cord has prevented death and paralysis that often ensues. No other therapy is better at reducing increased intracranial pressure. When head or spinal-cord trauma occurs because there is bone surrounding these two structures, the fluid from the inflammatory reaction greatly increases damage to the brain and cord.

Perhaps because DMSO is so cheap and natural, the FDA has only approved it for use as a preservative of organs for transplants and to treat interstitial cystitis. It has fallen out of the limelight and out of mainstream medical news almost completely, leading some people to believe that it has been discredited by drug companies. The truth is much more complicated. The famous punk-rock band Dead Kennedys, fronted by Jello Biafra, wrote a song called "DMSO" in the 1980s about its properties. It was rumored that hippies were going around with water pistols filled with a mix of DMSO and LSD and spraying them at cops. Just a few drops of DMSO mixed with LSD on an exposed bit of skin was said to make you trip for days.

The history of DMSO began in 1961, when Dr. Stanley Jacob, a pioneering researcher and the "Father of DMSO," was head of the organ transplant program at Oregon Health Sciences University. While investigating DMSO's potential as a preservative for organs, he discovered that it penetrated the skin quickly and deeply without damaging it, thus beginning his work with DMSO, which continues to this day. As the media soon got word of Dr. Jacob's discovery, it was not long before patients with a variety of medical complaints began using it. As it was available for industrial uses and is very cheap, patients could dose themselves. Why then does DMSO still sit on the sidelines of medicine, and why is it currently unable to be legally sold with the intention of its being used as a medical substance?

> It's a square peg being pushed into a round hole. It does not follow the rival approach of one agent against one disease entity. It is the aspirin of our era. If aspirin were to come along today, it would have the same problem. If someone gave you a little white pill and said take this and your headache will go away, your body temperature will go down, it will help prevent strokes and major heart problems—what would you think?*

Dr. Jacob believes the FDA suppressed DMSO to destroy interest in this natural drug, perhaps because it is so effective that it poses a

---

*www.dmso.org.

threat to many profitable synthetic drugs in today's pain-control market. As DMSO can carry other drugs with it across the membranes, it can be very successful even at lower doses, carrying drugs such as morphine, penicillin, steroids, cortisone, and many others into the body. This property would enable DMSO to act as a new drug-delivery system that would lower the risk of infection occurring whenever skin is penetrated while also sparing the digestive system from the toxic side effects of many of the common pain drugs.

Not only is DMSO possibly a natural wonder drug, it can also reduce the dose or need for many other synthetic drugs. Today DMSO is used most widely as a topical analgesic, as studies suggest that DMSO cuts pain by blocking peripheral nerves. Even burns, frostbite, cuts, sprains, and arthritic pain have been successfully treated, while a number of sports and Olympic athletes have used DMSO. Relief is reported to be almost immediate, lasting several hours.

It should be noted that DMSO (like aspirin) is not necessarily a cure-all, but rather a safe, natural symptomatic approach to controlling pain and reducing inflammation or as a delivery system for other nontoxic natural substances that can assist in healing.

MAGNESIUM AND TMT

Nowadays a deficiency of the mineral magnesium has become epidemic. Called the "antistress mineral," magnesium is vital for calcium absorption, muscle relaxation, nerve impulse, heart function, and several hundred other functions, while also preventing conditions like heart disease, hypertension, heart palpitations, arrhythmias, stroke, neurological dysfunction, and all types of pain. Adequate levels of magnesium are required for our bodies to utilize core antioxidant vitamins such as C and E. Without enough magnesium, insulin is not able to transfer glucose into cells, toxins are not properly eliminated, and your body ages prematurely. Magnesium is also needed for the removal of heavy metals, and along with iodine it helps to protect you from radiation. Glutathione, the mother of all antioxidants, is magnesium dependent. With all this a known scientific fact, allopathic doctors almost never prescribe magnesium when you are suffering from some condition or disease. Instead they prescribe pharmaceutical drugs, which deplete your magnesium levels even further.

According to Dr. Mark Sircus, author of *Transdermal Magnesium Therapy,* a number of studies show that more than half of the U.S. population is deficient in magnesium, and this is according to the current recommended dietary allowance, which many nutritional experts say is far too low and dated as well. Another concern is that we consume far too much calcium today. Yes, that's right. Most people are fed the lie that we don't get enough calcium, but it's magnesium we need more of, not calcium. Research has shown that our Paleolithic ancestors, who had extremely strong bones, had a calcium to magnesium ratio of 1:1; today that ratio is more in the 10:1. The list of diseases that can occur from this imbalance of calcium to magnesium is pages long. Many health practitioners are aware of the need for magnesium supplementation, and they prescribe semiabsorbable forms like magnesium citrate or magnesium oxide, which has almost no absorption. They do not realize that because magnesium has a mild laxative action, much of the oral magnesium we take doesn't get absorbed and passes out in the stools. Also, many people today suffer from leaky gut and Crohn's disease, while the elderly have poor absorption due to digestive weaknesses. This is why transdermal magnesium is a wonderfully effective way to supplement with magnesium, by bypassing the digestive system completely.

If you cannot afford to buy transdermal magnesium oil, you can make your own magnesium oil at home inexpensively and easily. Magnesium oil is simply magnesium chloride (crystal flakes) dissolved in a water solution. Magnesium chloride flakes can be purchased online, at health-food stores, and even at aquarium supply stores, where it's sold in bulk for saltwater tanks. In Japan it is called Nigari (E511) and used in the making of tofu. Make sure the source you use is pure, without any contaminants.

The best food sources of magnesium (depending, of course, on the soil) are buckwheat, almonds, Brazil nuts, and any organic green leafy vegetables.

Make Your Own Magnesium Oil

Ingredients: ½ cup of magnesium chloride crystals dissolved in ½ cup of boiling water will give you a (very generous) one-week supply. Once this mixture cools down, put it in a spray bottle or a plastic travel bottle.

Dosage: Apply liberally to arms or legs or both; eight sprays of the oil gives about 100 mg of magnesium.

Note: Magnesium oil can sting a little and feel oily to the touch. If it stings too much just dilute your mixture by adding more water. You'll need to wait twenty minutes before wiping off the excess that remains for all the magnesium to be absorbed.

THE MIRACLE OF UNPROCESSED, SUN-DRIED SEA SALT

In recent years salt has been demonized because of incorrect fad-dieting information and poor nutritional advice from the medical establishment. We have been encouraged to forget the amazing healing benefits and need for unprocessed sea salt in the diet. Sun-dried sea salt contains some of the most essential ingredients for our cells to survive.

As noted in the previous chapter, your body is not 70 percent water, it is 70 percent salt water. Most of the salt in the body is stored in the bones in the form of calcium and magnesium salt crystals. There is strong evidence that these salt crystals are vital for keeping the bones from breaking. This may well explain why Japanese women who consume little or no dairy products have the strongest bones in the world compared to women in the United States and the UK, who consume the highest amounts of dairy products and yet have the highest rates of osteoporosis. The Japanese claim that the reason they are less susceptible to osteoporosis is that their diet is both alkaline and high in natural forms of alkaline sea salt, like seaweed, tamari, and miso, all of which all contain unprocessed sea salt. Do not confuse high-grade sea salt with table salt or commercial supermarket sea salt, which is processed and chemically unbalanced.

What Is Unprocessed Sea Salt?

Unprocessed, sun-dried sea salt is sometimes called Celtic sea salt, macrobiotic sea salt, gray salt, and organic sea salt. Technically, salt is not organic because it's not carbon based (like all organic matter), although the word *organic* is used to loosely emphasize that this salt is unprocessed. Note that it is the imbalanced ratio of sodium to potassium, rather than sodium excess, that is related to many types of cancer.

Unprocessed sun-dried sea salt is very important for the acid-alkaline balance in the cells. A lack of natural sea salt in the body can contribute to overacidity, resulting in damage to the DNA and contributing to the proliferation of cancerous cells. It is important to note that when increasing your amount of drinking water it is advisable to also increase your natural sea salt intake. I have found in my clinical practice that the average adult needs anywhere from a half to over a teaspoon of unprocessed sea salt daily depending on the amount of exercise, which affects both water and salt loss. If you experience water retention, decreasing your processed salt intake and increasing your water intake along with the correct type of salt—unprocessed, sun-dried sea salt— can actually help you eliminate excess water. Also, you should take into account the fact that you may be eating a lot of naturally salty foods that contain a lot of the processed type of salt. The best form of salt is not table salt, low-sodium salt, or processed sea salt, as these products are processed, lacking in essential minerals, and chemically out of balance for our body. Salt is only beneficial in its natural, unprocessed, sun-dried raw state. The best by far are the Celtic, Normandy, and New Zealand sea salts, which are slightly gray in color, showing their distinct mineral content. These unrefined salts are still slightly moist when you buy by the bag and come coarse or finely ground.

If you experience cramps, muscle fatigue, joint deterioration, obesity, dizziness, and fainting, check your salt level first. Unprocessed, sun-dried sea salt, which is available in good health-food stores and online, can contain around seventy-plus trace minerals found in the sea, all of which are vital for our body's trace mineral balance. Again, do not confuse unprocessed sea salt with regular table salt or sodium chloride. They are totally different. The former is a medicine, the latter a poison.

Often when a doctor recommends cutting down on salt because of a heart problem or some other condition, what he or she is implying is that regular table salt will add to your present problem because it is chemically imbalanced, and this is correct. Unbeknownst to most allopathic doctors is the fact that unprocessed gray sea salt may well actually help to cure the problem. Today modern doctors do not study nutrition as a part of their general medical training, and therefore they do not understand the difference between processed salt and real salt, nor do they know about the many health benefits of unprocessed sea salt and its ability to heal and replace missing essential trace minerals.

VITAMIN B_{17}—THE MISSING VITAMIN

The nutritional power of certain seeds was known in ancient times and is attested to in the Bible: "And God said, 'Behold, I have given you every herb-bearing seed which is upon the face of all the earth, and every tree, in which is the fruit of a tree yielding seed; to you it shall be for meat'" (Genesis 1:9).

There are many chronic and metabolic diseases that have challenged modern medicine over the past years, and many of these diseases have been conquered. Only a few hundred years ago the metabolic disease scurvy killed hundreds of thousands of people, then the cure was found in good old-fashioned vitamin C. On the same note, other fatal diseases like pernicious anemia, pellagra, and beriberi were all found to be completely preventable and curable through specific dietary factors; specifically, essential nutrients. In time vitamin B_{17} may also be revealed to prevent and perhaps reverse many health conditions just as vitamins C and B have done in the past.

In 1950 biochemist Ernst T. Krebs Jr. isolated a new vitamin that he called B_{17}. As time progressed, many scientists became convinced that Krebs had finally found a successful cancer preventive or perhaps a cure. The pharmaceutical cartels at that time, unable to patent or claim exclusive rights to the vitamin, launched an attack of unprecedented aggression against the semisynthetic version "laetrile," despite the fact that the evidence for its efficacy in controlling most forms of cancer was impressive. Never before have pharmaceutical companies and the medical establishment done so much to prevent the public from knowing about the importance of a vital nutrient in the human diet.

B_{17} is found in the seeds of noncitrus fruits such as apples, peaches, and cherries and in both the leaves and unripe green fruit of the papaya tree (known as paw paw in Australia), with smaller amounts found in millet and the grasses of wheat and barley. Bitter almonds and apricot kernels are especially rich in B_{17}.

Fruit seeds that provide B_{17} are commonly eaten foods in cultures such as the Navajo, Hunza, and Abkhazians where people live long lives and cancer is extremely rare. Once upon a time, when cancer was not so common, people ate the whole fruit, chewing and enjoying the seeds or drying them and using them as an accompaniment to meals for nutritional purposes. Humans seem to have gotten into a very bad habit of eating the fruit and throwing away the most important nutritional cancer-fighting nutrient that is found within the seeds, vitamin B_{17}.

While apricot kernels don't contain cyanide or the semisynthetic version of B_{17} known as laetrile, as is often touted, they do contain amygdalin which is a more complex organic molecule that provides natural B_{17} and is safe in small quantities. Amygdalin is comprised of molecules of hydrocyanic acid and benzaldehyde (the chemical flavoring for marzipan) and two molecules of glucose. According to theoretical data and understanding about the toxicology of cyanide, medicine has made the assumption that any substance containing cyanic compounds is always toxic, even in small amounts, and gives no consideration to the natural ability of our bodies to utilize and metabolize cyanogenic glycosides in the small quantities found in our natural food chain.

We must understand that the longest-living cultures have always eaten small quantities of fruit seeds that contain this amazing complex molecule, which is detailed in the documentary *A World without Cancer* by Edward Griffin. That being said, we shouldn't make the apricot seed a main course, as overdosing can be toxic. While some doctors recommend 1 seed per 10 pounds of bodyweight for cancer treatment, we recommend no more than approximately 5–7 apricots seeds per day to play an important role as part of a comprehensive cancer wellness or prevention plan (see www.canceractive.com/cancer-active-page-link.aspx?n=512).

ENZYMES, THE FOUNTAIN OF LIFE

Enzymes are biologically active proteins found in all living cells, whether they be animal or vegetable. "Enzymes serve as the body's labor force to perform every single function required for our daily activities and are required to keep us alive," according to doctors D. A. Lopez, R. M. Williams, and K. Miehlke in their book *Enzymes: The Fountain of Life.* "They are responsible for all the functions of every organ system in our bodies. At the same time, they are most important in supporting our body defenses and immune system to protect us from harmful forces and specific dangers to our health. The immune system depends heavily on enzymes to conduct its protective functions."

There are two classes of enzymes, metabolic and digestive (food). Metabolic enzymes are produced by the cells of the body (the liver and pancreas) to speed up chemical reactions and for energy production, oxygen absorption, blood purification, and detoxification. All 100 trillion cells in the human body depend on metabolic enzymes to function. As we get older, our body produces fewer such enzymes, which contributes to the aging process, with the result being wrinkles, bone loss, and disease in general. Digestive enzymes are produced and secreted along the digestive tract by the digestive organs, such as the mouth (when chewing food), liver, gallbladder, pancreas, stomach, small intestine, and colon. They assist in breaking down proteins, fats, and carbohydrates, and they allow the nutrients in the food we eat to be absorbed into the bloodstream and the waste products to be removed.

Enzymes are composed of a protein base with an amino acid chain; functionally they're vital catalysts for every chemical reaction in the body, just as important as oxygen, water, salt, and minerals in the healing process. While metabolic enzymes help to build and repair the cellular structure of the body, digestive enzymes work the other way around, by breaking down food molecules into usable energy substances.

Food enzymes are introduced into the body only through raw foods—fresh uncooked fruits and vegetables, nuts and seeds, sprouted and whole grains, and also raw (unpasteurized) dairy products, raw eggs, and raw meat. All raw foods contain the exact amounts of enzymes necessary to digest that particular food, the only exception being the foods papaya (papain) and pineapple (bromelain), which contain more. Cooking or processing food destroys all of its vital enzymes. As many people eat only cooked or processed foods, our digestive system is then required to produce more digestive enzymes to aid the process. Humans are the only species that cooks food; all other animals naturally eat a 100 percent raw-food diet.

One of the most debatable subjects in the health field is how much raw food we should be eating. Well, for the majority of us, the answer is a lot more than you do now. Westerners in particular have become accustomed to eating only cooked, processed, and refined foods devoid of all enzymes. Our modern diet encourages digestive diseases because people tend to have incomplete digestion of fats, proteins, carbohydrates, and sugars due to the fact that cooking food destroys its natural enzymes. It only takes a temperature of approximately 120 degrees Fahrenheit to destroy enzymes. For example, pasteurizing milk destroys the enzyme lactase that aids in the digestion of the milk sugar lactose. One of the reasons so many people are lactose intolerant lately is not because there's something wrong with them, but because the milk is essentially dead. Before the widespread urban growth caused by industrialization, people kept dairy cows even in urban areas, and most towns and cities were served by a local dairy farmer (who delivered milk to your door), such that the short time period between production and consumption minimized the disease risk of drinking raw milk. Lactose intolerance, irritable bowel syndrome, Crohn's disease, and many other digestive disorders common today were almost unheard of. Then in 1973 the U.S. government mandated pasteurization of milk used in interstate commerce, and these diseases skyrocketed.

Almost all methods of cooking destroy enzyme quantities, but some are worse than others. The best methods of cooking that still retain some enzymes are sun-drying or dehydrating, light steaming, baking, or grilling. The worst are boiling and frying, while arguably the very worst method is microwaving. Don't look to allopathic medicine practitioners for advice on the benefits of incorporating raw foods into your diet, and even natural medicine experts continue to debate the subject of what ratio of raw-to-cooked food is best. If we were to say that 50 percent raw was generally the norm, then this percentage would increase in summer and decrease in winter.

If your digestive system is weak or if you are an older person and you commonly observe undigested food in your stool (a spleen or kidney yang deficiency in traditional Chinese medicine), you will likely find that raw food is difficult to digest, so in this case vegetable juices (not fruit juice) and raw soups are a far more effective way of getting the benefits of eating raw food. Add ginger and other warming digestive herbs to your vegetable juices and raw soups to help increase your digestive fire. Fruit juices are generally too high in sugar and can aggravate many people's blood-sugar levels. Fruit is best eaten raw and in its whole form, not as a juice, and be sure to eat a few of the seeds also. Nonsweet fruits such as citrus or nonsweet red grapes are usually tolerated in moderation by those with diabetes.

A diet of almost entirely raw foods was seen as the optimal diet decades ago, but now the tide is turning, and it is recognized that our Paleolithic ancestors were never completely 100 percent raw. While continuing to learn from traditional Chinese medicine (TCM), naturopathic medicine has realized that in some cases a 100 percent raw diet may not be optimal, especially in cases of digestive disorders like those previously mentioned. TCM has always encouraged people to eat according to the seasons, so during the summer months eat more raw vegetarian foods, and in winter months, eat more broths, soups, and warming herbs.

On many occasions I've seen the benefits of a raw-food program using vegetable juices and have witnessed medical miracles coming from periodic raw-vegetable juice fasting. Supplementing with enzymes also helps recovery from many illnesses, and not only digestive ailments. If you have a history of antibiotic use, have learning difficulties or autism, or you do not eat enough raw foods, enzyme supplementation may greatly benefit you. There are numerous enzyme formulas on the market, of varying quality. Supplementing with superfoods and fermented foods, skipping cooked meals and instead having a raw vegetable juice or soup is a sure way of keeping your enzyme levels where they should be. Another excellent way of increasing enzymes in your diet is through sprouting, as sprouts are rich in both protein and enzymes. Sprouting kits are available from most health-food stores, or you can very easily make your own sprouting container using a widemouthed canning jar and some cheesecloth, or a sprouting jar lid. Sprouting is super easy, and sprouts are very tasty on salads or as a garnish on cooked foods.

Juicing Your Way to Health

Dr. Joseph Mercola says about juicing, "I am convinced that this is one of the most powerful tools one can use to obtain high level vitality. All of us need raw foods every day, and this is an excellent technique to assure you receive large quantities of them."

If you are serious about recovering from an illness or if you just want to maintain good health, investing in a good juicer is a must. Everyone has heard about home juicers, juice bars, and natural juice supplements, but not many people understand exactly how beneficial juicing is for your health, let alone how relatively easy it is with a good juicer.

The Benefits of Juicing

- Is a source of organic vitamins, minerals, enzymes, and other micronutrients that are highly bioavailable
- Has a powerful blood-cleansing action
- Helps protect against degenerative disease and infection
- Increases the body's healing abilities
- Energizes the entire body
- Detoxifies the organs and tissues
- Reduces acidity in the joints and the blood

Recently, the National Cancer Institute has been looking at the specific chemicals in vegetables and fruits that provide protection against modern diseases like cancer and heart disease. One such class of phytochemicals that has been proven in numerous studies to provide protection against disease are the proanthocyanidins, which chemically are oligomeric flavonoids. These are found in large amounts in apples, grape seeds (especially red grapes) and grape skin, maritime pine bark, red wine, cranberries, and the leaves of the bilberry, birch, ginkgo, and hawthorn trees. Cinnamon, aronia fruit, black currants, green tea, and black tea also contain these proanthocyanidins, and cocoa beans contain the highest concentrations. Studies have shown that proanthocyanidins have an antioxidant power that is twenty times stronger than that of vitamin C, and fifty times stronger than that found in vitamin E. Grape seeds in particular have been shown to improve flexibility in joints, arteries, and body tissues such as the heart, helping to improve blood circulation by strengthening the capillaries, arteries, and veins.

To easily and inexpensively access all these nutrients without spending all your money on supplements, invest in a quality masticating home juicer that removes the indigestible fibers from vegetables and fruits, thereby making the healing nutrients more bioavailable and in much larger quantities than if you ate the fruit or vegetable whole. As most of the nutrients are trapped in the fiber, when you eat a raw carrot, for example, you only assimilate approximately 1 percent of the available beta carotene; however, when juiced, almost 100 percent of the beta-carotene in the carrot can be assimilated. Along with their many micronutrients, fruits and vegetables provide another vital nutrient essential for health: water. At least 70 percent of our cells are made of water, and some parts of the body such as the brain are 80 to 90 percent water. Cultures that consume diets high in water-rich foods—mainly fruits and vegetables—demonstrate better health and longer life spans.

Again, as fruit juices can contain large amounts of natural sugar and can aggravate people with blood-sugar problems, start by juicing vegetables initially and be careful with fruit. The best fruits to add to vegetable juices are apples, lemons or limes, and nonsweet grape varieties. Start with green vegetables and green leafy vegetables, and then go to carrots and other starchy vegetables. You can add a little apple, lemon, lime, grapes, or other fruits for flavor, and add some ginger or mint for more spice. Eventually you should begin adding seeds and grasses such as wheatgrass or barley grass for superior nutrition. Skipping meals and taking a juice as a replacement is actually quite healthy and aids in healthy weight loss. It also seems to regulate the appetite and reduce sugar cravings. If you haven't yet developed a taste for natural fresh juice, start slowly with the vegetables and fruits you like and begin developing a taste for more beneficial juices later. Here a juicing guide is highly recommended; most good juicers come with a simple guide, but these are often a bit limited. And remember, not all juicers are created equal. Superior juicers that professional juice bars use are available in home-model sizes. Today you can purchase an affordable home juicer that juices, grinds, and does grasses all in one.

If you are sensitive to sugars, you can make juices in a high-speed professional blender, which incorporates the fibers that help break down and metabolize the sugars in juices. But remember to add some water to make the juice more liquid. These high-speed blenders have a 1200–1500W motor and an RPM of 30,000 and are excellent for making hot raw soup also.

OMEGA RATIOS

Mahatma Gandhi famously followed a strict vegetarian diet, a belief deeply ingrained in Hindu and Jain traditions in India, especially in Gandhi's native Gujarat. Going all the way back to his early years as a barrister living in London, Gandhi studied what constitutes a proper vegetarian diet and concluded that "wherever flaxseed becomes a regular food item among people, there is better health."

The three types of omega-3 fatty acids involved in human physiology are alpha-linolenic acid, or ALA (found in plant oils); eicosapentaenoic acid, or EPA; and docosahexaenoic acid, or DHA (the latter two commonly found in marine oils). Scientists were first alerted to the many benefits of the omega 3 essential fatty acids ALA, EPA, and DHA in the early 1970s, when Danish physicians observed that the Inuit people of Greenland had a much lower incidence of heart disease and arthritis despite the fact that they consumed a high-fat, meat-only diet. Intensive research soon found that two of the fats (oils) they consumed in large quantities, EPA and DHA from seafood, played a key role in reducing arterial plaque and preventing heart disease and stroke. More recent research has established that fish oils (EPA and DHA) play a crucial role in the prevention of atherosclerosis, heart attack, depression, and even cancer.

It is estimated that 85 percent or more of people living in the West are deficient in omega-3 fatty acids, with most getting far too much of the omega-6 fatty acids, a family of pro-inflammatory and anti-inflammatory polyunsaturated fatty acids consumed mainly in the form of common vegetable oils. To understand the basics of which fats your body actually needs, let's put it in plain and simple terms: All food fats are a blend of two different types, saturated and unsaturated. Unsaturated fats include poly- and monounsaturated fats. Omega-3s and -6s are types of polyunsaturated fats; they are called "essential" because our bodies can't manufacture them from other fats, so we must obtain them from our diet. There are many kinds of fats in the body. Some of the most crucial ones are in the list of compounds that make up the body's cell walls. After isolating these fats, scientific studies determined that when the ratio of omega-6 to -3 fats exceeds 4:1, people suffer from myriad health problems. This is especially meaningful, since grain-fed beef can have ratios that exceed 20:1, whereas grass-fed beef is around 3:1.

Omega 3 Fatty Acids Are Essential for Normal Growth

Omega-3 fatty acids play an important role in the prevention and treatment of:

- Coronary artery disease
- Hypertension
- Arthritis
- Cancer
- Other inflammatory and autoimmune disorders

In the past hundred years there has been a rapid and unprecedented change in our diet. During this time the modern vegetable-oil industry was invented; these oils come primarily from plants rich in omega-6 fats and not omega-3s. Modern agriculture has also increased production of omega-6s by emphasizing grain feeds for domestic livestock, and grains are rich in omega-6 fats only. Therefore, aggressive, industrialized agricultural management techniques have decreased the omega-3 fat content in many foods, such as meat and farmed fish. This imbalance, in which omega-6 fat levels exceed omega-3 levels, can be seen by comparing wild edible plants and wild animals with products of modern agriculture. Products of modern agriculture frequently have drastically lower omega-3 levels. This imbalance has resulted in a wide range of problems: Udo Erasmus, author of *Fats That Heal, Fats That Kill,* says, "Omega-3 deficiency symptoms [include] growth retardation, vision and learning problems, motor co-ordination, weakness, tingling in the arms and legs, [and] behavioral changes. All except the first are symptoms used to diagnose MS."

Today, the modern diet of meat, fish, chicken, plus vegetable oils (especially olive oil), has a ratio estimated at around 20:1. Our healthy primal ancestors evolved on a diet with a ratio of omega-6 to omega-3 at approximately 1:1 to 2:1. Many nutritional scientists now believe that the major reason for the high incidence of heart disease, hypertension, diabetes, obesity, premature aging, and some forms of cancer may be due to incorrect ratios in our omega-6 to omega-3 essential fats.

Clinical trials have shown that fish oil supplementation is effective in the treatment of many disorders, including rheumatoid arthritis, diabetes, ulcerative colitis, and Raynaud's disease. Recognizing the unique benefits of omega-3s, especially EPA and DHA, and the serious consequences of an imbalance between omega-3s and omega-6s, the National Institutes of Health (NIH) recently published their recommended daily intake of fatty acids. This includes 650 mg of EPA and DHA, 2.22 grams daily of alpha-linolenic acid (ALA), and 4.44 grams of linoleic acid found in omega-6s. Natural fatty acids such as the omega-3s are found in high amounts in deep-sea fish (but you have to make sure that the fish is not contaminated with mercury), as well as grass-fed animals such as beef, bison, and ostrich. This type of fat does not make you fat; instead, it actually aids in slimming, cleaning the arteries, regulating blood pressure, and lowering cholesterol. The Inuit, who live entirely on meat and fat from sea life, actually have one of the lowest cholesterol levels of any culture, as they consume large amounts of fish oils (omega-3s), making their omega-3 and -6 ratio optimal. In short, the fewer inflammatory omega-6s you eat and the more omega-3s the better. Balancing your omega-3 and -6 ratios helps to combat disease by healing your nervous, immune, and hormonal systems and nourishing your brain. The optimal average ratio should be between 1:1 and 2:1 (omega-3s to omega-6s).

Vegetarian sources of omega-3 (alpha-linolenic acid) fats are found in flaxseed, chia, hemp, and perilla oil, while the predominant fatty acids found in fatty fish and fish oils contain both eicosapentaenoic acid (EPA) and docosahexaenoic acid (DHA). Alpha-linolenic acid contained in vegetarian sources must be converted to EPA and DHA in the body, and this conversion can be difficult in the elderly; hence, some nutritionists recommend using both vegetarian omega-3 oils and fish oils for maximum health benefits. Nevertheless, all these sources can deliver your body's needs for more omega-3s and less omega-6s.

THE AMAZING BENEFITS OF COCONUT

Jon Kabara, professor emeritus at Michigan State University, whose early pioneering work focused on the virucidal effects of monolaurin, says, "If there was an oil you could use for your daily cooking needs that helped protect you from heart disease, cancer, and other degenerative conditions, while improving your digestion, strengthening your immune system, and helping you to lose excess weight, would you be interested?"

Virgin cold-pressed coconut oil is exactly that. It is rich in lauric acid, a proven antiviral and antibacterial agent that is currently being used in the treatment of AIDS in many natural-medicine clinics. Monolaurin is a monoglyceride of lauric acid and is also found in human mother's milk; this is a key factor in providing us with a healthy immune system when we are babies. Extra-virgin cold-pressed coconut oil is both antibacterial and antiviral.

Virgin cold-pressed coconut oil is by far the best oil you can use for your cooking needs, due to its high temperature oxidation rate, while also increasing protection from heart disease, cancer, and other degenerative conditions and improving your digestion and strengthening your immune system. It has been shown to assist in weight loss by having a direct stimulating effect on the thyroid gland and metabolic organs such as the liver. In some quarters coconut oil has received a bad rap and is said to be high in saturated fats. Unfortunately, due to incorrect assumptions from the medical establishment, coconuts have been ranked right alongside beef fat and lard in terms of being unhealthy. The predated research that concluded that coconut oil was bad for you was done using hydrogenated (heat-processed) coconut oil, not extra-virgin coconut oil. To set the record straight, saturated fats from plants act in an entirely different way from saturated fats from animals. In fact, saturated fats from plants seem to be extremely healthy. Coconut oil does not contain cholesterol like animal fats do, so it will not raise your cholesterol levels; in fact, studies have shown that it lowers it. Nor does it promote blood platelet stickiness like animal fats do; instead, it helps prevent atherosclerosis and heart disease. Neither does it increase your risk of cancer; instead it seems to lower it.

Cold-pressed virgin coconut oil has been shown to have strong antiviral and antiparasitic action while simultaneously strengthening the immune system. It also has been shown to increase nutrient absorption and promote beautiful, soft skin. Coconut oil has a record of being used as healthy cooking oil for thousands of years. Even early in the 1900s, popular cookbooks advertised it. This all changed with the anti-saturated-fats campaign and the marketing and promotion of refined polyunsaturated fats such as genetically modified canola and soybean oils produced by American corporate food giants. What these large companies did not tell us is that Pacific Rim peoples who eat large amounts of coconut oil have considerably lower cholesterol levels than people living in the United States or Great Britain who eat processed vegetable oils from canola and soybean. Avoid both canola and soybean oil completely as they are both genetically modified and neither are healthful whether they are organic or not. The words *fat* and *oil* can sometimes be used interchangeably. Chemically speaking, *oil* refers to a substance that is liquid at room temperature, and *fat* is used if it's solid at room temperature. Coconut oil is solid at temperatures under 76 degrees Fahrenheit and liquid above this temperature. Always use virgin cold-pressed coconut oil for nutritional purposes.

The Miracle of Coconut Vinegar

You may have heard or read about the amazing health benefits and many cures of raw apple cider vinegar for numerous health conditions, but did you know coconut vinegar has all the same benefits and even more? Coconut vinegar is made from the coconut sap that is tapped from the branch arm of the coconut tree. Coconut sap is similar to fresh coconut water, but superconcentrated, containing a variety of nutrients. Naturally fermented for over six months in earthen clay pots, it is very high in alkalizing minerals and contains natural probiotic flora (FOS), unlike any other medicinal vinegars. This vinegar is organically produced, full of enzymes, and contains no added sugar or preservatives; it is chemical-free, gluten-free, and vegan as well. It can be used as medicinal vinegar for weight loss, diabetes, bloating, and acid reflux, as well as for stomach, liver, or spleen problems and numerous other related conditions caused by faulty digestion. Digestive imbalances have been linked to allergies, arthritis, asthma, weight gain, constipation, intestinal diseases, depression—the list goes on and on. One to two tablespoons can be taken diluted in a mug of warm-to-hot water or added to green tea, or taken in normal drinking water twice or three times daily for medicinal use. It also can be enjoyed as a culinary delight and works very well in salad dressings and homemade mayonnaise recipes.

When the coconut tree is tapped, it produces a nutrient-rich inflorescence, the nutrient-rich coconut sap (naturally flowing juice or "sap") that exudes from the coconut blossoms. It is naturally abundant in seventeen amino acids (the building blocks of protein), vitamin A (beta-carotene), B-complex vitamins (such as inositol, known for its effectiveness on depression, cholesterol, inflammation, and diabetes), and vitamin C (good for everything). It is rich in minerals like calcium, iron, and magnesium and also high in potassium (essential for electrolyte balance, blood pressure, and sugar metabolism). It also contains FOS in natural form, a prebiotic that promotes digestive health. The sap has a very low glycemic index (only 35). The most remarkable blessing about tapping a coconut tree is that once it is tapped, it flows its sap continuously for the next twenty years! From a sustainability viewpoint, the harvestable energy production from tapping coconut trees for their sap (which yields 5,000 liters per hectare), rather than allowing them to produce fruit, is five to seven times higher per hectare than coconut oil production from mature coconuts.

Coconut trees are grown in rich volcanic coastal soils, contributing to the sap's high mineral content. Apple cider vinegar enthusiasts document claims of a vast array of ailments that it can treat, which I have personally witnessed. Some enthusiasts say this is because it is full of nutrients. However, in truth, according to the USDA's nutrient database, nutritional analyses reveal that apple cider vinegar has no measurable vitamin A, vitamin B, vitamin C, or vitamin E, and the fiber (pectin) and amino-acid content is zero. In fact, other than potassium and acetic acid, it contains virtually no other nutrients. While apple cider vinegar still has numerous health benefits due to its potassium levels, malic acid content, and ability to balance stomach and liver functions, coconut vinegar has the same properties while also delivering many additional benefits from its increased nutrient levels, having up to ten to one hundred times more vitamins, minerals, and amino acids.*

ALOE VERA, AN ANCIENT HEALTH SECRET

Historically aloe vera was used in ayurvedic medicine externally for a number of skin ailments and internally as a body purifier and cleanser.

---

*For more specific information see www.superfoodly.com/benefits-of-coconut-vinegar
-vs-apple-cider-vinegar.

Aloe vera juice is an effective internal tonic for the liver; it is also a colon cleanser, as it has the ability to loosen and gently dispose of toxins in the intestines, allowing the body to absorb nutrients from food more effectively. It has been shown to be a helpful tonic for the female reproductive system, aiding during times of menopause and menstruation. Botanically, aloe vera is a member of the Asphodelaceae family and contains nutritional, immunomodulatory, and antioxidant properties while also showing effectiveness for antiaging. Taken as a nutritional supplement it contains polysaccharides (natural long-chain sugars), vitamins (A, B, C, and E), amino acids, enzymes, minerals (calcium, magnesium, manganese, zinc), and soluble fibers. It has been shown to assist in health ailments both internally and externally.

Aloe vera has the following applications:

- Internally: asthma, heartburn, acidity, peptic ulcer, digestive disorders, gas, constipation, piles, diabetes, blood pressure, arthritis, burns, urinary infections, kidney ailments, gout, fever, cough, sore throat, bronchitis, and as a general health tonic
- Externally: topical preparation for soothing skin irritations, including cuts, wounds, and insect stings; preventing hair loss by stimulating natural hair growth; dandruff, sunburn, natural sunscreen, postsurgery scars and stretch marks, foot cracks, joint and muscle pain, swellings, wrinkles, and dry skin

THE SWEETEST OF MEDICINES

Honey

An ancient Chinese proverb says, "In times of stress, sweeten the tea with honey." In almost all traditional medical systems raw, unprocessed honey has been regarded first as a medicine and second as a food. While for many centuries honey has played its role in providing both medical and nutritional benefits, today many are unaware of the healing benefits of this nectar. In fact, most commercial honey is so processed that only the sweet flavor is what remains. Yet honey, when raw and unprocessed, contains an array of nutritional elements, as well as therapeutic effects on digestion, assimilation, and elimination. It is antibacterial and anti-anemic and has fever-reducing qualities. It can stop the growth of bad bacteria in the intestines because of its natural sugar content, combined with its ability to release hydrogen peroxide from its glucose enzyme. The glucose enzymes in honey are also believed to increase the production of tryptophan, a very important amino acid that plays a key role in the production of serotonin, primarily found in the gastrointestinal tract, blood platelets, and the central nervous system and thought to be a contributor to feelings of well-being and happiness.

Unlike processed sugar, which provides only empty calories, raw honey is more easily metabolized by the pancreas than sugar is, and it breaks down easier in the small intestine. The hygroscopic properties of honey also make it an excellent additive to skin-care products because it has the ability to draw moisture from the air into the skin. Tension is often more effectively reduced by consuming a spoonful of raw honey than a chocolate bar; placing unprocessed honey on skin conditions overnight results in marked improvements. Several drinks of warm tea made of honey and lemon juice or apple cider vinegar has shown to assist in weight loss and immune-system benefits.

Molasses

The word *molasses* comes from the Portuguese word *melaço,* meaning "jammy," "honey sweet," and "sticky," all good descriptions of molasses. Molasses is regarded by many as just a by-product of sugarcane manufacturing. Some even think molasses is a by-product of refined sugar, but it is not. It comes from the first or second boiling of the sugarcane plant and can also be made from beets, sorghum, dates, and carob. It is packed with powerful nutrients like magnesium, calcium, potassium, iron, and B vitamins, as well as various beneficial unrefined sugars from the sugarcane juice. Its taste is probably more bitter than sweet, and this taste can easily grow on you. This superfood extract is often thrown out or sometimes given to cattle for health and nutrition and is probably one of the best-kept natural cures for numerous diseases, especially women's conditions. On a more prosaic level, molasses is used in beer making, in all kinds of baking, and in making natural licorice candy. In Australia molasses is fermented to produce ethanol and used as an alternative fuel in vehicles.

Molasses is a useful remedy for the following ailments:

- Anemia
- Mild depression
- Menstruation problems (cramps; irregular, excessive bleeding; poor blood flow)
- Ovarian cysts
- Fibroids
- Heart palpitations
- Diabetes and low blood sugar
- Acne
- Joint pain and cramps
- Constipation
- Edema
- Reducing gray hair

Adults should take one to two tablespoons once or twice daily; children should take one to two teaspoons once or twice daily. Make sure you use only organic, unsulfured molasses, which is high in minerals and low in sugar. Other types of molasses derived from beets, dates, or sorghum are available but are usually higher in sugar. Traditional blackstrap sugarcane molasses is what we recommend. We often combine molasses consumption with the use of aloe vera, carrot, and beet juice twice daily for curing many problems of the ovaries and menstruation. It is truly a wonderfully inexpensive, easy, and safe medicine for the whole family.

CANNABIS

It is amazing that most of the information on the healing benefits of cannabis has been systematically omitted from standard medical texts since the 1930s. In brief, here's why:

At one time cannabis was highly valued in terms of both its

medicinal properties and its industrial uses. In fact, between 1840 and 1900, more than a hundred U.S. newspapers recommended cannabis for various illnesses and for pain in general. During Herbert Hoover's presidency, from 1929 to 1933, however, Andrew Mellon became Hoover's Secretary of the Treasury and the primary investor in the chemical company Dupont. He appointed his future nephew-in-law, Harry J. Anslinger, to head the Federal Bureau of Narcotics and Dangerous Drugs. Secret meetings were held by these financial tycoons. Cannabis was declared dangerous and a threat to their billion-dollar enterprises. For their dynasties to remain intact, it had to go. Not long after this plan was set in place, the media began a blitz of yellow journalism in the late 1920s and 1930s. On April 14, 1937, the prohibitive Marihuana Tax Law—the bill that outlawed cannabis—was brought directly to the House Ways and Means Committee. In September of 1937, cannabis and hemp (a variety of non-THC *Cannabis sativa* used mainly for materials like cloth and rope) prohibition began. Arguably the most useful plant known to humankind thus became illegal to grow and use, both in its non-THC strain, as hemp, and its THC strain, called by the then-derogatory Mexican slang word *marijuana.*

The public at that time was without the benefit of access to information as found on the Internet today and had to base their opinions and beliefs on the mainstream, corporate-controlled news media. Congress banned hemp because it was said to be a violent and dangerous drug. In reality, hemp does nothing more than act as an amazing resource to virtually any industry and any product. As you can imagine, this was also a big reason for the banning of hemp, as it posed a serious threat to many of the big industries that were pushing mainly plastics, oil, and paper. Unfortunately, as big business squashed the use of hemp, so too were the nutritional and health benefits of the cannabis plant erased from medical texts for reasons that seem to be political rather than based on a sincere caring for the health of human beings. To this day, this valuable plant is still illegal to grow in the United States, and most of the hemp products and hemp oil found in the market here today come from Canada.

The cannabis plant has many varieties and plant relations. Some varieties contain the chemical THC and are smoked or eaten for medical or recreational use; some non-THC varieties, known as *hemp,* are used for fabrics and textiles, or for purely nutritional purposes. Nearly all forms of cannabis can be used in some way for assisting in healing the body. The CBD oil, and not the THC contained within cannabis, is the main therapeutic agent within this medicinal plant, with a strong and successful history in most countries. No records of death have ever been reported from cannabis use, whereas other legal recreational drugs such as alcohol and tobacco kill thousands each year. The National Institute on Drug Abuse (NIDA) ranks cannabis as the safest drug used today, well above tobacco and alcohol for tolerance, dependence, and intoxication.

Cannabis grows virtually everywhere on the planet and is actually one of our oldest medicines, with a remarkable record of safety and efficacy in the treatment of more than a hundred illnesses. It is one of the most tested therapeutic drugs in history, being used and studied as far back as 2700 BCE, when the physician to the ancient Chinese emperor Shen prescribed cannabis to the ruler as a medicine. It is a fact that if any other drug showed the various flexible medical properties of cannabis, it would be labeled a miracle drug.

Cannabis is two to three times more effective than allopathic medicines that are currently used for reducing ocular pressure, yet without the harmful side effects associated with today's approved glaucoma drugs. It has also been estimated that 80 percent of asthmatics can benefit largely from using cannabis as a highly effective bronchial dilator. One of its greatest advantages is its unusual safety, estimated at 20,000:1 in terms of its risk of lethalness. Today cannabis is used in the treatment of hundreds of illnesses, including migraine, multiple sclerosis, cancer, epilepsy, emphysema, arthritis, anorexia nervosa, back pain and spasms, asthma, AIDS, depression, insomnia, and many more.

The big question is, what is the healthiest way to administer cannabis? I do not recommend smoking this herb, as inhaling any kind of burning substance can be bad for the lungs—although smoking it in small quantities is far less harmful than smoking tobacco. Also, eating the drug has certain risks, as tolerance via the digestive system varies on an individual basis according to what we eat on a daily basis. By far the best way to consume cannabis is via a modern infuser or vaporizer. In this way the drug is not heated directly or burned, as in smoking; rather it is heated, releasing the plant oils. These machines can be purchased easily from medical marijuana shops or online.

Cold-Pressed Hemp Seed Oil

The nutritional and healing benefits of hemp seed oil, which contains virtually no THC or drug-related compounds, is truly profound. As nutritional research is proving the body's cells require a ratio of 2:1 omega-6s to omega-3s, hemp seed oil is the only food to perfectly match this ratio. It also contains small amounts of GLA (alpha-galactosidase, a glycoside hydrolase enzyme), which is also found in evening primrose and black currant seed oils. Hemp's ideal ratio of fatty acids makes it a vital food addition for healthy brain, nerve, and blood functions. Hemp as a food, and especially hemp oil, was once a part of the worldwide dietary intake, as hemp was one of the first crops ever cultivated by humankind. Cold-pressed hemp seed oil is a complete essential fatty acid supplement that can be used in combination with other superior omega-3-rich oils such as flaxseed and perilla. It has exceptional benefits, such as normalizing blood pressure and lowering bad cholesterol in the arteries and reducing brain degeneration in old age, such as that found in Alzheimer's disease. With its nutty taste it can be used as an enjoyable food and in salad dressings, mayonnaise, and dips, or poured over fresh whole-grain breads to replace butter and processed oil spreads.

A Healthy Butter Suggestion

A far healthier alternative to fake butter and certainly to dangerous vegetable oils is to mix half a cup of real butter with a quarter cup of virgin olive oil and a quarter cup of hemp or flaxseed oil in a container, keeping it refrigerated. Spread it on natural whole-grain, gluten-free breads with a touch of unprocessed sea salt and black pepper. Or if you have dangerously high levels of bad cholesterol, focus on increasing your intake of omega-3 fats and use cold-pressed flaxseed or hemp oils only and skip omega-6-rich olive oil, which will help to reduce your cholesterol levels by shifting your omega-3 to -6 ratios.

REDUCING OR ELIMINATING MEAT

The Bible warns against the consumption of animal flesh: "But flesh with the life thereof, which is the blood thereof, shall ye not eat. And surely your blood of your lives will I require, at the hand of every beast will I require it" (Genesis 9:4–5). Whether or not to consume meat is a question that befuddles many people today, including health professionals, who often give out incorrect advice on this sensitive but important subject. Certainly the reduction of meat consumption has many health benefits, including the following:

Physiological reasons: As our bodies are built with a vegetarian digestive system approximately thirty feet long (like our vegetarian primates), meat is simply not an ideal food, as it cannot fully pass through the digestive system fast enough without releasing fermented toxins. If nature had intended us to eat large quantities of meat, she would have given us razor-sharp teeth and claws like all other meat-eating animals in the world (tigers, cats, dogs, etc.), and not flat, vegetable-chewing teeth and fingernails. The average intestinal length of meat-eating animals such as large dogs, tigers, and lions, which are about the size of the human body, is seven feet long.

Nutritional reasons: Approximately 40 percent of the antibiotics produced by Big Pharma today are fed to our livestock; in turn fed to us via the food chain. Many people give me strange looks after I tell them that their tests reveal an overuse of antibiotics in their system. They are amazed, as some have not taken oral antibiotics for years. They then admit that on a daily basis they eat meat that is not organic and grass-fed. Meat today, unless certified organic, is full of antibiotics, synthetic hormones, and steroids that are used to increase growth and limit diseases in animals, which then become absorbed when you eat it, causing serious health problems, especially for women because of their more sensitive hormonal systems during the childbearing and menopause years. Meat is not the only source of protein. Pulses (thick soups usually based on edible seeds of plants in the legume family), sprouts, nuts, seeds, and algae contain the same high levels of protein. In fact, meat is actually a second-class protein, meaning that animals eat grass or some kind of plant protein to obtain its protein, and then we eat the animal flesh for its protein. In this way we are consuming the protein secondhand instead of going straight to the source and consuming firsthand proteins such as nuts, seeds, and pulses. Meat, much like cow's milk, is very high in phosphorous, causing negative effects on calcium and magnesium, pulling them from the bones and tissues into the blood, causing mineral imbalances.

Spiritual reasons: Many world religions advocate a vegetarian diet, claiming that these dietary practices are aligned with our spiritual evolution. Much information about this is recorded in the origins of Christianity, among other world religions. The Bible contains many statements concerning vegetarianism, such as "Thou shalt not kill" (Exodus 22:13). It could not be stated more clearly there. The exact Hebrew translation is *lo tirtzach*. One of the greatest scholars of Hebrew linguistics in the twentieth century, Dr. Reuben Alcalay, in his book *The Complete Hebrew-English Dictionary,* states that *tirtzach* refers to "any kind of killing whatsoever." The word *lo,* as you might suspect, means "thou shalt not." It seems quite clear that the Bible means the killing of animals and not just humans. Buddhism advocates the practice of ahimsa, which also means nonintentional harming of all sentient beings, certainly animals. In the Vedanta tradition, meat closes the heart chakra and agitates the mind and feeds our egoistic nature.

Environmental reasons: Right now, as there are almost six billion people on planet Earth, she cannot possibly handle the environmental effects of everyone's hunger for dead flesh. Much of our rainforest and trees are now being cut down to make way for raising cattle for our hamburgers. The eating of plants for the same population is far less damaging to the earth's natural ecosystem. The amount of water it takes to clean, feed, and maintain animals destined for meat is more than ten times what it takes to grow vegetables and grains on the same land, not to mention the amount of waste that is produced by the cattle, which pollute the atmosphere and our water supplies. If the Western world continues to eat meat at its current rate, our forests and waterways will be completely destroyed. These environmental facts must not be ignored for the sake of our children's future as we bank on the hope that they, and not us, will lead us out of the environmental mess we've made over the last century. At least for the sake of your children and grandchildren, reduce or cut out meat. As Albert Einstein said, "It is my view that the vegetarian manner of living, by its purely physical effect on the human temperament, would most beneficially influence the lot of mankind."

So given all this, the question is: can I get all that I need from a vegetarian diet? It seems that strict veganism is not ideal, as many vegans are lacking in some essential amino acids and vitamin B_{12} that small amounts of meat can deliver. I recommend organic eggs or raw goat milk, which do not involve the killing of animals, to easily get these missing nutrients. For those who are not ready to give up eating dead flesh, organic, grass-fed meat or wild game consumed in moderate quantities once or twice a week is fine, especially for O blood types. As well, fresh, unpolluted, nonfarmed fish contains many vitamins and essential fatty acids for proper brain and nerve function and is an easily digested form of meat for human systems, especially when eaten raw or lightly steamed or grilled. Fish has a cholesterol-lowering effect due to its omega-3 fatty acids, which naturally thin the blood and keep the arteries from clogging. The only problem today is that much of our fish is contaminated with mercury, so you can't be sure what you're eating; also, overfishing practices are destroying ocean environments.

Is Chicken a Healthy Alternative to Red Meat?

Dr. Richard Schulze, author of a number of books on natural health and the creator of a comprehensive line of supplements that go by his name, says, "If you think chicken is a health alternative, every day in America, ten people die from food poisoning directly related to eating chicken, and an additional 10,000 get sick. Chicken is often billed as the healthy white meat alternative to red meat by TV advertising, but this could not be a bigger lie. White meat chicken has just as much cholesterol as full-fat hamburger meat. Chicken also causes more poisoning than any other type of meat consumed."

Many people today are turning away from red meat and eating more chicken than ever before, thinking it is healthier. But unless you are eating organic, free-range chicken, this meat is one of the most questionable sources of nutrition consumed today. The chicken you buy in the average supermarket undergoes extensive hormonal treatments, living in tiny cages, never, ever being able to walk or even use their legs. This increase in chicken consumption is an underlying cause in many hormonal and weight-gain cases, as well as overdeveloped breasts in both men and women. The synthetic hormones that chickens consume are absorbed into your bloodstream, playing havoc with your hormonal system, especially sensitive female systems. When eating chicken, only choose organic, free-range chicken.

B$_{12}$, the Missing Link in a Plant-Based Diet

Deficiency in vitamin B$_{12}$ is not only common in vegetarians and vegans, but in meat eaters as well, and there are many reasons for this. The widespread use of pesticides in our food, water fluoridation, reliance on antibiotics, and coffee drinking all mean that this important vitamin is poorly absorbed. Therefore, it is very important that this nutrient be added to your diet or checked regularly using modern tests. For those not wanting to eat sentient beings, there are nonsentient sources of B$_{12}$, such as fermented vegetables, kefir, eggs, and bivalves (the last three of which are obviously not vegan sources). Bivalves include oysters, mussels, clams, and scallops; they have no head, eyes, mouth, or central nervous system, with a limited ability to feel pain or experience consciousness and are therefore sometimes regarded as being nonsentient. Bivalve veganism is gaining in popularity because it is a healthy and natural way to obtain the same B$_{12}$ and iron found in sentient land or sea animals. It's not a vegan diet per say, rather a vegan-based diet that eats bivalves, so one does not have to supplement the diet with B$_{12}$ artificially.

Ancient Oriental Vegan No-Bone Broth for Healing your Gut and Skin

Bone broths have become popular recently with the popularity of the GAPS diet and other gut-healing protocols aimed at the strong connection between our guts and our minds. In fact, cultures worldwide have been boiling up the bones, cartilage, and connective tissue of animals for thousands of years for medicinal benefits in addition to a healthy diet. Bone broths are rich sources of collagen, which heal the lining of the gut, reduce inflammation, remineralize the tissues, promote immune-system function, repair joints, and feed the hair, skin, and nails. The vegan version of bone broth does the same thing, being rich in collagen and elastin and promoting elements such as hyaluronic acid, which is the main nutrient needed for collagen formation in the body. In fact, the body may absorb collagen-enhancing nutrients from plants more easily than those decocted from an animal carcass.

Instructions: Place the following ingredients and water in a slow cooker for several hours, then blend and serve. Serve as a soup with a side of raw, fermented vegetables or a side salad. There is no exact level of ingredients in this recipe, so I encourage you to approach cooking with reckless abandon. Just make sure you put in plenty of seaweed (as much as you can comfortably handle), tempeh, and shiitake, as these three are key ingredients for collagen production.

- Miso paste (unpasteurized) or tamari soy sauce
- Tempeh pieces (fermented soybeans)
- Seaweed (available from Asian grocery shops), such as wakame or arame, or several handfuls of broken nori sheets
- Shiitake dried mushroom
- Vegetables (sweet potato, celery, beets, cabbage, wild greens, asparagus, brussels sprouts)
- Cilantro or parsley
- Spices (thyme, oregano, turmeric, ginger, galangal, sumac)
- Coconut oil and macadamia oil
- Apple cider vinegar to taste

Soy Products

When soy is not fermented, as in tofu and soy milk, chemicals remain that can cause serious health problems. Traditionally, the Japanese and the Chinese did not eat soybeans unfermented. Soy has been promoted by the health-food industry in recent years with claims that it is a healthy alternative to meat and milk for protein and minerals. It is frequently advertised that Asians eat large quantities of soy every day, and so we should, too. From my extensive travels and research on the Asian diet, this is far from true; in fact, strong evidence proves otherwise.

That most of the soy today is genetically modified is just one of the reasons that we need to be careful when consuming large quantities of unfermented soy. The so-called soy health miracle is truly an example of modern marketing skills and blatant lies. It was only a few decades ago that the soybean was considered unfit to eat, even in Asia.

To dip into a spot of history, it was the Chou Dynasty (1134–246 BCE) that first designated the soybean as one of the five sacred grains, along with barley, wheat, millet, and rice. However, the picture graph for the soybean, which dates from those times, indicates that it was not used as a food at all. The picture graphs for the other four grains show the seed and stem structure of the plant, while the pictograph for the soybean emphasizes the root structure only. Agricultural literature around that period speaks frequently of the soybean and its use in crop rotation. It seems apparent that soy was initially used as a method of fixing nitrogen into the soil and not as food at all, so the Asians did not eat that much soy after all.

The soybean did not serve as a food until the discovery of fermentation techniques, sometime during the end of the Chou Dynasty. The first soy foods were fermented products such as tempeh, natto, miso, and traditionally fermented soy sauce, or tamari (which is not to be confused with the many commercial and cheaply made soy sauces that are not fermented). It seems that around the second century BCE Chinese scientists discovered that a puree of cooked soybeans could be precipitated with calcium sulfate (i.e., plaster of Paris) and small amounts of magnesium sulfate (Epsom salts) or magnesium chloride to make a smooth, pale curd known today as tofu (bean curd). The use of fermented and precipitated soy products soon spread to other parts of Asia, notably Japan, Korea, Vietnam, Thailand, and Indonesia. The Chinese did not eat unfermented soybeans as they did other beans because they somehow knew that soybeans contain large quantities of antinutrients that deplete the body's mineral reservoirs. Among them are potent enzyme inhibitors that block the action of trypsin and other enzymes needed for protein digestion. Such inhibitors are large, tightly folded proteins that are not completely deactivated during ordinary cooking. These have been known to produce gastric distress and reduce protein digestion, leading to chronic deficiencies in amino acid uptake.

Furthermore, in laboratory experiments it has been shown that diets high in trypsin inhibitors cause enlargement and pathological conditions of the pancreas, including cancer. Soy also contains small amounts of goitrogens, which are substances that depress thyroid function, resulting in hypothyroidism and weight gain. When soy is not properly fermented, chemicals remain that can cause serious health problems. Traditionally Asians didn't eat soybeans unfermented; hence they always fermented the bean before eating it, which we now know destroys harmful chemicals that can cause so many health problems. People who consume large amounts of unfermented soy suffer from many health complaints, from hormonal to digestive.

Because of this, I believe that one should avoid eating large amounts of unfermented soybeans in the form of soy milk, tofu, and various soy-based meat alternatives, especially if one is sensitive to estrogens. There are many nuts, grains, and pulses that can be eaten instead of soy. The best source of nutrients comes from almonds and hemp seeds, which both make an excellent milk and cream or can be used in vegetarian dishes to replace both unfermented soy and meat.

High-Protein Plant-Based Foods

The following foods are full of nutrition and are also aligned with Taoist teachings:

Pulses/legumes: black beans; broad beans; fava beans; fermented soybeans (tempeh, miso, natto, tamari); kidney beans; butter beans; adzuki beans; yellow, orange, and green split peas; chick peas; red, green, and brown lentils; peanuts; carob or locust beans (Note that some pulses can be soaked and then sprouted and eaten raw.)

Green beans and peas: green string beans, snap or snow peas, green peas. These are peas and beans we eat as vegetables, usually raw or lightly cooked, unlike pulses, which we usually cook or sprout.

Nuts: almonds, walnuts, Brazils, cashews, pecans, macadamias

Seeds: sunflower, sesame, pumpkin, flax, chia, hemp, buckwheat, quinoa, wild rice (considered a seed)

Gluten-free whole grains: rice (brown, red, black), oats,* millet, amaranth, sorghum, corn, quinoa and kaniwa,† teff, Montina (a fermented brown rice protein powder)

Mushrooms: buttons, portobellos, porcinis, chanterelles, oysters, shiitakes, maitake

Green leafy vegetables: spinach, kale, silver beets, broccoli, brussels sprouts, moringa tree (leaves and seed pods), etc.

Grasses: wheatgrass, barley grass

Freshwater blue-green algae: spirulina, chlorella, AFA (*Aphanizomenon flos-squae*)

---

*Oats are technically gluten-free since they aren't a type of wheat, barley, or rye grain, the three groups of whole grains that naturally contain the protein gluten. Instead of containing gluten, oats actually have proteins called avenins. Oats are considered safe for those with a gluten allergy, easier for most people to digest, and safe even for someone with celiac disease. It's also very common for oats to be handled in the same facilities that manufacture wheat-containing products, so there's always a chance that oats can become contaminated with gluten during the packaging process. Organic labeling doesn't tell you anything about gluten content, so be sure that even if you buy organic oats, you check that they're certified gluten-free, too.

†Like quinoa, kaniwa also hails from South America. Cultivated in Peru and Bolivia, kaniwa is the seed from a flowering plant called goosefoot (*Chenopodium pallidicaule*). Quinoa is from the same genus (*Chenopodium*) but is a different species (*quinoa*), with slightly different properties. Quinoa consists of small seed grains that may be red, dark brown, or white in appearance. Kaniwa seeds are smaller than quinoa seeds—about half the size—and are dark red or brownish in color. Both quinoa and kaniwa have a delicious nutty flavor, although kaniwa is slightly sweeter than quinoa. Additionally, kaniwa has a slightly crunchy texture, while quinoa is fluffy and soft.

Red marine algae: Dumontiaceae, gigartina, dilwyn, nothogenia (known for its antiviral activity)

Seaweeds: kelp, Irish moss, bladderwrack, kombu, wakame, arame, dulse, bird's nest, etc.

Marine phytoplankton

Nutritional yeast

Lemon Eggs, an Inexpensive Calcium-Deficiency Remedy

If you're needing a calcium boost and do not want to buy costly calcium supplements, which in most cases are not absorbed well, try this lemon eggs recipe. Here is my version of this traditional calcium remedy:

Take three eggshells crushed (clean with boiling water and then wash with hydrogen peroxide; discard any ink stamp), place in empty glass jar (one-cup size), and fill the jar with lemon juice completely. Place the lid on, and store in the fridge for approximately three days (the contents will bubble a little bit). After three days the eggshells will be somewhat dissolved (filter out any leftover shells), forming a calcium-citrate-lemon mix, which is usually good for about one week. Take one tablespoon daily to boost your calcium levels. Shake well before taking.

A Word about Garlic

Dr. Bob Beck, who created the Beck Protocol, a natural health, bio-electric protocol designed to help the body heal itself, says, "Most people have heard most of their lives that garlic is good for you. We put those people in the same class of ignorance as the mothers who at the turn of the century would buy morphine sulfate from the drugstore and give it to their babies to put them to sleep at night."

Many herbalists rave about the health properties of garlic, accrediting it with lowering cholesterol (the herb guggul is over five times more effective), immune-building (echinacea is much more effective), and antibiotic (turmeric is far superior). There was a person with terminal cancer who was eating several cloves every hour because some health practitioner gave her a book that said it would cure her cancer. Unfortunately, she died a few months later, and likely the garlic poisoning didn't help her in her chances of survival. What most people do not realize is that, among these slightly distorted facts, garlic's negative effects when taken alone and not with other immune-building and detoxification herbs can far outweigh its positive effects. What you need to know is that there are many herbs and nutritional supplements that lower cholesterol, strengthen the immune system, and kill parasites much better than garlic does. The reason garlic can be toxic if consumed every day for extended periods of time is actually due to the chemicals that it is famous for. One of garlic's bacteria-killing chemicals, the sulfone hydroxyl ion, can penetrate the blood-brain barrier. Bob Beck discovered this fact, much to his and many people's amazement, when he was the world's largest manufacturer of ethical EEG feedback equipment such as the encephalograph.

Organic gardeners commonly know that if you do not want to use the toxic agricultural spray DDT, garlic will kill anything in the way of insects and other agricultural pests. Garlic has long been regarded as a powerful herb. In fact, in ayurveda, garlic is regarded as a tamasic food (i.e., increasing passion and ignorance), in the same category as red meat, alcohol, and tobacco. This is why garlic has long been taboo in ayurveda and forbidden in all ashrams, temples, and holy places in India where meditation is practiced, as ayurveda states that garlic irritates the brain and disturbs meditation. This was first recorded in Vedic scriptures over two thousand years ago; somehow health scholars knew way back then that garlic is not a healthy food for humans on a daily basis. Garlic can be used without any permanent damage to the brain and often combines well with other immune and antiparasitic herbs as most of us know, but we do not recommend taking it all the time as a food ingredient.

It is noteworthy that fighter pilots are advised to not eat garlic seventy-two hours before flying, because it can slow their reaction time by double or even triple. You might say you are three times slower when you eat garlic. Garlic has actually been found to desynchronize brain waves, and a research study at Stanford University found that garlic is actually poisonous in large quantities. If you can rub a clove of garlic on your foot, you will be able to smell it shortly afterward on your wrists. This is why the chemical DMSO (a cruder, organic form of MSM that is highly effective in pain control) smells a lot like garlic—the sulfone hydroxyl ion penetrates the corpus callosum in the brain.

Many people who have low-grade headaches, attention-deficit disorder, or difficulty focusing on the computer in the afternoon can be affected by excessive garlic consumption. If this sounds like you, and you do eat a lot of garlic (or take garlic supplements), limit your garlic intake and see how you feel. The subtle dangers of garlic also include the deskunked varieties such as odorless garlic tablets and similar products sold at health-food stores. Many detoxification and antiparasitic herbal formulas contain garlic and seem to show no problems but only if taken intensely over short periods of time. One could say garlic is safe in short, sharp bursts when needed. If one is looking for a long-term herbal program to detoxify and cleanse, lower cholesterol, and improve immunity, try olive leaf, which is much more effective over extended periods.

FOOD COMBINING

Harvey and Marilyn Diamond, authors of the best-selling book *Fit for Life,* say, "It may seem as if eating great food, not counting calories, not locking up your refrigerator, and not dieting are impossible dreams, but let us assure you, it is no dream—it works." Such is the power of correctly combining your foods for optimum health and weight. The relatively recent discovery of correct food combining is actually a retread of an old idea, as the ancient art of food combining for better digestion, assimilation, and health was first developed around two thousand years ago by Chinese doctors and is still regarded as one of the five keys to health and longevity. Although they did not know about carbohydrates and proteins like we do today, ancient Chinese physicians, through careful observation and intuition, developed the first groupings of foods for good digestion that we still use today.

Certain macronutrient food groups like fruits, vegetables, proteins, and carbohydrates require totally different enzymes to be properly digested, and they digest in different parts of the digestive system. For this reason there can be problems when we persistently combine the different groups at the same meal. Take meat for example: this protein food needs the enzyme pepsin to digest it. And potatoes, a common carbohydrate, needs ptyalin for digestion. When these two foods are eaten at the same meal, both enzymes are produced by the stomach in an attempt to digest them both. Unfortunately, these two important enzymes neutralize each other, rendering them both ineffective and leaving both foods poorly digested in the stomach and then in the bowels. This leads to health problems like weight gain, irritable bowel, bloating, and sluggish digestion. It can even contribute to hiatal hernia and other serious stomach problems. Fruits, for example, digest completely differently from proteins and carbohydrates. Proteins sit in the stomach for up to three hours to digest, while fruits, on the other hand, pass quickly into the small intestine for digestion. Therefore, when these two food groups are eaten at the same sitting or close together, the fruits will stay in the stomach, with the protein overfermenting and causing irritation to the bowels and intestines when it finally reaches it. This causes poor digestion, irritable bowel syndrome, weight problems, and related digestive disorders.

Points to Remember for Food Combining

- Avoid eating high-protein foods along with high-starch carbohydrates in the same meal or within three hours.
- Low-carb vegetables combine with all food groups except fruits.
- Pure fats like butter/oil don't combine well with high-starch carbohydrates.
- Fruits combine with nothing else; eat fruit alone or leave it alone; best at beginning of the day. Especially do not eat fruits after a main meal of proteins or carbohydrates.

- Bananas, although fruits, seem to do well with starches/carbohydrates.
- Melons, like fruits, digest primarily in the small intestines and not the stomach because they are their own food group and have their own food enzymes and need to be eaten alone.
- Milk enzymes such as rennin and other digestive enzymes coagulate in the stomach, preventing digestion. Milk does not combine well with other food groups.

An example of main-meal planning with correct food combining would be eating rice (a carbohydrate) with vegetables or salad for one meal, and fish (a protein) with low-carb vegetables and salad for another meal (see page 386).

How Much Food?

Most health studies in the past century have revealed that overeating is a major health problem. As the ancient Greek philosopher Diogenes attested, "As the houses well-stored with provisions are likely to be full of mice, so the bodies of those who eat much are full of diseases."

The habit of eating less, or undereating, needs to be a basic rule for superior health to occur. This means leave the table when you're 80 percent full, and not full to the brim. Over the last century there have been many studies on the health and eating habits of long-living people, those who in many cases live to the ripe old age of a hundred or even older. In an early 1910 British study, Charles de Lacy Evans wrote:

> We generally find some peculiarity of diet or habits to account for the alleged longevity; we find some were living amongst all the luxuries life could afford, others in the most abject poverty, begging their bread, some were samples of symmetry and physique, while others were cripples, some drank large quantities of water, others little; some were total abstainers from alcoholic drinks, others drunkards; some smoked tobacco, others did not; some lived entirely on vegetables, others ate a great deal of animal foods; some led active lives, others working more

with their brains, others with their hands; some ate one meal a day, others four or five; we notice great divergence in both habits and diet, but in those cases where we have been able to obtain a reliable account of the diet, we find one great cause which accounts for the majority of cases of longevity; moderation in the quantity of food!*

During World War II, health studies in Europe revealed that during major food shortages the health of people was at its best, and degenerating diseases at their lowest. Although chronic malnutrition did cause some diseases during wartime, in general reduced caloric intake alone massively reduced degenerative diseases during that period because undereating was experienced by most Europeans. It seems that the body needs fewer calories than most people think. As Benjamin Franklin famously said, "To lengthen thy life, lessen thy meals." This maxim also demonstrates that the body prefers to thrive on a simple diet rather than mixing too many different foods together in one meal.

How Often?

Doctors of traditional Chinese medicine have long advised against the theory of eating every few hours because they believe that this practice injures the spleen, pancreas, and stomach, causing long-term damage that can lead to diabetes or other digestive illnesses in later life. Furthermore, starting the day with a big breakfast, as is often advised, would not necessarily help you lose weight by reducing your appetite later in the day, making you eat less. A study published in 2011 found that "higher energy intake at breakfast is highly associated with greater whole-day energy intake in normal weight and obese subjects. Therefore low-energy intake at breakfast can be helpful to lower daily intake and improve the energy balance during treatment of obesity."† Researchers

---

*From *How to Prolong Life: An Enquiry into the Cause of "Old Age" and "Natural Death."* (London: Chas. W. Sawyer, 1910). Available online.

†V. Schusdziarra, M. Hausmann, C. Wittke, et al., "Impact of breakfast on daily energy intake: An analysis of absolute versus relative breakfast calories," *Nutrition Journal* 10, no. 5 (2011).

involved in this study who examined the eating habits of around three hundred people discovered that they also had a big lunch and a big dinner, along with their big breakfast. So if you want to lose weight, reduced breakfast intake is associated with reduced overall intake at lunch and dinner. The word *breakfast* means exactly that, to "break the fast," and this breaking of the fast does not have to be in the morning; it can be done as late in the day as possible. Personally I have my breakfast well into the afternoon each day, and it is not a big meal. Then I have my next meal, which is my major meal, in the early evening.

Taoists have always recommended having two meals a day rather than three (excluding those who are underweight) and to eat those meals as close together as possible. This results in maximum fasting time each day, and only now is this practice being widely studied by modern science and getting approval in health and fitness arenas. This process of daily intermittent fasting is now referred to as "Cyclical Intermittent Fasting" and gaining more popularity in recent years, thanks to Dr. Amen Ra, who has used this practice as a foundation for becoming a world dead-lifting champion.

A 2003 study by investigators at the National Institute on Aging found that "decreasing meal frequency and caloric intake protects nerve cells from genetically induced damage, delays the onset of Huntington's disease-like symptoms in mice, and prolongs the lives of affected rodents."* These findings suggest that humans may benefit from skipping a meal now and then, though the researchers noted that going an entire day without food is not the best option either. This and other, similar studies seem to contradict the generally accepted notion that humans should eat regularly throughout the day and in fact may not even need to eat three meals a day. As some people's blood-sugar levels are very sensitive, mainly due to liver toxicity, they become extremely anxious and weak if they do not eat every few hours. This can often be overcome by cleansing the liver and taking vegetable juices, molasses, and apple cider vinegar throughout the day instead of meals. Small

---

*"Fasting forestalls Huntington's disease in mice," National Institute on Aging, NIA Press Office, Feb. 10, 2003.

snacks of dried raw food or dried fruits or nuts and seeds serve as healthy snacks to help get you through to your main meals of the day.

THE MYTH OF THE FOOD PYRAMID

Dr. Joseph Mercola, author of *The No-Grain Diet,* says, "According to the latest research, the current USDA food pyramid is misleading and incorrect; it is primarily carbohydrates, and not fats, that contribute to increased weight gain and lead to a variety of illnesses and disorders."

Just as cars and music equipment outdate themselves because of better technology and more research, so too do medical theories, especially nutritional ones. One of the biggest outdated theories to date is the FDA's food pyramid, which was created in 1992, when someone behind a government desk with little to no understanding of nutrition thought that we need six to eleven servings of bread and grains each day! Things change, fortunately, but sometimes they do not, so you need to change them yourself, and in this case it's the dictates of the food pyramid. One could even go so far as to say that these recommendations have contributed to the increase in diabetes, heart disease, and cancer. So if you want to be obese, unhealthy, and depressed like so many people are today, then by all means follow the advice laid out by folks who seemingly know nothing about nutrition and even less about food combining.

Remember that grains are mainly carbohydrates, which are converted into simple sugars when digested by the body. Meat does not make you fat; refined carbohydrates, sugar, poor food combining, no exercise, acidic diets, and parasites make you fat. If 50 percent of our food intake consists of vegetables and salads (a balance of raw and cooked, according to your needs), you'll have a good result in both your health and your weight management very quickly. Choose vegetable protein over meat protein and whole grains over refined carbohydrates, and you are really making a big step toward obtaining optimal health on a nutritional level.

Eating a high-protein meat diet exclusively will only clog up your skin with wastes and fill your bowels full of toxins. Do not be fooled by fad diets; the Japanese eat lots of grains, and they have the highest health and longevity in the world. It is the refining of food and the consumption of processed food, and too much of it, that causes poor health. While whole grains can be eaten fairly well by those who tolerate carbohydrates, some people do have a metabolic type that is more protein-based, so it's best to reduce even cooked whole grains such as brown rice. Alternatively, grains can be sprouted and eaten raw by those who are sensitive to carbs. Moreover, sprouted grains are rich in enzymes, which help in their assimilation.

FIVE EASY WAYS TO HEALTHY WEIGHT LOSS

The truth is simple: diet pills do not work. Correct weight loss takes time. If you are looking for a fast way out, forget it. Fad diets simply do not work, and the majority of people who follow them end up gaining more weight back in the long run. The secret to gaining a trim, healthy figure means changing your eating habits, combined with regular exercise. It doesn't always mean eating less but does means eating differently. From my own experience I do not recommend or believe in diet pills, meal-replacement drinks, or expensive fad diet programs, because none work long-term. They only deplete your bank account, leaving you at your original weight or with more weight after the diet ends. As most people who are overweight are desperate and uncomfortable, many companies that make diet products prey on this fact, encouraging you to buy their "miracle" products.

One of the biggest enemies of weight loss is hunger, and using the steps outlined here can assist you in minimizing the desire to overeat and snack constantly by minimizing your hunger.

Oxygen, water, and unrefined sea salt: Water and cell salts from organic unprocessed sea salt activate sleeping metabolisms and remove fluid stagnation. When the body is starved of sufficient water and optimal levels of oxygen over a period of time, we eat more. Also, our bodies begin to store water as a survival function if we are not getting enough of it, just like our camel friends. Deficiency in trace mineral and cell salts is especially common in obesity, with fluid retention being largely a result of a combination of trace mineral deficiency and dehydration. Water is also the cheapest and safest appetite suppressant. Regularly drinking water throughout the day suppresses the appetite naturally. Drinking while eating does not help and may hinder digestion, although if food is prepared with water as in soups, it satisfies the appetite. Introducing unprocessed sea salt into the diet can help regulate urinary function, reduce fluid retention, and strengthen the kidneys. On the other hand, consuming regular table salt and products containing processed salt will only add to the weight-gain problem. Replacing processed salt with unprocessed sea salt also aids in alkalizing the tissues and restoring lost tissue salts, especially in the bones. In addition, if there was one main nutrient you had to choose to aid in metabolism and to naturally suppress the appetite, it's oxygen. Increasing oxygen levels by adding oxygen to your water (see chapter 1), combined with deep-breathing exercises, are an effective slimming aid, along with ingesting unprocessed sea salt and getting proper hydration.

Use an effective eating plan: Follow a complete nutritional system (acid/alkaline, blood type, food combining, nutritional supplementation) that takes into consideration the specific needs of your own body. Following the eating advice laid out in this chapter is a sure way of nourishing your body and shedding unneeded weight. Focusing on alkalizing foods while correctly combining food is a proven method that has been used for centuries to restore proper metabolism and reduce excess weight. Remember to avoid all the "nonfoods" listed in this chapter, as all these deplete nutrients, reduce metabolism, and encourage overeating. Also, slow down when eating. Getting into the habit of chewing food longer increases the metabolism of fats and overall digestive power because of the increase in the production of enzymes in the mouth; it also causes us to eat less and feel full faster. Supplementing one's diet with superfoods that include minerals such as chromium reduces appetite and sugar cravings and nourishes depleted nutrients. Four foods that can be increased in the diet because they specifically aid in weight loss by increasing metabolism or reducing hunger pangs are citrus-fruit peels, virgin coconut oil, raw apple cider or coconut vinegar, and green or oolong tea. In fact, most expensive diet pills often contain some or all of these four as their main ingredients, so it's better to go straight for the real thing.

Detoxification of the internal organs: Correct detoxification of the intestines, kidneys, liver, and lymphatic system allows for complete elimination of metabolic wastes and the parasites that suppress the metabolism. Juicing and cleansing the digestive system is one of the most important and underrated areas of weight and metabolic control. A sluggish bowel results in sluggish metabolism of fats and unusual weight gain. The average person holds approximately ten pounds of undigested food matter in the bowels, so when this organ is properly cleaned, instant weight loss occurs along with steady weight loss thereafter. As we are all unique, some people do not gain weight when their bowels are unclean; instead they lose it. Although rarer, this is mainly due to the presence of parasites. Cleaning out the bowels is a must for any holistic weight-reduction program. Usually a seven- to ten-day program may need to be repeated monthly for three to six months minimum for proper cleansing to occur. Juice fasting is often combined with internal cleansing for best results.

Exercise (internal and external): Calorie-burning external exercises such as sports and especially internal exercises like Tai Chi, Chi Kung, and yoga all balance the internal meridian system. Exercise increases metabolism and activates metabolic organs, burning fats and calories, and is vital in a holistic weight-reduction plan. Combine external exercises such as sports with internal exercises (yoga and Chi Kung) for best results—thirty minutes of internal exercise and thirty minutes of high-intensity external exercise daily is sufficient to bring about beneficial results. External exercises differ from internal exercises (more on this in chapter 6), primarily because gymnastics and associated gym exercises stimulate the muscles and burn fat, while internal exercises, although often passive and gentle, stimulate and balance glandular functions, which is important for correct long-term weight loss. Overweight persons who have problems burning fat with normal cardio fitness programs often suffer from sluggish metabolic glands such as the pancreas and thyroid, and these kinds of internal exercises wake up those organs.

Mental and emotional aspects: Often overeating and obesity are a result of emotional imbalances, so it is vital that these be addressed and transformed. Mental discipline involves the reprogramming of old habits, thoughts, and limiting beliefs about looking good and gaining a healthy, trim figure. The simple techniques outlined in chapter 6 provide powerful ways to transform negative emotions that pollute the body and contribute to excess weight gain. Rather than choosing to "lose weight," it is more advantageous to think of it in terms of "gaining a healthy, trim figure," because you do not really lose anything. The concept of getting trim is most often associated with the word *loss*, which triggers the subconscious to think that it is losing something valuable, when in reality shedding pounds has only a healthy outcome for those who are overweight.

Stevia, a Healthy Sugar Alternative

Instead of sugar, try stevia, nature's gift in terms of natural sweeteners. This Amazonian plant is many times sweeter than sugar and has no calories and many health-giving properties, unlike sugar. It is extracted by boiling the leaves to make a liquid; this can be easily carried in a small dropper bottle in the pocket and added to beverages anywhere you go. It is also great for cooking in place of processed sugar. Stevia is such a powerful and safe natural sweetener that the U.S. government attempted to ban it, as it was feared that it would completely destroy the multimillion-dollar artificial-sweetener industry (controlled by large pharmaceutical companies) that makes toxic substances like aspartame. Stevia can be found online and at most health-food stores. At present, it makes up approximately 40 percent of the sweetener market in Japan because the Japanese have found it to be a much safer and healthier alternative.

THE ACID-ALKALINE BALANCE

In his book *Alkalize or Die,* Dr. Theodore A. Baroody says, "The countless names attached to illness do not really matter. What does matter is that they are all from the same root cause . . . too much tissue acid waste in the body."

As our cells and tissues are made up of the same elements that we ingest from our food and the earth in which it is grown, so are we bound by the same laws of chemistry as the soil. This commandment of health has sadly been omitted from the modern orthodox medical system for many reasons. The law of correct pH of the blood (approximately 7.4) is one of the most fundamental laws of the human body, because unless proper chemistry is present inside the body, all chemical reactions are compromised in one way or another, especially cellular respiration. Virtually all degenerative diseases such as cancer, heart disease, arthritis, osteoporosis, diabetes, kidney disease, and gallstones, and especially tooth decay, are associated with a diet or lifestyle that is too acid and causes depletion in one's alkaline reserves.

Acid-Alkaline Levels

When water ions are separated, water (H_2O) ionizes into hydrogen (H+) and hydroxyl (OH−) ions. If these ions are in equal amounts, the pH is a neutral 7; if more H+ ions than OH− ions occur, the water is called acidic. If OH− ions outnumber the H+ ions, the water is then alkaline. The pH scale goes from 0 to 14, and most importantly this scale is logarithmic. This means that each step is ten times the previous step. In other words, a pH of 4.5 is ten times more acid than 5.5, a hundred times more acid than 6.5, and a thousand times more acid than 7.5. So you can see how even minor changes in the pH can affect your body's chemistry and lead to serious health problems. As the body is a constant chemical reaction, the pH levels inside our body's cells must remain within the desired range for homeostasis to occur. There is not a single human being who can escape this vital law of chemistry. Just as Mother Earth and her soils must have a balanced pH for producing good foods for eating, so does the body need them for health. Just like the soil or the swimming pool, so too are many human illnesses directly or indirectly related to changes is the chemistry (overacidity) of the body. Overacidity accounts for 99 percent of pH imbalances, and the other 1 percent occurs during overdoses of alkalizing drugs.

The main reason we have overlooked this simple yet vital commandment of health is because of our insistence on ignoring the fact that so many different illnesses in different people all boil down to the same thing: overacidity. As humans are determined to search for complex cures for their even more complex ills, we overlook the most basic law of good medicine, calling it old-fashioned. That two different people with totally different diseases that are caused by the same cause—overacidity—is just too simple and straightforward for modern medicine to acknowledge. It has to be more complex than that! When modern medicine became a highly profitable industry, the simple cures became totally ignored, for obvious reasons.

Overacidity attacks your weakest organs and tissues, creating different illnesses in different people. Cancer in particular is closely linked to excessive acidity in the tissues, which affects cellular DNA and RNA. Thus, depending on each person's genetic predisposition and weakness, overacidity tends to attack our weakest parts. The body's finely tuned hormonal system, from the pituitary to the reproductive glands, can be strongly affected by excess acid waste in the tissues. As blood is the vital component of the body, supplying oxygen and nutrients to every cell via chemical reactions, we can see how overacidity of the tissues, which weakens the metabolic organs, can manifest in a wide variety of diseases. If acid wastes tend to store in the joints first, stiffness in the joints, including the back, and arthritis are signs that the body is storing excess acid wastes due to overacidity. Depending on the person's unique makeup, arthritis may not develop at all, yet he or she can still be suffering badly from overacidity as acid wastes accumulate in the blood, causing the kidneys to work overtime to maintain a perfect pH. The signs are wide and varied according to the person's weakest areas.

Let's look at cancer, for example. Just as a low oxygen state must exist for cancer to exist, so too must it have an acid environment to survive. Amazingly, your doctor may never tell you this as he or she may not have been educated in this simple fact. Biochemist and Nobel laureate Linus Pauling acknowledged that modern medicine lacks any clear understanding of basic body chemistry laws when he said, "Everyone should know that the 'war on cancer' is largely a fraud." Cancer cannot and does not exist inside a properly alkalized body. One does not simply get very unlucky and get cancer; one creates a breeding ground for it and other diseases through one's diet, lifestyle, and emotional habits. I say diet, lifestyle, and emotions because all can affect the pH level and are the major governors of it. The study of food and how it influences the acid-alkaline balance is now heavily researched in natural medicine, as are the studies that confirm that certain emotional states immediately affect the pH of the body. It seems logical that stress increases pH levels via hormonal reactions in the liver and kidneys, which are both involved in cleaning the blood of acidic wastes. It seems even more obvious that prayer, mediation, and relaxation have an alkalizing effect.

Overacidity's Effect on the Immune System

Viral infections such as HIV cannot thrive in a well-oxygenated, alkaline body. Immediate oxygenation and alkalization can have a profound effect on preventing viral infections, because for any virus to thrive, low oxygen and an overacid environment are needed—it's like a playground for them. The immune system deteriorates quickly when the body has too many acid wastes. Overacidity also causes oxygen depletion in the body, as it impairs the red blood cells' oxygen-carrying capacity, so an oversensitive autoimmune system is a true sign that the body has too many acid wastes. Autoimmune illnesses such as asthma, allergies, and even arthritis are usually related to overacidity and are improved significantly by alkalizing the body alone. One such place where acid wastes accumulate and contribute to many diseases is the colon; hence proper bowel cleansing assists the body in emptying acid residue from undigested acid-forming foods.

Stress Linked to Increased Blood Acidity Levels

Stress increases the production of acid-forming hormones, hormones that otherwise allow us to deal with stressful situations. Many of us are suffering from unusually high levels of stress due to our modern lifestyle and environmental stress. These things can literally kill you by acidifying your system. As well, our emotions have a very strong impact on the food we are eating. Even if you eat alkaline-forming foods, they can turn acidic in your gut if you eat while under stress. Eating when angry, watching TV, or otherwise being in an emotional state can also cause alkaline foods to turn acidic. This is why it's important to create some time each day to enjoy your food in a relaxed fashion, chewing it very, very well, and without the distraction of watching TV or the computer. Overeating also causes acidity, even if one is eating alkaline-forming foods.

Overeating Alkaline Food Creates Acid Wastes

Improper food combining has a huge effect on the acid levels in the tissues. Even if consuming 100 percent alkaline foods in a single sitting, if they do not combine well together as described previously in this chapter they will produce an acid residue. This is why we must incorporate food combining along with acid-alkaline balancing for optimal health. This practice was common in many traditional dietary guidelines. It's no wonder that gluttony was considered one of the major sins listed in the Bible—overeating is so dangerous for one's health because the body releases acid wastes in an attempt to counter the excess food that is unneeded by the body. Even if we are sitting down to a nice alkaline meal of wholesome foods, overeating can turn good food into bad in the stomach. Moderation in one's food intake is one of the ancient secrets to longevity that was taught by the ancient Chinese Taoists and Indian yogis.

Testing Your Acid-Alkaline Level

Using body fluids such as saliva and urine to test your pH level is problematic because urine and saliva can change daily from the foods we eat. Measuring the saliva and urine first in the morning on a daily basis over several weeks while beginning to follow the nutritional guidelines outlined in this chapter will yield an approximate reading at home, which is very useful. This is done with pH litmus paper (5.5 to 8), available at health-food stores or some pharmacies. A saliva test indicates one's overall state of health and digestive enzyme function. Simply swallow existing saliva, then wait a few minutes for new saliva to accumulate in the mouth, place the litmus paper in the mouth for a few seconds, and then check it. Urine is tested first thing in the morning using the midstream part of the urine. Dip the litmus paper into a half-cup of urine, or simply urinate on the strip. Generally, urine should not go below an average of 6.4, and for saliva it should be 6.8. Take the daily averages over each week and monitor the changes. If it is below this, then the body is too acid, and you should begin alkalizing through diet while also using the lemon and bicarbonate solution given below. Overalkaline urine may indicate urinary-tract infection or urinary-system problems, so see your doctor immediately and get checked out.

The use of bicarbonate (baking soda) in the treatment of diseases related to acidity, such as arthritis, cancer, asthma, autoimmune, and many other conditions, has been around for many years in natural medicine and was once commonly used by allopathic medicine before Big Pharma took over. These days it has been totally removed from the allopathic medical toolbox because it's cheap, nonpatentable, and therefore nonprofitable. More recently, Dr. Tullio Simoncini from Italy has popularized the awareness of sodium bicarbonate with his use of it in highly successful treatments of cancer. Moreover, a 2009 study involving 134 patients with advanced kidney disease found that taking baking soda daily dramatically slowed down the progression of kidney disease, resulting in no need for dialysis.* Currently an estimated 37,800 patients in the UK alone receive renal replacement therapy, which involves dialysis or a kidney transplant.

Those with cancer, fungal or viral infections, or renal disease, and anyone with acidity-related diseases (the list is endless), as well as every health care practitioner, should understand that the oral intake of

---

*I. Brito-Ashurst, M. Varagunam, M. J. Raftery, and M. M. Yaqoob, "Bicarbonate supplementation slows progression of CKD and improves nutritional status," *Journal of the American Society of Nephrology* 20, no. 9 (2009): 2075–84.

sodium bicarbonate offers an *immediate* change of the blood pH into the alkaline range. So powerful is the effect that athletes notice the difference in their breathing, as more oxygen is carried throughout the system as more acids are neutralized.

Lemon and Baking Soda Alkalizer

This simple formula may help balance biological parameters, pH, ORP (oxidation/reduction potential), phosphates, bicarbonates, and antioxidants of vitamin C, making it a potential life-saving miracle water. There have been studies that show that sodium bicarbonate (simple baking soda) may also be beneficial for the removal of radiation from the body.

Directions: Add 2 tablespoons of lemon or lime juice to a glass. Then add water to three-quarters full (this is your lemon water). Then add one-third of a level teaspoon of baking soda, stir, and wait for any fizz to stop or bubble over. To be taken one to three times daily on an empty stomach. This should be taken for one month, or however long is needed, and can be stopped at any time according to your body's needs. Make sure you work with your health care practitioner or doctor, and be sure to test your own pH to avoid the danger of alkalosis.

Note: Pure baking soda (sodium bicarbonate) is *not* the same as baking powder. Baking powder contains other impure ingredients that are used in the making of bread. Make sure you use pure 100 percent sodium bicarbonate. For those with hypertension and sodium issues, you can offset the sodium increase by taking unpasteurized apple cider vinegar in warm water twice daily at different times from the baking soda solution to increase potassium and offset the sodium; as well, eat a plant-based diet high in potassium foods and reduce salt intake through any processed foods. Our experience has been that the lemon and bicarbonate works more for the kidneys, while the apple cider vinegar and bicarbonate works better for liver concerns; both are effective. It is recommended that you take either formula on an empty stomach and avoid food for one hour afterward.

Acid and Alkaline Food List

Any substance can be determined as being either acid or alkaline by measuring its pH (potential of hydrogen), which is the measurement of force between the hydroxyl (OH−) ions, which are alkaline-forming, and hydrogen (H+) ions, which are acid-forming. Simply speaking it is the measurement of force of the negative and the positive ions against each other. When food enters the body, chemical reactions take place that cause a highly organized group of electrical reactions. To determine the acid or alkaline levels of certain foods, a certain food matter is burned, and the ash is then mixed with water. The pH of the water solution will then determine if the food is either acid or alkaline. Foods that contain mostly alkaline minerals such as fruits, vegetables, and grasses, turn out to be mostly alkaline.

The largest cause of overacidity for most of us is probably found in the food we eat and the thoughts we think. When we digest a particular food, it creates either an acid or alkaline residue that is absorbed into the bloodstream via the digestive system. We must realize that not only do nutrients from food absorb into our blood, but so do acid residues.

Approximately two thousand years ago the Chinese developed a list of foods that were said to be either yang (acid) or yin (alkaline). These foods are almost identical to modern scientific testing of foods and their pH levels today. Please understand that some foods that you may think are acid-forming actually form an alkaline residue after being fully digested, such as citrus fruits and apple cider vinegar.. Many of our clients say that their allopathic doctor told them to stop eating citrus fruits, but this is not entirely correct. Even though citrus fruits are acid to the taste, when they digest they form an alkaline ash and are in fact very alkaline-forming and quite often benefit many health conditions. Simply diluting your fruit juices 50:50 with water will prevent most stomach upsets, but most citrus are best avoided if you have an ulcer, as they aggravate the surface of the ulcer.

During times of illness it is advisable to follow a diet of 100 percent alkaline-forming foods, and then apply the 80/20 rule for general health after the illness has been successfully cured. For health maintenance, 80 percent alkaline and 20 percent acid is most often recommended; this ratio varies slightly for those in extremely hot or cold climates. In extremely cold climates, a higher ratio such as 30 percent acid-forming foods may be needed, as acid-forming foods can increase body temperature. In extremely hot climates around the equator, the 95 percent alkaline diet may be most beneficial. I personally find it best to follow a program of 100 percent alkaline-forming foods for one week every three months for health maintenance. Often coinciding with this week of alkaline foods one can also do a bowel, liver, or tissue cleansing assisted by herbal remedies all at the same time.

Highly Acid-Forming Foods (Avoid):

- Land animal meats of all types (red meat, chicken, lamb, etc.)
- Seafood and shellfish
- Coffee (instant coffee very acidic; organic coffee best in moderation, limit to one cup daily during healthy times and avoid during illness)
- Alcoholic beverages (spirits are more acidic than wines; limit to three to four glasses of wine weekly)
- Commercial dairy products (acid- and mucous-forming)
- Fried food (dangerous heated fats for the heart and arteries)
- Soda (soft) drinks, carbonated and processed beverages
- Sugar (white, brown, sucrose, and other label names, highly dangerous nonfoods)
- Sweetened fruit juices (not 100 percent juice)
- Processed or hydrogenated vegetable oils, margarines, and artificial butter spreads made from refined vegetable oils
- White bread, white (wheat) flour, baker's flour (often bleached with chemicals added)
- White rice and other grains that have had the fiber removed
- All processed foods (packet, canned, preserved, and pickled)

- Artificial sweeteners
- Tobacco smoking or chewing (not recommended under any circumstances)

Lightly Acid-Forming to Neutral (Eat Moderately):
- Whole-grain breads
- Brown and red rice and whole grains
- Pulses (beans, peas, and lentils)
- Nuts and seeds (except almonds and Brazil nuts)
- Unprocessed raw dairy products

Alkaline-Forming (Highly Recommended):
- Fresh vegetables, fruits, and herbs
- Millet, buckwheat, quinoa, and amaranth (gluten-free whole grains)
- Sprouted pulses and Essene bread (sprouted bread)
- Almonds and Brazil nuts
- Cold-pressed vegetable oils
- Fermented soy such as miso, tamari, natto, tempeh, etc.

MODERN NUTRITIONAL SCIENCE FOR LONGEVITY

When the subject of longevity is raised, most of us think of centenarians, the common term used to describe people who live to one hundred years or more. As you probably have realized by now, many factors cause humans to live long lives, namely diet and lifestyle and of course a mental aptitude to deal with stress. As Japan today holds the record with the highest percentage of centenarians per population, it makes common sense to study the dietary and lifestyle practices of this culture, especial the regions in southern Japan where this is most common. In doing this, researchers have discovered not one single secret to these longer life spans, but rather several general factors as mentioned above. One study of 1,500 centenarians found that their diets, activity levels, and even

smoking habits varied widely. It was noted that nearly all of them pos-
sessed a good sense of humor and did not waste time worrying. Thomas
T. Perls, assistant professor of medicine at Harvard Medical School, ger-
iatrician at Beth Israel Deaconess Medical Center, founder and director
of the New England Centenarian Study, and author of *Living to 100:
Lessons in Living to Your Maximum Potential at Any Age,* says, "Perhaps
rather than having survived disease, centenarians were more likely to
have altogether avoided the chronic and acute diseases associated with
aging in order to live to 100. What emerged from this sudden intuitive
realization was the hypothesis that has become the study's guiding light
ever since: One must stay healthy the vast majority of one's life in order
to live to 100."

DHEA

A recent nutritional trend has people taking hormones such as HGH
(human growth hormone) or DHEA (dehydroepiandrosterone), both
often said to be "fountain-of-youth" hormones. One must consider
the risk in taking a hormone that our body already produces. Our
glands decrease in function as we get older, causing us to age. This has
triggered many clinics to offer hormone injections to the aging population of baby boomers, a lucrative proposition. Some reports have
dubbed DHEA "the mother of all hormones" and a "super hormone,"
a magic pill that can help us live longer, erase wrinkles, lose weight,
and prevent cancer, heart disease, and even Alzheimer's, all the while
combating infectious diseases. Unfortunately, most of the hype often
drowns out the facts. DHEA is a steroid hormone, a chemical cousin
of testosterone and estrogen, and is produced by the adrenal glands.
In our initial first few years of life, the adrenals make very little of
this substance; then at age six or seven they begin pouring out larger
amounts. Production peaks in the midtwenties, making DHEA the
most abundant hormone in circulation at that time. From one's early
thirties onward, there is a steady decline in DHEA production; in fact,
the average seventy-five-year-old has only 20 percent of the DHEA in
circulation that he or she had fifty years earlier. Ray Sahelian, M.D.,

author of *Mind Boosters,* believes that DHEA supplementation carries many risks:

> Over the past two years I have come across many cases of heart-rhythm disturbances associated with high-dose use of DHEA and pregnenolone. I reported one such case in a man taking 50 mg per day in the October 1998 issue of the *Annals of Internal Medicine* (volume 129, page 588). Other side effects include acne, unwanted hair growth, scalp hair loss, menstrual irregularities, irritability, and aggression. In my opinion, DHEA, androstenedione, or pregnenolone should not be sold over the counter in doses greater than 5 mg.

When DHEA is taken over longer periods it has been shown to actually reduce the body's own natural DHEA production. Dr. John Nestler, a professor of endocrinology and metabolism at Virginia Commonwealth University who has studied DHEA effects extensively, says that "no one should take DHEA except under the supervision of a physician, who should routinely check steroid and cholesterol levels, glucose tolerance, and prostate health in men." Dr. Elizabeth Barrett-Connor, chairperson of the department of family and preventive medicine at the University of California, San Diego, who has studied natural DHEA levels in older people, states unequivocally: "DHEA is snake oil. It makes me very nervous that people are using a drug we do not know anything about. We would not recommend it." DHEA has side effects, some of which may be irreversible. Since it's converted into testosterone, some women who take it grow body or facial hair, and if they are under age fifty, can stop menstruating. DHEA has also been shown to decrease levels of HDL "good" cholesterol in women and could thus increase their risk of heart disease.

HGH

There are some studies demonstrating the antiaging and disease-reversing capabilities of somatotropin, commonly known as growth hormone, or HGH. Growth-hormone injections, carefully monitored by a physician, may initially have benefits, while those sold in sprays or homeopathic form have shown little to no results other than placebo. The question is whether HGH is really safe in the long term. Many of the studies promoting HGH can be found in Dr. Ronald Klatz's book *Grow Young with HGH,* which documents the very powerful antiaging benefits of injectable HGH, costing as much as $20,000 per year. Not surprisingly, he is also the founder of many clinics that offer these injections.

HGH is a protein naturally secreted by the pituitary gland that promotes cell growth. Today HGH injections are the latest in fountain-of-youth crazes; they are said to prevent physical and mental deterioration, among many other claims, including longevity. However, the risks are considerable. Growth hormones can cause fluid retention, high blood pressure, and blood-sugar problems that lead to diabetes. They may also stimulate the growth of existing cancer tumors, so if you have a tiny tumor you do not know of you could be turning a treatable situation into a serious stage IV cancer. HGH injections and DHEA supplementation are dubious long term. There are other options for avoiding disease and increasing your life span that are less damaging to the body and the wallet.

Enter the Missing Trace Element Indium

Indium is a soft, silvery metal and the third heaviest molecular element, known to be useful in nutrition. It is element number 49 on the periodic table. Interestingly, it is never found in food or water or in our bodies after the age of twenty-five to thirty and is close to being the tenth most scarce of all available elements on the periodic table. Indium sulfate, the form that we recommend and have tested for more than ten years on myself and then on clients, is totally safe and has not demonstrated any toxic effects to humans or animals, even using several thousand times the recommended dosage. Dr. Morton Walker, in his book *Indium: The Age-Reversing Trace Element,* says, "Just one daily drop of this completely overlooked nutrient can turn back the aging clock by stimulating a cascade of youth-promoting hormones . . . more energy . . . more stamina . . . better vision . . . improved bodily functions, and relief from myriad maladies associated with aging."

Indium's most important function is its connection with longevity and its ability to affect the function and production of age-reducing hormones of the hypothalamus and pituitary gland, releasing a cascade of over thirty beneficial hormones. Indium in this form is an aqueous solution containing pure .9999 percent indium sulfate anhydrous and distilled water as the sole ingredients. It has a clean, strong, and metallic taste but is not unbearable, and many people actually enjoy the taste. Its benefits include:

- Long-term reduction of the appearances of aging
- Greatly elevated immunity activity
- Reduced severity and duration of colds and bruising
- Faster-working memory
- Less sleep requirements
- A greater sense of well-being

Some other studies reported by Dr. Walker have shown that indium can improve both high and low blood pressure and increase libido in both men and women, while other investigations have reported the return of hair growth in people who are balding. Many seniors report that their sense of smell and taste improves greatly in a matter of days. Anecdotal reports of its benefits include a reduction of addictions and the normalization of body fat. Indium can also reduce intraocular pressure (IOP) in cases of glaucoma. Dr. Henry Schroeder, a research toxicologist, found that mice demonstrated 42 percent fewer cancers and malignant tumors with indium supplementation. Indium may be anti-carcinogenic in mice, but what about humans?

As indium is a nonpatentable substance that comes directly from nature, drug companies are not doing any expensive testing any time soon to prove its effectiveness, so the mystery continues as to what indium can really do. In the meantime we suggest you test this safe, nontoxic, completely natural trace mineral on yourself. Indium in aqueous form is best taken as one drop on the top of the tongue upon awakening, before brushing teeth, with no food, beverages, or medicine for at least the next twenty minutes. This is because undigested food residue in the stomach, even after eight hours of sleep, may decrease its effectiveness, so it is best to follow these directions.

ELECTRICAL NUTRITION

In the late 1930s, scientists made an amazing discovery, telling us that the smallest thing in the universe had been found. The atom was said to be the building block of all things, including molecules (the basic building blocks of matter) and thus humans. The question was asked as to what then would happen if we split the atom, and the rest is history. When we look at the atom closely, we see that it is more than an atomic structure that becomes the building block of our structure. The atom is composed of—you guessed it—more atoms. Even protons, neutrons, and electrons are composed of atoms. In fact, scientists have been able to keep dividing and subdividing these atoms until their equipment runs out of space or the technology is not finite enough to measure any further.

When we add the total physical density of the supposedly solid atom we find that it is 99.9 percent empty space, and that the reason it *appears* solid is due to the rate at which the electrons spin around its core. But when we look closer at each proton or electron, the real structural part of the atom, we see that they too are made up of protons and electrons like the atom they form and are also basically 99.9 percent empty space. With the advancement of electron microscopes and computer technology, the world's top nuclear physicists are yet to narrow anything down that confirms that we actually exist on a solid, physical level. It seems that the once-heralded discovery of the atom, the building block of humankind, is leading us to one of the oldest discoveries that has been put forward for millennia by metaphysicians: that we are made up of pure energy. To fully understand the potential of this realization we need to look at quantum physics and explore it further. The new way of looking at nutrition is often referred to as *quantum nutrition,* and it is being pioneered by some amazing research-ers in the field of nutrition. When we understand that our body is made of atoms that are held together by a force of energy forming a physical body, medical treatment takes on a whole new, exciting direction. The concept of drugs and even modern surgery seems far away, and medical treatment begins to move away from primitive treatment and toward electricity, sound, frequency, harmonics, light (laser), and other forms of newly discovered energy.

Nutritional supplements that are electrically or harmonically bal-anced are of course likely to be more beneficial that those that are not. When buying a vitamin supplement we usually just look at what vita-mins it has and perhaps how many milligrams it has. We do not really think to ask if it is electrically active the way our body is. It is possible that two supplements containing the same amount of a vitamin could perform very differently in the body if one of these two supplements is more electrically active, in turn being more bioavailable, which brings us to the next obvious question.

Natural or Synthetic Supplements?

More than 97 percent of the vitamin and mineral supplements found in the typical retail health-food store are synthetics or made from fraction-ated and isolated nutrients. These products cannot hope to perform the important task of healthy cell regeneration. With long-term use, these poorer sources can often lead to additional health problems.

Some believe that ascorbic acid, for example, is the same as vitamin C, but ascorbic acid is actually the antioxidant ring that sur-rounds the vitamin C complex. Since its initial discovery during the last century it has been found to have many other vital compounds that compose its totality. Other compounds such as rutin, bioflavonoids, the K factor, the J factor, tyrosinase (an organic copper), and ascorbi-gen all work together to be fully used by the body as what we know as vitamin C. Moreover, it has been found that while natural vitamin C from acerola berries and citrus peel can reverse scurvy (a once-common vitamin C deficiency disease suffered by sailors), ascorbic acid alone cannot do this. Humans are organic beings based on complex carbon molecules; therefore, when we constantly ingest inorganic synthetic molecules or bits of an original organic molecule we disrupt the electrical and metabolic functions that run every function in our body.

Many people have heard the debate over natural versus synthetic. This is interesting, as not many people realize how many synthetic chemicals (molecules) they eat or ingest every day. For example, we see vitamin supplements advertised as "natural." This merely means that they have kept the original structure of the molecules when making that particular vitamin, but there is usually none of the original substance left from what it was extracted from. Perhaps a very small quantity is from natural source with the rest of it being totally manufactured.

When a drug is formed, it is most often based on naturally occurring organic chemicals that have been observed in a plant. This then is extracted and chemically synthesized, concentrated, and duplicated in a laboratory. The original idea is there, only now one particular chemical has been extracted, synthesized, patented, and marketed. The downside of this is that other naturally occurring chemicals inside the original plant where the original chemical was found in the first place have very special properties that balance the effects of the extracted chemical and reduce any side effects. This is the beauty of Mother Nature. So let us eat the whole plant as we have done for centuries instead of extracting individual chemicals and synthesizing them in a laboratory.

There is a large debate between nutritional scientists and naturalists concerning whether there are side effects to ingesting synthetic vitamin substances over the long term. We know that drugs have numerous side effects, yet pure herbs used as medicine do not have such dangerous side effects. That said, they can interact with pharmaceutical drugs, so please check with drug-herb interaction lists online. So do man-made vitamins affect us in the long term? From clinical tests we know that man-made vitamins are thousands of times safer for the body than pharmaceutical drugs, as people do not die from taking vitamins like they do from taking pharmaceutical drugs. So how does taking man-made vitamins or mineral supplements fit in with a healthy lifestyle, and should they be part of a daily program? Clinically manufactured supplements are great for correcting chronic deficiencies quickly and are much safer than drugs while also treating the cause, but in the long run we much prefer to use herbs and superfoods rather than synthesized vitamins as a part of a daily health program whenever and wherever possible. As Robert Marshall, Ph.D., founder of Quantum Nutrition Labs and host of the radio show *HealthLine Live,* says, "When whole-food phytonutrients are combined together synergistically, their effect is far greater than the sum of individual vitamins and minerals. This geometric increase, by a factor of 100-fold or more, is called the *quantum effect.*"

Our final word on this subject is this: do not expect to get informed nutritional advice from your allopathic medical doctor. For the most part, getting information on nutrition from your next-door neighbor would be safer than getting it from your doctor. This is because there is a greater chance the average person has done more research on the subject than the general practitioner of Western medicine. Nutrition is the new frontier of modern health care and the future in the treatment and prevention of degenerative diseases, yet our medical system, for various reasons, has been slow to realize this fact.

Dr. Michael Colgan, founder and director of the Colgan Institute, which is concerned primarily with the effects of nutrition and exercise on aging, athletic performance, and the prevention of degenerative disease, says, "Nutrition is the most important science in medicine." Unfortunately, these days most of the five or more years of education that allopathic doctors undergo to gain an M.D. degree is intensely focused on the workings of human anatomy, physiology, pathology, drug pharmacology, and surgery, and not on the advancements of twenty-first-century nutrition science. Teaching from outdated nutritional texts and old-fashioned food pyramid diagrams, medical schools' classes on nutrition are so brief that one could not possibly learn or understand the immense possibilities of healing through nutrition. During the five years of allopathic medical school most medical students are lucky if they attend one forty-five-minute lecture on basic nutritional principles, and this information is relatively prehistoric in terms of what's known about the role of nutrition in health. A recently convened panel of U.S. nutrition experts, the Intersociety Professional Nutrition Education Consortium, concluded that "American physicians are undertrained when it comes to issues of nutrition and health. The authority whom patients most wish to consult for information on health—their physician—remains insufficiently informed about the role of diet in the prevention and treatment of disease." The report concluded that less than 6 percent of medical school graduates receive adequate training in nutrition.

This may be why a growing number of people are less likely to see a general practitioner for minor ailments and are flocking to natural medicine—because most of us have begun to realize that the majority of our health problems are related to what we put into our bodies in the form of our food. Almost a hundred years ago Dr. Alexis Carrel, 1912 Nobel Prize winner for physiology, asserted that "if the doctor of today does not become the dietician of tomorrow, the dietician of today will become the doctor of tomorrow."

Fourth Immortal Healer—Ho Hsien-Ku

Cleanse Your Organs and Glands

No physician can ever say that any disease is incurable.
To say so blasphemes God, blasphemes nature, and
depreciates the great architect of creation. The disease
does not exist, regardless of how terrible it may be, for
which God has not provided the corresponding cure.

PARACELSUS

The healing of internal cleansing is symbolized by Ho Hsien-Ku, who is often regarded as the only female among the Immortals. Legend has it she was born in the seventh century CE. She became an Immortal at the age of fourteen after meeting fellow Immortal Lu Tung-Pin, who taught her internal alchemy, giving her the precious, rare peach of Immortality. She achieved great fame and was summoned to present herself to the Chinese empress Wu. She ignored the royal command and instead ascended to heaven in full daylight, disappearing from Earth.

This female Taoist Immortal represents the Earth Mother, our source in nature, which is also our cleansing force. She is our nurturer and represents the pristine cleanliness of nature herself through her "Internal Alchemy" of internal cleansing. She is often described as a morally pure woman, an ideal daughter, and a selfless seeker after spiritual freedom. In iconography she is typically pictured bearing a lotus flower that improves one's health, both mental and physical. She also is shown carrying the peach of Immortality, and is sometimes shown with the musical instrument known as *sheng*, or a *fenghuang*, to accompany her. She may also carry a bamboo ladle or fly whisk.

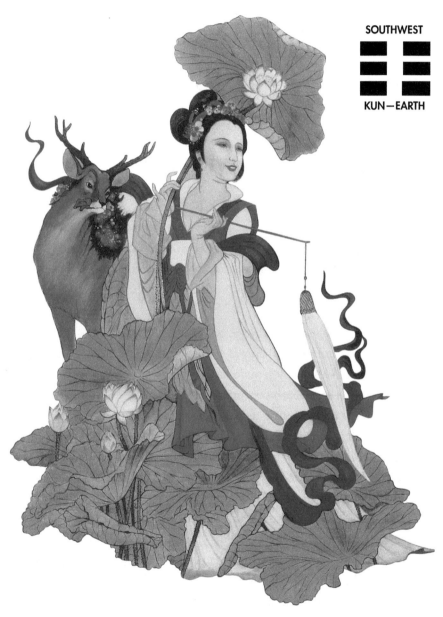

SOUTHWEST

KUN—EARTH

Fig. 4.1. Ho Hsien-Ku (He Xian Gu)

CLEANSING AND DETOXIFYING THE BODY

The Bible, like many ancient sources, is full of allusions to the path of health through cleanliness. Matthew 23:27 says, "You are like white-washed tombs which indeed appear beautiful outwardly, but inside are full of dead men's bones and all uncleanness."

From toothpaste to shampoo to skin-care products, we spend thousands of dollars on products that cleanse and beautify our external body, but most of us do not realize the importance of cleansing the internal organs. Over time, toxins build up in the body as a result of our exposure to environmental pollutants in the air we breathe and the food and water we eat and drink. Our bodies are designed to eliminate these toxins from our daily life, but over time they build up anyway, burdening the eliminatory organs and in turn overwhelming our ability to remove them naturally and efficiently. Using healing foods and herbs to cleanse the organs and tissues of acid wastes and other impurities is an excellent way of healing the body and optimizing health. Cleansing is as simple as following an optimal healing diet, usually 100 percent alkaline foods, combined with natural supplements and herbs that assist in the cleansing process.

Internal cleansing involves the following:

- Cleansing of the liver, colon, kidneys, and other organs
- Increasing tissue oxygenation
- Purifying the blood
- Reducing the buildup of body toxins
- Releasing chemicals stored in body fat and tissues
- Losing excess weight and fluid retention

Internal cleansing brings about the following benefits:

- Smoother digestion and elimination
- Renewed energy
- Improved ability to adsorb and utilize nutrients from food
- Clearer thinking and better focus

- Correct elimination, including two to three bowel movements daily

FASTING, AN ANCIENT WAY TO REJUVENATE YOUR HEALTH

Religious fasting is a duty required by various spiritual traditions. The Bible records Jesus telling his Apostles, "When you fast, anoint your head and wash your face so that you do not appear to others to be fasting . . . but your Father, who sees in secret, will reward you openly" (Matthew 6:16–18). The prophet Mohammed said, "She or he who does well of her or his own accord shall be rewarded, but to fast is better for you, if you but knew it." In more recent times, Mahatma Gandhi, speaking from the Hindu tradition, said, "Fasting will bring spiritual rebirth to those of you who cleanse and purify your bodies. The light of the world will illuminate within you when you fast and purify yourself. What the eyes are for the outer world, fasts are for the inner."

Fasting as a way of restoring health and reversing the aging process is one of the oldest and still most effective methods of detoxifying the body's tissues and healing. All the great spiritual prophets and sages promoted fasting to gain mastery of the body and mind. Jesus is said to have fasted for forty days and nights (which is highly possible), and Buddha fasted extensively on his path to enlightenment. Fasting is a science and needs to be treated as one. We do not recommend fasting straight away, and one needs to have a solid grounding in the laws of fasting before attempting it successfully. Although there have been many stories of people fasting without being taught how to do so correctly and achieving great results anyway, it is better to first school yourself in the correct way to fast.

Preparing to Fast

To start out, we recommend one-day fasts each week for a month before your first real seven-day fast. This helps you build confidence and prepare the body for longer fasts. During this one-day-a-week fasting day, drink plenty of lemon water and feel free to take some herbal fiber or magnesium oxide to cleanse the bowels. Dry skin brushing in the morning and at night is also advised to activate lymphatic drainage and detoxification. It has always been taboo to fast during the winter season for many reasons, particularly because the cold affects the metabolism, making fasting dangerous and difficult. By far the best times to fast are the spring and summer months. When you have picked a good week to have your seven-day fast you will need to ease off any drugs and alcohol a week beforehand so that your detoxification is not so intense. In particular, eat light meals the day before you begin. It may be best to suspend all but the most essential herb and vitamin supplements during a fast, so your system doesn't become overloaded and is allowed to detoxify.

First Three Days of Fasting

The first three days of fasting are the most difficult, both emotionally and physically. What we mean here is that you can have detoxification reactions such as headaches, bad breath, and body aches during this time as poisons are eliminated from the tissues and organs. As it takes approximately seventy-two hours for the body to change over from digestive mode (the usual body mode) to metabolic mode (the cleansing mode), the first three days can be irritating to say the least. There is one great piece of advice that has been given to me by masters of the fasting discipline that has gotten me and many others through these trying first three days, and that is to simply "grin and bear it."

Fourth Day of a Fast

By the fourth day of a fast one usually wakes up feeling clearheaded and on a natural high. Also, the hunger pangs are usually gone and the thought of going without food for four more days is not a concern anymore. In fact, your hunger has usually completely dissipated by the fourth day, and you feel light and energized, which is encouraging. Your eyes will look brighter and even change color for some. The skin begins to shine and the mind clears. During this time it is advisable to do some mild exercise to assist in lymphatic circulation, providing further detoxification of the tissues.

Breaking Your Fast on the Eighth Day

The word *breakfast* actually means "to break the fast"; i.e., the fast of not eating at night while you sleep. This is why we have always promoted a light breakfast based on fruit and vegetables and their juices, and not animal proteins or refined carbohydrates in the form of breakfast cereals. It is important on the morning of the eighth day to begin by eating only fruits and/or vegetables; then on the ninth day you can slowly introduce some whole grains, and on the tenth day, nuts and seeds. If you try to eat heavy food right after a seven-day fast, your stomach will go into severe shock. As most people overeat anyway, as explained in the previous chapter, what happens during a fast is that the stomach, which is largely muscle tissue, shrinks to about the size of your fist, so when you sit down to eat what is considered a normal-size meal, you can only eat half of it.

Things to Remember When Fasting

We have seen fasting performed successfully by the old and young, and by those who are healthy as well as those who are very ill. Obviously, fasting could be dangerous if performed by someone taking heavy pharmaceutical drugs or by those suffering from eating disorders like anorexia or bulimia. It is important to listen to your body while fasting and drink plenty of water and take bowel- and blood-cleansing herbs to keep the bowels regular during the fast. Some people like to have a vegetable or fruit juice daily during a fast, as these can actually assist in detoxification and help to satisfy you and make the fast easier. Others prefer to only take water and cleansing herbs. Some practitioners of regular fasting also believe in taking enemas or colonic irrigation several times during the fast to deeply cleanse the bowels, although we do not do this and prefer to cleanse the bowels from the other end, by orally taking the bowel-cleansing herbs or magnesium powder. We encourage people to try both ways to see what works best for them. If you find yourself getting extremely weak and you feel like you are going to faint or your blood sugar or blood pressure drops, simply eat an apple or some other fresh fruit or take pinch of sea salt on your tongue to stabilize yourself. Fasting is not a competition; it's a way of giving your body the time and space it needs to clean itself. So listen to your body.

How to Deal with Adverse Reactions

Dr. Richard Schulze says, "Everyone wants a quick cleanse or a 24-hour detox. Sure, party for a decade and then try to clean up the whole mess in a few minutes—it's not going to happen. Any cleansing or detoxification program is a total joke unless you do a thorough bowel cleansing for a few weeks first."

As the path of transforming poor health into good health can be a challenging path, rocks are bound to be found on the road along the way. Often when one embarks on a journey to improve one's health either by changing one's diet or lifestyle or quitting a habit of some kind, it results in a minor illness developing, whether it be a lingering cold or flu, a sore throat, or poor, lusterless skin. The Herxheimer reaction, named after German physician Karl Herxheimer, is the term used in modern medicine, while some people simply call it a healing crisis. I prefer the term *healing process,* as it can sometimes be a physical and emotional test that you must go through when committing yourself to becoming well.

These temporary pathological symptoms can be triggered if you begin to suddenly eat healthy, fast for more than three days, or take herbal medicines to detoxify and cleanse the tissues. As well as being related to the process of detoxification, this healing process can also be a result of the die-off period that occurs when herbal medicines and other therapies stimulate the immune system, which in turn destroys large numbers of harmful germs and pathogens in the body. We can and do absorb toxic wastes from these dead and dying microorganisms. The large amounts of foreign antigens triggered from this die-off causes a sudden shock to the immune system, which can temporarily worsen your initial symptoms. Usually this healing process only lasts several days to two weeks depending on the amount of toxins in the body. This not-so-nice process can be minimized by increasing your water intake and using herbs that assist in speeding up elimination of the bowels. Also, dry skin brushing, hot and cold showers, deep-breathing exercises, mild to moderate exercise, and massage can greatly help to ease the process. Like the old saying goes, two steps forward, one step backward; the healing process can feel like a rocky road during the first months of healing from an illness. It's most intense if one is working on healing a chronic illness such as cancer, heart disease, or diabetes.

The body begins to do what it does best—self-heal—when given the correct foods and thoughts. It does this by clearing wastes stored in the tissues and dumping them into the blood, in turn being eliminated by the four main eliminatory organs: the colon, kidneys, lungs, and skin. In addition, one of the hundreds of jobs your liver performs is to clean the blood, which can become pretty "dirty" when your body begins to detoxify and cleanse itself. Someone who usually does not get migraines could suddenly get them, or your skin could suddenly look grayish or unhealthy, or you could find yourself with a sudden cold, fever, or swollen glands. All these and many other acute symptoms are a result of your body attempting to clean itself out. It is often during this kind of healing process that those taking the natural-medicine route (by choosing to treat the cause rather than the symptoms) lose faith and have second thoughts about the natural approach. The temptation is to go back to taking painkillers, anti-inflammatory drugs, or steroids to deal with uncomfortable symptoms. Unfortunately, this will never cure any chronic health problem, as detoxification is necessary for true healing to occur. With the help of a good natural practitioner this uncomfortable process can be controlled so that the person's life is not in serious risk as a result of clearing out toxins. Generally, it is controlled by adjusting one's program gradually and drinking plenty of water, combined with keeping the eliminatory organs open and fully functional to allow the complete elimination of wastes coming from within the tissues and organs. The speed at which you eliminate must be tailored to your individual personal health needs according to your age and overall strength. That is why working under the close guidance of your natural-medicine practitioner is highly recommended when fasting or tissue cleansing, especially if there is chronic disease.

PARASITES ARE THE UNDERLYING CAUSE OF MANY DISEASES

Dr. Hermann R. Bueno, a fellow of the Royal Society of Tropical Medicine and Hygiene in London, says, "Parasites are the missing diagnosis in the genesis of many chronic health problems, including diseases of the gastrointestinal tract and endocrine system. Most individuals would be truly amazed if they knew the extraordinarily high number of people who are unknowingly infected by parasites." According to the World Health Organization, 3.5 billion people suffer from some type of parasitic infection. Many people are under the impression that parasitic diseases are a problem of developing countries or of tropical climates and that they don't really pose a threat to people living in developed nations such as the United States and Western European countries. This couldn't be further from the truth. Some studies estimate that as many as 50 million American children are infected with parasites, but only a small percentage of these are actually detected and reported. So it's completely false that parasites are rare in Western countries, and more the case that they are a hugely misdiagnosed problem.

A parasite is a general term for a microorganism that feeds off the tissues and body fluids of its host, stealing the host's nutrients and creating metabolic wastes. Just as our body contains microorganisms such as good bacteria that are beneficial, it also contains microorganisms that cause disease. Some parasites are large enough to be seen with the human eye, while others can only be seen with a microscope.

There are eight major sources of parasitic infections:

1. Insects, especially mosquitos
2. Physical contact with others
3. Contaminated water, especially bottled water

4. Unclean foods, especially meat and dairy products
5. Airborne contact
6. Our pets
7. The soil
8. Our own toxic body that allows parasites to proliferate

Signs of parasitic infection include various digestive symptoms, including bloating, diarrhea, flatulence, constipation, and cramps, and less frequently bleeding, irritable bowels, leaky gut, and excess mucus secretion. Parasites also cause nondigestive symptoms, including allergies, fatigue, nausea, nervous-sensory disorders, skin diseases (eczema and psoriasis), muscle problems, fever, headache, immune deficiencies, insomnia, and weight loss or weight gain. It is now speculated that serious diseases such as cancer, arthritis, and diabetes also have parasitic involvement, in turn being an underlying causative factor. When the immune system is suppressed or when one suffers from a serious health ailment, parasites run rampant, further burdening the body's immune system, making it almost impossible to cure the illness without addressing the parasite issue. It is important to know that if left untreated, parasites can remain in the body for a lifetime and eventually cause death through horrendous ailments that are often blamed as the cause of death instead of the parasites. As Dr. Richard Shulze grimly observes, "When you die, the worms actually crawl out, not in."

Natural medicine has always used herbal remedies to treat parasitic infections because many chronic ailments are an end result of parasites in the body. Unfortunately, of the six hundred different disease-causing microorganisms, Western medicine only tests for a few of them and has adequate medicine for even fewer; and stool samples, the commonly accepted way to test for parasites in allopathic medicine, are a highly ineffective way to determine whether there are parasites in the organs and blood. Flatworms known as *flukes* go totally unnoticed in orthodox medicinal blood tests, and it is these that seem to do the most damage in terms of suppressing the immune system and causing serious illness. Recent scientific research has revealed that our immune systems are primarily built for one main function: to seek out and destroy parasites.

This simple yet profound discovery supports the idea that the underlying causes of many diseases are related to parasites that go undetected by modern allopathic medicine's tests.

Traditionally, Native Americans used black walnut hulls for parasites, while ancient Greek doctors like Hippocrates used olive leaf. Asian physicians used wormwood and the Egyptians used black seed (*Nigella sativa*). There are many other traditional cultures that use similar remedies to treat a variety of diseases such as cancer and diabetes, which they believed to be linked to parasites or viruses that lie dormant in the system and then suddenly attack the body when the immune system becomes too tired and overloaded to cope. This fact has been acknowledged in some parts of the scientific community, notably by Dr. Robert J. Huebner, chief of the Laboratory of Infectious Diseases of the National Institute of Health: "There isn't the slightest doubt in our minds that human cancers are caused by viruses," he says. "To this extent they are simply infectious diseases."

As far back as 1911, Nobel Prize–winning virologist Francis Peyton Rous extracted cancerous tissue from a hen and then removed all the cancer cells from the extract and injected the remaining fluid (minus any cancer cells) into other healthy hens. He then noticed that all the hens injected developed cancer. This evidence was further supported in the December 1956 issue of the *Journal of the American Medical Association* in an article written by Dr. Ludwik Gross: "Experimental data began to accumulate pointing more and more to the possibility that many, if not all, malignant tumors may be caused by viruses. Thus, a large number of malignant tumors of different morphology and in different species of animals could be transmitted from one host to others by filtered extracts."

Pioneering researchers were heavily criticized and even jailed for these unorthodox medical views: scientist and inventor Royal Rife was an early exponent of high-magnification time-lapse cinemicrography, who in the 1930s used a specially designed optical microscope to observe microbes that were too small to visualize with previously existing technology; and Dr. Hulda Clark, a naturopath, found that all human disease had a connection to parasitic infection. Once again it all boils down to money, for if most diseases that plague humankind do involve parasites, and the elimination of parasites is relatively easy to accomplish, then Big Pharma would be out of business. Ideas around "fringe medicine" as practiced by Rife and Clark seem to have their origin in a Senate bill passed way back in the 1930s that involved the influence of drug companies. As a result, the use of microcurrents and high-frequency equipment to kill parasites in order to heal cancer is totally prohibited. For example, Royal Rife, like many doctors who went in search of a simple cure for cancer, believed that safe levels of frequencies and currents could be used to eliminate pathogens in the body and stimulate the immune system, which in turn allows the body to self-heal from cancer.

ANTIPARASITIC HERBAL REMEDIES

There are three commonly used herbs that can rid you of over a hundred different types of parasites, and they do this without interfering with most prescription medications that people take for their disease. These are black walnut hulls (green-hulled), wormwood (*Artemisia* spp.), and freshly ground cloves. These three herbs should be used together for best results. While black walnut hulls and wormwood destroy the developing and mature parasites, the freshly ground cloves destroy the parasite eggs. Remember to use green-hulled black walnut hulls, which are much stronger and very effective, because once the hull turns black the natural parasite-destroying chemicals are reduced. Many diseases and lingering ills have shown remarkable results after correct parasite cleansing. Rather than wait till you get sick and develop a serious illness, do a parasite cleanse twice yearly. Whether you are a doctor, lawyer, or housemaid, whether you are rich, famous, or poor, we are all equally at risk of developing a parasite-related illness.

COLLOIDAL SILVER—ANTIBIOTIC, ANTIPARASITIC, AND ANTIVIRAL

The most powerful and safest method I have found to kill harmful bacteria and microbes in water as well as in our body's tissues (which are

70+ percent water) is by using colloidal silver. The ancient Greeks and Romans used silver in water after they observed that liquid remained fresher longer when placed in silver containers. These silver-infused liquids were taken solely to rid the body of disease-causing parasites. Dr. Robert O. Becker, author of a number of books on natural healing, including the best-selling *The Body Electric,* says, "What we have actually done was rediscover that silver killed bacteria, which had been known for centuries . . . When antibiotics were discovered, clinical uses for silver as an antibiotic were discarded."

The word *colloidal* means that a mineral—in this case silver—is suspended in water (not dissolved); its ionic properties mean that it has a common positive charge, causing the mineral to remain repelled and dissolved in water, usually with a smaller particle size. Colloidal silver is simply a universal antibiotic. No known disease-causing organism can live in the presence of even trace amounts of the element silver. In 1834, a German obstetrician, Dr. Carl Siegmund Credé, administered 2 percent silver nitrate as an antiseptic into the eyes of newborns, thereby eliminating the incidence of ophthalmia neonatorum, a cause of blindness in newborns. Later, the solution was diluted to 1 percent silver nitrate, and what is now known as *Credé's prophylaxis* has since become a standard practice in obstetrics. In fact, colloidal silver was used successfully in mainstream medicine up to the early 1930s, when silver became increasingly expensive, and pharmaceutical companies developed antibiotics, which were far more profitable. These antibiotics were heavily promoted to the medical establishment, and silver suddenly took a backseat. Yet as often happens when we deviate from nature, we only revert back to natural methods after realizing our mistakes. Decades after the advent of antibiotics, many types of disease-causing organisms have built a strong immunity to their action, making our immune systems weaker. Recently, the medical establishment has reported on the new strains of "super bugs" that cannot be destroyed by any type of antibiotic. *Newsweek* reported on March 28, 1994, that in 1992, 13,000 hospital patients died of infections that resisted every drug doctors tried.

Many people are aware of the antibiotic properties of garlic, which can destroy several common strains of bacteria and parasites. However, silver has demonstrated effectiveness on 650 strains of pathogens. Simply applying the correct electrical charge to 99.9 percent silver plates or wire while they are submerged in distilled water produces colloidal silver water. The microsilver particles have a charge that exerts more force than gravity. The charged particles of silver range from 0.01 to 0.001 microns in size; these detach themselves from the silver plates and are electrically suspended in the water. Colloidal silver, when made correctly, is ionic and completely nontoxic; it exerts a mild action on the essential beneficial bacteria inside our intestinal tract that acts as a second immune system, leaving it completely intact. While most antibiotics, including even the so-called broad-spectrum antibiotics, have an optimal effectiveness against only a few different disease-causing organisms, they still do not eliminate fungus, yeasts, protozoa and other parasites, or viruses. And since virtually all known viruses are immune to antibiotics, colloidal silver is quite effective in the treatment of both viruses and parasites. Dr. Bjorn Nordstrom, of the Karolinska Institutet, Sweden, has successfully used silver in his cancer treatment protocol for many years and believes that it has brought remission in many cancer patients whom conventional medical doctors have given up on.

According to the latest research out of the Silver Institute, which explores all the various applications of silver, both medical and industrial, silver seems to work by disabling a particular enzyme that bacteria, fungi, and viruses use for their own oxygen metabolism. Unlike modern antibiotics, silver has no known recorded side effects or adverse drug interactions and is not addictive. The body does not build a natural tolerance to it, unlike common antibiotics, which tend to make the immune system weaker with continual use. Colloidal silver has been shown to be safe for use by pregnant women, small children, babies, and even our beloved pets.

Silver is unique among antimicrobial agents because of its broad spectrum. It effectively kills germs of all major types, including gram-positive and gram-negative bacteria, spore-forming bacteria, fungi and yeasts, viruses, and protozoa parasites. Furthermore, according to Dr. Becker, "Silver [does] more than kill disease-causing organisms. It promotes major growth of bone and accelerated the healing of injured tissues by over 50 percent." And as far as any adverse side effects, Dr. M. Paul Farber, author of *The Micro Silver Bullet,* says, "There has not been a single case of argyria [graying of the skin] from a properly manufactured modern-day colloidal silver product. The cases of argyria reported in the 1920s and 1930s resulted because the technology of the day was unable to produce a colloidal silver product with a small enough particle size."

Colloidal silver can be used in so many ways it's amazing that everyone doesn't use it. It can be added to your drinking water when traveling or camping to purify the water or sprayed directly onto burns to assist in rapid healing with minimal scarring. You can also sterilize anything with it, from toothbrushes to surgical instruments, and use it topically on cuts, wounds, abrasions, rashes, sunburn, razor nicks, and bandages. It can be sprayed on the garbage to prevent odors and used on kitchen sponges, towels, or chopping boards to eliminate *E. coli* and salmonella bacteria, in turn preventing food poisoning, gastrointestinal inflammation, and genital-tract infections. It can also be used when canning, preserving, and bottling and used like peroxide on acne. It can be added to juices and milk to delay spoiling, fermenting, deterioration or curdling. Spray inside shoes and between the toes and legs to stop the itching of athlete's foot and fungus, including genital itching. Use it in natural creams and shampoos to treat dandruff, psoriasis, and skin rashes. Use in bathwater and gargle with it; use it in douches, colonic irrigation, nasal sprays, and dental solutions. Using it can dramatically cut down the time needed to recover from colds, flu, pneumonia, staphylococci infection, strep, respiratory infections, and rhinoviruses.

The uses of colloidal silver are so many it seems that it's effective for almost anything. Most skin conditions, eye and ear infections, and some moles and warts vanish when silver colloid is sprayed onto the body after bathing. Use with a cotton swab on fingernails, toenails, and ear fungus. You can spray it in the mouth and add it to natural toothpaste to neutralize tooth decay and bad breath. Silver colloid stops halitosis by eliminating bacteria deep in the throat and on the back of the tongue. Unlike pharmaceutical antibiotics, colloidal silver never permits strain-resistant pathogens to evolve. Put a few drops on bandages to shorten healing times. Toothaches, mouth sores, and bacterial irritations are diminished with its use. Soak dentures in it. Spray refrigerators, freezers, and food-storage containers with it. Stop mildew and wood rot with it. Try it in the dishwater and in cleaning and mopping solutions. Spray pet bedding with it and let dry. Spray it on top of the contents of opened jam, jelly, and condiment containers and inside lids before replacing. Mix a little in pet water, birdbaths, and cut-flower vases. Spray air-conditioner filters after cleaning with it. Swab air ducts and vents to prevent breeding sites for mold. Use routinely in laundry final rinse water and always before packing away seasonal clothes. Damp clothes or towels and washcloths will not sour or mildew when used in the laundry. Eliminate unwanted microorganisms in planter soils and hydroponics systems. Spray plant foliage to stop fungi, mold, rot, and most plant diseases. Use colloidal silver in pools, fountains, humidifiers, Jacuzzis, hot tubs, baths, dishwashers, gymnasium foot baths, and on bath and shower mats. Spray it inside shoes, watchbands, and gloves and under fingernails periodically. Treat shower stalls, bathtubs, and animal watering troughs. Rinse fruit and vegetables before storing or using. Put in cooking water. Human and animal shampoos become disinfectants when silver is added. Prevent carpets, curtains, and wallpaper from mildewing. Wipe telephone mouthpieces, pipe stems, headphones, hearing aids, eyeglass frames, hairbrushes, and combs with it. Colloidal silver is excellent for diapers and diaper rash and for cleaning toilet seats, bowls, tile floors, sinks, urinals, and doorknobs. It also successfully kills persistent odors.

The uses for this inexpensive, odorless, and easily produced, powerful, nontoxic disinfectant and healing agent are virtually limitless. You will find that a spray or misting bottle of silver colloid solution may be the most useful health enhancement you have ever used.

Making Colloidal Silver Safely at Home

Buying colloidal silver can be expensive (and even banned in some European countries), yet making it yourself is inexpensive and safe. There are many colloidal silver makers commercially available, such as the one made by Dr. Bob Beck that we discuss in chapter 7. To find safe and effective colloidial silver manufacturing units for home use we recommend the Simple Truths Foundation, www.simpletruths.me.uk. When making colloidal silver with distilled or reverse osmosis water, which has a zero or very low mineral content, there is no chance of any side effects such as argyria. This condition, in which the skin turns gray, is used as a scare tactic by pharmaceutical lobbies; it does not come from consuming the type of silver product we are dealing with here. Reported cases of argyria known as the "blue man" and "blue woman" did not from consuming pure colloidal silver, but rather from silver nitrate and silver chloride compounds. Using any of the commercially marketed colloidal silver makers, you can be assured of getting a safe, nontoxic, highly beneficial product.

MMS (MASTER MINERAL SUPPLEMENT)

One supplement that has recently gained popularity, especially in my own clinic, is MMS, thanks to the pioneering work of Jim Humble, the inventor of this germicide. Like many stabilized oxygen and pH-alkalizing supplements, MMS contains sodium chlorite, but in higher amounts than normal oxygen supplements. MMS is 72 percent distilled water, 22.4 percent sodium chlorite, and 5.32 percent sodium chloride, with some additional nontoxic stabilizing agents. Jim's testing found that the main ingredient in stabilized oxygen drops, sodium chlorite, produced not only oxygen but small amounts of chlorine dioxide, one of the most powerful and yet safe pathogen killers known to man. Jim says, "MMS is not a cure . . . it's really just a killer."

While the amount of chlorine dioxide released by most stabilized oxygen supplements is small, Jim found that by mixing MMS with lemon juice (citric acid) for a few minutes before diluting the drops, it causes this reaction to be maximized. Over 75,000 successful malaria cures later, MMS is becoming a household name among natural medicine enthusiasts. MMS could be a twenty-first-century panacea, and best of all it is inexpensive and safer than any drug designed for the same purpose. Once disease-causing pathogens are destroyed with the help of MMS, the body's own immune system has a chance to recover and do the final healing. MMS has been used recently in the treatment of a host of diseases such as MS, HIV, viral hepatitis, swine flu, pneumonia, Lyme disease, herpes, parasitic infestations, and a whole range of infectious bacteria.

Like so many safe, inexpensive supplements that are gaining popularity, MMS is undergoing intense resistance from the pharmaceutical lobby. Although claims that MMS is a cure have been downplayed by Jim, who prefers to see it as a pathogen killer, Big Pharma is extremely nervous that it could cause a massive downturn in drug sales, especially antibiotics and vaccines. So do not expect your local doctor to offer you good news about MMS; it's more likely he or she will give you the same scare tactics issued by the drug companies. So do your own research and watch some of the videos and testimonies online for the latest information on the safety and effectiveness of MMS. Although there are no known side effects except for the general detox reaction, MMS may reduce iodine levels in the body; therefore, it's a good idea to add some SSKI (potassium iodide) or seaweed to your diet while taking it.

Two Useful MMS Formulas

MMS Oral Dosage: Mix three drops of MMS with fifteen drops of lemon juice, wait for three minutes (for reaction to occur), and then simply add water or noncitrus juice such as diluted apple juice and drink three to eight times daily.

Topical MMS/DMSO Protocol for Transdermal Therapy: Place three drops of MMS mixed with fifteen drops of lemon juice, wait for three minutes, and then add three drops of DMSO liquid. Apply topically anywhere. A slight burning sensation may follow for only several minutes after application.

SSKI, POTASSIUM IODIDE

Nobel laureate Albert Szent-Györgyi (1893–1986), the Hungarian-American physiologist who discovered vitamin C, said: "When I was a medical student, iodine in the form of KI was the universal medicine. Nobody knew what it did, but it did something and did something good. We students used to sum up the situation in this little rhyme: 'If ye don't know where, what, and why, prescribe ye then K and I.'"

SSKI, saturated solution of potassium iodide, is commonly known for killing pathogens and for water purification, treatment of thyroid disease (hyper or hypo, but not Hashimoto's), and also for protection from radiation poisoning during the Chernobyl and Fukushima nuclear disasters. What many people don't know is that it's also a great home remedy for many other conditions such as arteriosclerosis, COPD, asthma, ovarian cysts, and fibrocystic breast disease. It also helps your body metabolize estrone (slightly carcinogenic human estrogen) and 16-alpha-hydroxyestrone (a more dangerous metabolite of human estrogen) into estriol, the anticarcinogenic form of human estrogens. This amazing substance can also be mixed with DMSO (50:50) and applied topically to cure hemorrhoids (it does sting), parotid duct stone, herpes sores, swollen glands, and cysts, and to reduce keloid scars and treat thickening or hardening of the tendons, tissues, or skin such as in Dupuytren's contracture and Peyronie's disease, all without side effects. It can effectively treat respiratory infections or used short-term (a few weeks) as a natural antibiotic or antiviral medicine.

Traditional iodine tincture (USP) is a combination of SSKI and elemental iodine in a base of pure alcohol (ethanol) and is not the best source for internal consumption, as some people are high in elemental iodine and low in SSKI; but it's okay in an emergency or in short-term use by those with normal liver function. Although some say this is very dangerous to take internally, you are only using several drops daily, and most people consume a lot more ethanol in alcoholic beverages than from the small amount ingested from internal use of iodine tincture. Iodine tincture does not contain methanol (wood alcohol), which some people mistakenly think is toxic in even small amounts. I suspect that tincture of iodine is not recommended internally because it may have something to do with Big Pharma's fear of the many diseases it can cure.

Iodine tincture USP can be used very well for iodine foot painting as a way to introduce SSKI into the body; this form is great for treating warts, toenail fungus, and a host of skin diseases. Lugol's iodine is the same product, but without the alcohol, and can safely be used internally, but with the same caution for long-term use. Other forms of iodine include nascent iodine and detoxified (atomic) iodine, which are more expensive yet seem to yield the same results as pure SSKI in our experience.

SSKI Recommended Dosage

Depending on the strength of the product, take anywhere from five to ten drops daily, or as directed by the product manufacturer or your doctor.

Note: Although rare, sometimes side effects or allergies to iodine can occur such as nausea, diarrhea, or skin rash. Avoid if pregnant, and always monitor your thyroid and have checkups with your doctor, as high doses can suppress the thyroid if taken for extended periods.

OLIVE LEAF

Olive leaf has had a place in human life since the beginning of recorded history. The Bible records that "the leaves of the olive tree shall be for the healing of the nations" (Revelation 22:2). Olive leaf was the first botanical medicine mentioned by God in the Book of Genesis, and it was the dove that brought back the olive leaf to Noah to show the existence of new forms of life following the Flood. Olive leaf was a common medicine in the Middle Eastern Mediterranean region for thousands of years, and the ancient Egyptians used it in the process of mummification of royalty.

The olive tree belongs to the same family of plants as jasmine and lilac, with cultivated olives being harvested from the tree known botanically as *Olea europaea,* a plant native to the southeast Mediterranean area. According to Greek mythology, the olive tree was created by Athena. The goddess initially planted it around the rocks of the Acropolis, giving it physical powers to create nourishment and heal sickness and wounds, combined with spiritual powers to transform evil into goodness. In Ezekiel 47:12, God speaks of a tree "the fruit thereof shall be for meat, and the leaf thereof for medicine."

The medicinal properties of olive leaves first gained attention in the field of modern allopathic medicine early in the 1800s, thanks to a French colonel and physician by the name of Etiene Pallas, who took note of the healthful effects that olive-leaf tea had on those who consumed it. He examined the leaf's constituents and isolated a compound he named *vauqueline,* a bitter substance to which he credited most of the plant's febrifuge (fever-reducing) properties. Yet even back then, with limited knowledge and scientific instruments, Pallas acknowledged that the fever-reducing characteristics of olive leaves represented only a small portion of their therapeutic components. French biologists have more recently discovered that an extract from the olive leaf renders many viruses and bacteria harmless, including the herpes virus. Subsequent research has now demonstrated that an extract of the leaves of the olive tree (not the fruit) also destroys other viruses, bacteria, and fungi.

Olive leaf has a number of health benefits:

- Enhances immune-system function
- Increases energy
- Has an internal cleansing action
- Antiviral, antifungal, antibacterial, and antiparasitic
- Lowers blood pressure and cholesterol
- Reduces blood sugar and acts as a pancreatic tonic

Olive leaf extract strengthens the immune system and is invaluable to people with low resistance to disease, as well as being a natural immune stimulant in time of colds and flu. The recent explosion of antibiotic-resistant microorganisms increases the relevance and importance of natural products with antibiotic properties; this is why olive leaf extract is a handy remedy in today's natural medicine pharmacopeia. American biochemist Arnold Takemoto has found that olive leaf extract is a "valuable addition against chronic fatigue syndrome," and sufferers are said to be greatly helped by its energy-giving, antiviral properties. Other researchers have discovered that olive leaf extract can relieve heartbeat irregularities and improve blood flow to the heart. Olive leaf extract does not necessarily cure disease but is rather a cold-blooded killer of disease-causing parasites and other viral pathogens that are the underlying causes of a vast number of health conditions. Once these disease-causing microorganisms have been killed off, the immune system can then begin rebuilding itself to allow the body to self-heal.

Olive leaf has been found to be beneficial in cases of candidiasis and other fungal infections. In his book *Olive Leaf Extract,* Dr. Morton Walker documents HIV/AIDS cases in which olive leaf extract was used therapeutically. The results were quite favorable, far more so than any results from AZT. In the case of retroviruses, olive leaf is able to neutralize the production of reverse transcriptase and protease, which are essential enzymes that enable the alteration of the RNA of a healthy cell. Olive leaf extract has been shown to dramatically increase phagocytosis, which is an immune-system response whereby the cells ingest harmful microorganisms. In Spain, pharmacologists have learned that olive leaf extract causes relaxation of the artery walls, suggesting a possible benefit for hypertension. Italian researchers found it beneficial for lowering blood sugar and uric acid levels in animals, indicating its potential in cases of heart disease and diabetes. Olive leaf extract is a natural, nontoxic immune-system builder. It is a safe, highly effective food supplement with potent, proven antimicrobial action with no toxic or other evident side effects, even in high doses. It is widely available at most health-food stores and online.

TURMERIC

Turmeric (*Curcuma longa*) is one of the most powerful healing spices available today. A relative of the ginger family, turmeric has been used in Asian cooking for thousands of years and is especially valued in ayurvedic medicine as an anti-inflammatory, antibiotic, probiotic, and detoxifier suitable for all body types. Turmeric is a nonspicy, surprisingly bland spice with a very light sour, earthy, pungent flavor. Most Westerners consume tiny amounts of turmeric without knowing it in products like classic American yellow mustard, the nonspicy variety commonly added to hot dogs and hamburgers. Although only 2 percent of the product contains the spice turmeric, it's what gives yellow mustard its bright color.

Turmeric is not only an excellent antibiotic useful in treating candida infections, it is also an amazing probiotic that strengthens digestion by increasing the production of bile and boosting the production of beneficial bacteria in the colon. Like garlic and onions, which are rich in FOS (fructooligosaccharides) and promote probiotic bacteria in your gut, turmeric contains rich sources of other beneficial compounds that boost beneficial bacteria. According to the November 23, 2010, issue of the *International Journal of Food Science and Technology*, three lactic acid bacteria strains (LAB), namely *Enterococcus faecium, Lactococcus lactis lactis,* and *Lactobacillus plantarum,* were isolated from turmeric rhizomes. These microorganisms showed similar characteristics as probiotic organisms.

One of the main medicinal compounds in turmeric is curcumin, which inhibits the cancer-causing bacteria *H. pylori,* according to a 2002 study conducted at the University of Chicago.[*] Turmeric also contains tumor-shrinking properties,[†] with human clinical trials indicating no dose-limiting toxicity when administered at doses up to 10 grams daily. These and numerous other studies suggest that curcumin has enormous potential in the prevention and treatment of cancer.[‡] Turmeric is also well known in ayurvedic and traditional Chinese medicine for its ability to heal bruises, sprains, wounds, and infections of the throat. Recent research indicates that it is also beneficial for diseases such as MS, Parkinson's, and Alzheimer's, which may have links to systemic mycotoxin bacteria. The antioxidant, anti-inflammatory, anticarcinogenic, and blood-thinning properties of turmeric are becoming widely known, and nowadays health-food stores stock the herb in capsule, powder, and fresh root form and promote its benefits for arthritis and other autoimmune conditions.

---

[*]G. B. Mahady, S. L. Pendland, G. Yun, and Z. Z. Lu, "Turmeric (*Curcuma longa*) and curcumin inhibit the growth of *Helicobacter pylori,* a group 1 carcinogen," *Anticancer Research* 22, no. 6C (2002): 4179–81.

[†]A. Gescher, U. Pastorino, S. M. Plummer, and M. M. Manson, "Suppression of tumour development by substances derived from the diet—mechanisms and clinical implications," *British Journal of Clinical Pharmacology* 45, no. 1 (1998): 1–12.

[‡]For example, B. B. Aggarwal, A. Kumar, and A. C. Bharti, "Anticancer potential of curcumin: Preclinical and clinical studies," *Anticancer Research* 23, no. 1A (2003): 363–98.

Turmeric can be taken in capsules or in powdered form mixed with raw honey to make a paste for internal consumption. Start with one teaspoon of turmeric and honey paste two to three times a day. The fresh root and powder can also be added to juices, teas, soups, and salads.

Note: Although turmeric is considered safe even at high doses, it should be used with caution by those with gallstones or gastric ulcers. Women taking turmeric in anything other than normal culinary doses should consult their doctor first, as turmeric can be a uterine stimulant in larger doses.

GRAPEFRUIT SEED EXTRACT

Grapefruit seed extract (GSE), also known as *citricidal,* is a safe and excellent home remedy for treating many diseases that are related to infectious bacterial diseases or parasites. We have seen it work successfully on staph infections even after several courses of antibiotics did not work, and on cases of dysentery and amebiasis when all drugs failed. It also cures young children's massively swollen stomachs due to parasites. GSE is effective on many drug-resistant bacteria, viruses, parasites, protozoa, and fungi; it has no side effects and is safe for kids. It does not interact with most other medicines, and taking it is as simple as adding it to your drinking water. Dr. Louis Parish, an investigator for the Department of Health and Human Services of the U.S. Food and Drug Administration, found that GSE is as effective as, if not more so than, any other amoebicide now available, yet without any side effects.

GSE is bitter to the taste but not disgustingly so, and it is mild to the skin and sensitive areas, making it great for use as a mouthwash, throat gargle, and ear and nose cleanser. It is also very mild yet effective as a vaginal douche and helps treat thrush and yeast infections. Many people have reported successful treatment of autoimmune diseases such as rheumatoid arthritis, which may be related to bacterial strep infection as with *Proteus vulgaris* and *Klebsiella pneumoniae,* with GSE. There are also successful reports regarding Crohn's disease, which may be linked to *Mycobacterium avium* subspecies *paratuberculosis,* and Hashimoto's disease, which may be caused by a *Yersinia enterocolitica* infection.

The recommended dosage of GSE is five to fifteen drops in a glass of warm water, taken three to five times daily or as recommended by your health care practitioner.

VITAMIN C

Physiologist Albert Szent-Györgyi, awarded the Nobel Prize in 1937 for his discovery of vitamin C, related the following anecdote: "Mr. X has a lack of vitamin C and contracts a cold. The cold leads to pneumonia. Mr. X dies and his body is taken to the mortuary . . . not with the diagnosis 'lack of vitamin C,' but with the diagnosis 'pneumonia.' This does not matter for him anymore, but it matters for the rest of mankind, which is misleading in its thinking and judgment about vitamins."

Many of us may be aware that getting the World Health Organization's recommended (since the 1970s) daily dose of only 45 mg of vitamin C does nothing to protect us from common colds and degenerative diseases, nor do we get any real antioxidant protection or disease-preventing capabilities. This small amount is really only the bare minimum needed to prevent scurvy, a vitamin C deficiency disease that eighteenth-century sailors died of when sailing on long voyages around the world. At one time scurvy was one of the major limiting factors of marine travel. This was due to a lack of perishable fruits and vegetables onboard, so many sailors existed only on cured meats or dried bread and therefore died of vitamin C deficiency.

Vitamin C strengthens the capillaries and cell walls, enabling the body to manufacture the maximum amount of collagen, which forms the connective tissue of the vascular system. Until the isolation and discovery of vitamin C in 1932 and even earlier, the successful experiments with citrus fruits to prevent scurvy by Sir James Lind, an officer of the Royal Navy who served during the American War of Independence and the French Revolutionary and Napoleonic Wars, there was little understanding about scurvy and why people died during long sea voyages. Humans, unlike most other animals on the planet, do not manufacture vitamin C and must take it from food sources for survival. For example, goats, like almost all other animals, make their own vitamin C. An adult goat weighing approximately 70 kg (approximately 150 pounds) will manufacture more than 13,000 mg of vitamin C a day.

Today, even with our advanced technology, we are once again dying of diseases that involve chronic, long-term vitamin C deficiency. Vitamin C is destroyed during pasteurization (therefore babies consuming only bottled milk can suffer from scurvy) and from cooking food. As many people consume primarily cooked and processed foods, combined with a stressful and toxic lifestyle (both of which deplete vitamin C from the tissues), heart disease is on the rise. Linus Pauling, the only man to win two unshared Nobel Prizes, observed that "10,000 infants die every year needlessly from cot-death," while Australian physician Archie Kalokerinos, a supporter of Linus Pauling's theory that many diseases result from overproduction of free radicals and can accordingly be prevented or cured by vitamin C, which led him to treat many conditions with high intravenous doses of vitamin C, stated, "We know the cause of SIDS [crib death]. We can and have prevented them. It's all done with a compound called acerbate [vitamin C]. Not to use it means deaths will continue. There is no other answer. There never will be, for our findings are based on scientific facts, not medical opinion."

According to the medical establishment as reflected in the current Wikipedia entry, scurvy is a disease of the past. But according to leading vitamin C researchers such as Linus Pauling, Matthias Rath, Andrew Saul, and a host of other doctors of nutrition, all testify that megadoses (i.e., orthomolecular) of vitamin C can reverse heart disease and treat many forms of cancer far better than chemo and radiation therapy. Most prominent researchers and naturopaths recommend 2 to 3 grams of vitamin C daily for antiaging and the prevention of serious disease while simultaneously helping to detoxify environmental pollutants such as heavy metals. In a 1994 interview shortly before his death, Dr. Pauling said, "If you are at risk of heart disease, or if there is a history of heart disease in your family, if your father or other members of the family died of a heart attack or stroke or whatever, or if you have a mild heart attack yourself, then you had better be taking vitamin C and lysine." In times like now, when cancer, heart disease, and diabetes have become the leading killers, it is recommended that even higher doses such as 8 to 12 grams orally, spread throughout the day, or even IV injections be taken.

Like most natural-medicine therapies, vitamin C therapy is inexpensive and nonpatentable (excluding the forms Ester-C and Lypo-Spheric vitamin C), so it is not surprising that drug companies are doing nothing to research the power of IV or oral megadoses of vitamin C. Most people think they are doing well when they take 500 mg, but vitamin C is so cheap and scientifically effective that most of us could be taking much larger doses. While modern medical studies confirm the effectiveness of supplementing with 2 to 3 grams of vitamin C daily to prevent serious diseases such as cancer and heart disease, conventional medicine claims that megadoses are flushed out through the urine (as reflected in color changes seen in the urine), therefore wasted. What they don't tell you is the whole story, which is that vitamin C is not stored in the body and is water soluble, and thus washes out of the body every day, and along with it are many toxins, heavy metals, and pollutants. Today vitamin C is safely used therapeutically for antiaging and as an antioxidant and antibiotic, to treat allergies and inflammatory conditions, to boost immunity, to detoxify, to relieve heart disease and reduce cholesterol, in chelation (removal of heavy metals), and to prevent diseases of all kinds.

Major Types of Synthesized Vitamin C

We do not discount that natural forms of vitamin C are always best, available in foods like camu camu (a Brazilian fruit), acerola, rose hips, and certain fresh fruits. As well, food sources of vitamin C contain valuable amounts of bioflavonoids that are naturally partnered with vitamin C in nature and complement the effectiveness of vitamin C. In additional to taking these natural superfoods to increase your intake of vitamin C, orthomolecular vitamin C doses can be taken in the following forms:

Ascorbic acid: This is the original and crudest form of vitamin C that is still recommended by many researchers today as being just as good as other forms and the least expensive. It has a sharp taste and is a cheap and cheerful way to take vitamin C. It can cause gastric irritation in those with sensitive stomachs. This form may be difficult to take orally in large doses by the elderly and those suffering already from gastric distress or diarrhea. Ascorbic acid tablets are not meant as a source of megadoses of vitamin C, since dozens of tablets per day would introduce excessive amounts of excipients (tablet-binding and filling agents) into the body, to which some persons may be sensitive. Instead, always choose pure ascorbic acid powder or crystals for mega (orthomolecular) dosing.

Mineral acerbates: These are salts of ascorbic acid bound to minerals such calcium, magnesium, potassium, sodium, and zinc. The most common are sodium and calcium acerbate; the others are more likely to be found in mineral acerbate formulas. They provide a nonacidic form of vitamin C that is more gentle on the digestive system as well as providing supplemental minerals that compensate for the chelating effects of vitamin C. Though it is mainly the sodium in sodium chloride (table salt) that aggravates and contributes to heart disease, those who have hypertension should be cautious when taking large amounts of sodium acerbate, as every 500 mg tablet of sodium acerbate contains 60 mg of sodium.

Ester-C: Esterified vitamin C is a more expensive form of nonacidic (gentler on your stomach) vitamin C. It is mainly calcium acerbate plus small amounts of vitamin C metabolites dehydrate-ascorbic acid (oxidized ascorbic acid), calcium threonine, and trace levels of xylonite and limonite. The manufacturers of this patented form of the vitamin state that the metabolites, especially threonine, increase the bioavailability of the vitamin C. While some studies do claim that it is better absorbed, these studies are not conclusive according to unbiased expert vitamin C researchers.

Lyposomal vitamin C: Often referred to as "vitamin C on steroids," this new form uses liposomal encapsulation technology, which combines the latest in nanotechnology and biotechnology to deliver minute amounts of therapeutic substances to the tissues without being altered or affected by other parts of the body. Lyposomal particles are approximately 100 to 150 nanometers in diameter (a nanometer is one-billionth of a meter) and move quickly and efficiently to their targets before releasing their contents; therefore, less is required for the same effect. This means less gastric upset (diarrhea) occurs with taking such large amounts of vitamin C. There are many recipes found online on how to make your own lyposomal vitamin C, which is much cheaper than buying it.

OIL PULLING

The ancient foundational text on ayurveda, the Charaka Samhita, advocates the practice of oil pulling: "It is beneficial for strength of jaws, depth of voice, flabbiness of face, improving gustatory sensation and good taste for food. One used to this practice never gets dryness of throat, nor do his lips ever get cracked; his teeth will never be carious and will be deep-rooted; he will not have any toothache, nor will his teeth set on edge by sour intake; his teeth can chew even the hardest eatables."

Oil pulling is a safe and effective way of treating many infections, especially in the mouth and surrounding areas, but that's not all; it seems to have myriad health benefits, as thousands around the world are now discovering. More recently, oil pulling has been repopularized thanks to the research of F. Karach, a Ukrainian doctor who in the 1990s presented what he called a remarkable treatment at a conference of the Ukranische Union of Oncologists and Bacteriologists, a part of the Academy of Sciences of the USSR. His talk involved a super-simple healing process for the human body, oil pulling.

Oil pulling involves swishing ("pulling" back and forth) oil in the mouth for up to twenty minutes a day, and then spitting the oil out and rinsing out your mouth. It's estimated that more than half the population of the world has gum disease and doesn't know about it, so this ancient treatment is indeed helpful in maintaining the health of the teeth and mouth. But many in the natural-health field claim that oil pulling is a cure, or at least helpful, in addressing many other health conditions, including asthma, digestive ulcers, liver problems, arthritis, diabetes, and anxiety. Some theorize that oil pulling removes toxins from the mouth and the body, while others state that toxins are removed due to the antibacterial properties of the oil used. Exactly how oil pulling works is yet to be scientifically proven; what we do know is that it is safe and does yield results for many people. In our clinic we recommend using hemp or coconut oil because both oils contain highly beneficial antibacterial and immune-strengthening properties. In ayurveda, sesame oil is used for oil pulling, but Dr. Karach recommends cold-pressed sunflower oil, mostly because this oil was easily available in Ukraine during his research. Many people today use virgin olive oil and other types of pure, clean vegetable oil.

Oil-Pulling Procedure

First thing in the morning, on an empty stomach, take one tablespoon of oil of your choice and swish it back and forth in your mouth and between your teeth (do not gargle or tilt your head too much). The oil will become more liquid as saliva mixes with it during the swishing. Do this for ten to twenty minutes. Then spit the oil out in the toilet* and rinse your mouth with warm water several times. Never swallow the oil, as it contains toxins and bad bacteria. Afterward you can rinse your mouth out with 1.5 to 3 percent hydrogen peroxide. Depending on the condition being addressed, this procedure can be done once in the morning and perhaps again later in the day. Hydrate with plenty of water after this procedure.

*If you are using coconut oil spit it out in the trash as it will solidify in the pipes.

COLON CLEANSING

Norman Walker (1886–1985), a pioneer in the field of vegetable juicing and nutritional health, the author of a half-dozen books on this subject, and the inventor of one of the first modern juicers (the Norwalk hydraulic press juicer is still sold today), said, "The colon is the most neglected part of the body. Colon health emphasizes prevention rather than cure. It is the most important step in maintaining or regaining vital health." When you study the anatomy of the colon you can see why every traditional medicine system emphasizes the importance of cleaning the bowels for the initial treatment of any disease, as well as for disease prevention.

The colon is at the end of the digestive tract and is where all the wastes from the body are dumped and also where much of our good bacteria and blood (from nutrients in food) are formed. As the walls of the colon are highly permeable to its contents, if there's fermenting food in the colon it will get into your blood. Dr. Richard Schulze states that "the average American stores from six to ten pounds of fecal waste in their colon, which is not healthy. As far as the record-breaking accumulation of fecal matter, I had one man in Hawaii who got his dosage up to forty-six capsules of my Intestinal Formula #1, a record in itself, before his bowels moved. Then that night, sitting on the toilet, he evacuated fifty-six pounds of fecal matter."

It's hard to believe that the colon can accumulate such enormous amounts of food wastes, but so it is seen on many occasions. This can be due to numerous reasons: improper toilet technique, a low-fiber diet, the eating of processed (dead) foods, a lack of sufficient hydration, and eating too quickly, all of which are common today. The colon is largely pocketed in its anatomy, and the ascending colon is the only part of the digestive system that goes directly upward, against gravity. In this part of the bowel the smooth muscles of the colon must use peristaltic action to push food against gravity. During times of stress and if the diet is lacking in fiber, essential fatty acids, or sufficient fluids, the bowel becomes sluggish, and the function known as peristalsis becomes weakened, resulting in a slower transit time. Colon-cleansing products contain bowel-specific herbs and some mild herbal laxatives. These herbs, when combined, gently cleanse and strengthen the bowels.

There are a variety of natural remedies that assist in elimination and the proper functioning of the colon:

- Flax meal has many medicinal fats and nutrients for brain and joint health, but it's also a great source of gentle fibers.

- Psyllium husks are much more intense than the flax, and some people do not tolerate them as well, yet they are powerful for cleaning the pockets of the bowels and removing deposits.
- Cascara sacrada, a plant-based laxative, increases peristalsis, tones the bowel, and loosens fecal matter naturally, while also moving the other bulking, fiber-based herbs along their way.
- Slippery elm is a mucilage herb that aids in detoxification as well as healing damaged tissues of the colon wall.
- Cayenne pepper is an amazing herb for improving the circulation to the muscles of the bowel as well as improving the effectiveness of all other herbs when used in combination.
- Ginger can soothe and heal bowel lesions and ulcers and prevents the griping pain that sometimes occurs during bowel cleansing.
- Black walnut, wormwood, and cloves clean up wastes and kill parasitic infestations, including their eggs located in bowel pockets.

Cleansing the Intestines with Oxygen

The use of oxygen-releasing tablets delivered in the form of magnesium peroxide (MgO_2) is fast becoming an alternative way of colon cleansing. As candida and other infections of the bowel cannot live in high levels of oxygen, these products can greatly assist bowel detoxification and healing without the use of herbs. Some folks cannot tolerate psyllium and other strong bowel-cleansing herbs, especially in cases of irritable bowel syndrome and Crohn's disease, so using a more gentle technique in the form of oxygen-releasing capsules or powder can assist in eliminating wastes, curing constipation, and increasing regularity. Magnesium peroxide is an odorless and tasteless white powder or tablet that reacts to changes in pH inside the digestive tract. These pH changes cause magnesium peroxide to gently release oxygen in the form of hydrogen peroxide. Notably, the same process that occurs inside the body can also be used in oxygenating the lower parts of artificial or natural lakes, as well as wastewater and effluent facilities. MgO_2 can also work in coating seeds to improve germination and seedling survival rates, or in oxygenating the roots of plants.

Magnesium peroxide, when hydrated, releases oxygen per the following chemical reaction: $MgO_2 + H_2O \rightarrow \frac{1}{2} O_2 + Mg(OH)_2$. This gentle process not only inhibits the growth and survival of bad bacteria and other anaerobic disease-causing organisms in the gut, but also works to discharge the bowel plaque that builds up on the walls and inside pockets of the colon. Unlike fiber herbs, which act to literally peel off plaque from the walls of the colon, MgO_2 gently uses oxygen. After magnesium hydroxide breaks down into hydrogen peroxide and enters the bloodstream, a catalase enzyme immediately breaks it down into water and atomic or single oxygen. This single atom of oxygen does not exist long enough in the body to harm cells or cause oxidation, although many assume that oxygen is an oxidant. Hydrogen peroxide is actually produced normally on a daily basis by healthy white blood cells to destroy invading bacteria and stimulate the oxidation-reduction cycle. This cycle incorporates detoxification functions with the body as well as the destruction of anaerobic pathogens.

This form of magnesium also seems to work efficiently in reducing stomach upsets, acid reflux, heartburn, and other digestive complaints. Many of the convenient drugs like antacids do not cure, and often increase the chances of your problem remaining and causing more harm in the long term. This is simply because it's your stomach's logical reaction to produce more acid in an attempt to digest food, so the more antacids you take, the worse the problem gets. Correcting your dietary practices and taking MgO_2 with meals may help to correct this problem while also cleansing the bowels, which can be a common underlying cause of even upper-digestive complaints. The colon is like a rubbish bin—it may empty daily, but it doesn't clean itself. Going to the toilet is not cleaning the bowel, but rather emptying the meal you had yesterday. Correct management of the colon is the key to preventing bowel or intestinal cancer.

Digestive Transit Time

Bernard Jensen, an international authority on digestive health, iridology, and tissue cleansing, says, "The definition of regularity is two to three bowel movements per day." Transit time is the amount of time it takes your food to get from your mouth (when you eat it) to the time when it leaves your body (eliminating that meal with a bowel movement). The average human bowel is thirty-plus feet in length, and the correct transit time for a meal to pass through the bowel is twelve to fourteen hours. If food does not pass in this amount of time, food nutrients quickly ferment due to high acid temperatures in the digestive canal. The impacted fecal matter then begins releasing toxins that are absorbed into the body via the bowels, which are permeable to these toxins, a phenomenon called *autointoxication*. This can be a regular occurrence for most people who suffer from fatigue, headaches, and myriad other ills.

One easy way to test your transit time is to drink a cup of fresh beet juice or pureed beets along with the evening meal, noting the exact time of your meal. The next day (and for some days following) closely observe the color of your bowel movements each time you use the toilet. When the beetroot meal passes, it will be a very distinct red color, looking like blood. When you have this bowel movement, note the exact time and do the math. The hours between eating the beet meal and passing it is your transit time. Although this test does reveal your peristaltic transit time, it does not tell us the condition of the bowel wall in terms of tissue health. For example, in cases of chronic bowel disease the colon becomes so irritated and diseased that diarrhea occurs, resulting in extremely fast transit times, such as in Crohn's disease. This is usually after a history of constipation and poor bowel health. This is where advancements in modern medicine using visual cameras inserted into the intestines can tell us exactly what's going on inside. If your transit time is slower than twelve to fourteen hours, I urge you to follow the practices laid out in this book, from nutritional to lifestyle changes. These will help strengthen your internal organs, resulting in correct transit time and curbing the autointoxication problem that is a major cause of disease in today's world. Colon cancer is fast becoming the most common form of fatal cancer, and proper bowel health can be achieved with this practice.

Toilet Etiquette

At least half the world's population (especially in Asia) goes to the toilet in a squatting position. This isn't because they can't afford the modern toilet; namely, the "English throne." The reason people have traditionally emptied their bowels while squatting is that our bodies are designed that way. This is why all our primate cousins who have a similar bowel anatomy squat when moving their bowels. When you squat (or sit on a regular toilet with the knees raised approximately one foot in height with a footstool), the colon totally opens. When you sit on a regular toilet chair, the end of the colon is kinked, just like when you bend a garden hose so that the water only trickles out. In Chinese medicine, incorrect toilet practices are seen as a major cause of colon disease and many other digestive illnesses.

According to various historical studies, the sudden appearance of common appendicitis is a direct result of the introduction of sitting toilets. When one has a bowel movement in the upright "royal" fashion, the muscles of the colon must work harder, straining them and making them weaker over time. It also produces an incomplete bowel movement that results in fecal stagnation. This in turn leads to hemorrhoids, constipation, and sluggish transit time, increasing the risk of colon cancer, which not surprisingly is much more common in Western countries. For those who do not want to install a traditional squat toilet, I recommend purchasing a small wooden or plastic footstool and placing it front of the toilet so that you can raise your legs to just below the toilet rim, which allows a clear passageway for the colon so it can be fully open and relaxed during a bowel movement.

Squatting has many benefits:

- It makes elimination faster, easier, and more complete, preventing fecal stagnation.
- It protects the nerves that control the prostate, bladder, and uterus from being strained.
- It reduces the onset of hemorrhoids.
- It seals the ileocecal valve (the valve between the colon and the

small intestine). In the conventional sitting-upright position, this valve (theoretically a one-way valve) is unsupported and can leak during evacuation, backing up into the small intestine.

Probiotics

In times past most people ate fermented foods on a daily basis because refrigeration was not around, and this was a common way of preserving foods. It turns out that this is one of the best ways to balance intestinal bacteria. Products like organic unpasteurized yogurt contains broad-spectrum beneficial bacteria, as does sourdough bread and sauerkraut. The daily intake of beneficial bacteria, called *probiotics,* is essential, especially after cleansing the colon. A healthy human intestinal tract can contain up to three pounds of "good" bacteria. When we think of preventing or healing illness and disease, the immune system comes to mind first. What many of us do not know is that the immune system is not always our first line of defense; our good gut bacteria are.

Our bodies contain more bacterial cells than our own human cells. Inside the digestive tract is what we call "friendly" bacteria. These are bacteria that fight off the bad bacteria such as candida and keep our intestinal tracts healthy. They also aid in breaking down food and even in manufacturing vitamins A, K, B_1, B_2, B_3, B_5, B_6, and B_{12}. When friendly bacteria becomes overrun with bad bacteria such as *E. coli,* health problems emerge. Symptoms include gas, bloating, intestinal toxicity, constipation, irritable bowel, and malabsorption of food nutrients, all of which lead to a host of ills. Good intestinal flora can easily be destroyed by poor health habits such as drinking chlorinated water, taking antibiotics (including residues of antibiotics in nonorganic meat and dairy products), and ingesting sugar or a diet high in refined, processed foods. The use of modern antibiotics over natural, God-given ones like colloidal silver and olive leaf extract often results in increased susceptibility to infection in the colon by fungi, yeasts, bacteria, viruses, and parasites, leading to myriad health complaints. While modern antibiotics harm beneficial bacteria, plant-based herbal antibiotics seem to have little to no harmful effect on them.

The benefits of probiotic supplementation have been documented in a number of scientific journals. These include:

- Alleviating the symptoms of lactose intolerance
- Increasing natural resistance to infectious diseases of the intestinal tract
- Cancer prevention
- Reduction in serum cholesterol concentrations
- Improved digestion
- Stimulation of gastrointestinal immunity

Unlike viruses and parasites, which are anaerobic (low-oxygen species), probiotics are aerobic—they love oxygen and quickly respond to changes in pH in the digestive system (so you can see how a poor diet and low oxygen levels can create a breeding ground for bad bacteria and resulting health problems). Many species of these beneficial bacteria produce their own antibiotics also, called "replacement antibiotics," which scare the bad bacteria away. Some of these good bacteria actually have antiviral effects as well. Although it's not exactly known how they do this, it is suspected that they produce hydrogen peroxide, which is antiviral, antibacterial, and antiparasitic.

Lactobacillus constitutes a significant component of the beneficial microbiota at a number of body sites and comes in many different species; it is one of the most important strands of good, friendly bacteria in the intestines. The term comes from the suffix *lacto,* meaning they are able to turn milk sugar into lactic acid (thereby playing a key role in the production of yogurt and cheese products). The "father of lactobacilli," Dr. Elie Metchnikoff, a Russian zoologist best known for his pioneering research on immunology, for which he won the Nobel Prize in 1908, was the first person to note the benefits of lactobacilli. While studying Bulgaria's long-living (and yogurt-eating) people, he discovered that lactobacilli could transform milk sugar into lactic acid. Metchnikoff was the first to hypothesize that the slight acidity produced in the intestines by this bacteria provides a hostile environment for unfriendly bacteria, which was later proved correct. There are many strands of beneficial bacteria in our intestine, so it is very beneficial to supplement with probiotics after bowel cleansing while also increasing probiotic foods. There is firm medical evidence to support the idea that unbalanced bacteria levels can contribute to depression because the amino acid tryptophan, which is produced by lactobacilli, serves as an antidepressant.

KIDNEY CLEANSING

Dr. Homer Smith (1895–1962) was an American physiologist who spent most of his career at New York University School of Medicine, where his 1930s experiments on the kidneys proved beyond any doubt that they operated according to physical principles, both as filters and as secretory organs. His research resulted in his best-known 1953 book *From Fish to Philosopher: The Story of Our Internal Environment*. Dr. Smith said, "Recognizing that we have the kind of blood we have because we have the kind of kidneys we have, we must acknowledge that our kidneys constitute the major foundation of our philosophical freedom. Only because they work the way they do has it become possible for us to have bones, muscles, glands and brains. Superficially, it might be said that the function of the kidneys is to make urine; but in a more considered view one can say that the kidneys make the stuff of philosophy itself."

The kidneys are approximately the size of a fist; these two vital organs never stop working, and if they do, you'll die unless you get on kidney dialysis or get a kidney transplant, and that's not fun. The kidneys' main function is to filter the blood and remove urea, excess salts and minerals, toxic chemicals, and other wastes from the blood through a complex network of filtration, providing you with the final product, urine. This is why urine has so many external benefits and why so many traditional aboriginal cultures used urine for skin diseases, bites, and stings.

The trouble that oftentimes occurs with the kidneys is that like any filtration network in nature, when they get polluted they get congested and stop working correctly. All the tiny little tubules that compose the kidneys accumulate a toxic waste buildup, causing urinary infections, back pain, kidney stones, or mineral imbalances in the body, leading to myriad health problems. The kidneys filter about 1,000 liters a day, maintaining the critical water and electrolyte balance that is essential for proper metabolism. This is why oftentimes weight problems and fluid retention can be helped with a kidney cleanse. When the colon does not eliminate wastes efficiently or when the digestive system is impaired, the undigested proteins and other toxins that build up as a result enter the bloodstream, creating ever more work for the kidneys. It's simply too much for them to handle, and they eventually decide to stop doing the work of other organs and just pack it in. So you can see how important it is to first begin cleansing the colon and eliminating parasites before you go on to cleanse the kidneys and liver. Cleansing the kidneys is done simply by following a pristine nutritional program while taking a kidney-cleansing herbal formula. It can also be done by juice fasting with kidney-cleansing juices.

Kidney-Cleansing Herbs

- Cleavers (*Galium aparine*) is one of the greatest herbs I have ever worked with. Famous for assisting the lymph system, it is even better for the urinary system. When one places kidney stones or gallstones in a glass of cleavers tea for twenty-four hours, they dissolve.
- *Tribulus terrestris,* which goes by the common name goat's head, a common weedy species that grows in dry climates, is no doubt the best herb in ayurvedic medicine for all sorts of urinary dysfunction and cleansing. It is also a tonic that can be used to treat deficiency conditions, which are common with the kidneys.
- Corn silk shows remarkable effects on kidney stones and other waste deposits that build up in the kidney tubules.
- Parsley and coriander are great common household diuretics and kidney cleansers and great sources of vanadium, iron, and vitamin C, while also helping to destroy infections.
- The root of *Rehmannia,* commonly known as Chinese foxglove, is a classic Chinese herb that supports kidney function and calms the adrenal glands, harmonizing the effects of other herbs while also

increasing low libido, a common sign of low kidney function.

- *Phyllanthus niruri,* also known as *chanca piedra,* is a well-researched herb that shows excellent results. Common names for this herb include stone breaker, as it is well known for dissolving both gallstones and kidney stones.
- Uva ursi (bearberry) herb is a urinary astringent that has been used for centuries to correct bed-wetting. It also can help dissolve kidney stones and remove excess deposits.

Performing a juice fast is also a good way to cleanse the kidneys without herbal medicine. Juices that aid in kidney cleansing include carrot, apple, celery, cucumber, cilantro, parsley, lemon, and grape.

Modern medicine has been feeding us bogus theories on the cause of renal stones, such as eating too many tomatoes, eggplant, spinach, tea, nuts, chocolate, beets, rhubarb, or strawberries, all considered high-oxalate foods. The truth is that renal calculi (calcium oxalate stones account for 80 percent of stones) is mostly caused by overacidity of the blood due to an overly acidic diet and lifestyle, combined with an incorrect type of salt intake and dehydration. When the body becomes overacidic it uses calcium, an alkaline mineral that is stored in massive amounts in the bones. It takes this calcium from the "bone bank" and puts it into the bloodstream to buffer the acidity. The body's blood must maintain a constant pH of approximately 7.4; otherwise death can occur. Once the calcium has done its job of neutralizing the acids in the blood, like all blood elements they are filtered by the kidneys. The excessive calcium is then extracted and ends up building up calculi in the renal tubules, forming kidney stones. Hence renal acidosis and mineral surplus in the blood are the real causes of kidney stones.

Kidney Stone Remedies

Lemon Water Cure
Like apple cider vinegar, lemons too are highly alkaline, not acid as one might think. They both form an alkaline ash once digested, although both are acidic to the taste (and best avoided if suffer-

ing from ulcers). Lemons are very beneficial in detoxifying acidic wastes and helping to prevent osteoporosis. Drinking fresh lemon juice diluted in water is an excellent treatment for cleaning the kidneys. Drinking lemon water not only prevents renal acidosis, it also has the effect of dissolving calculi.

Three-Day Kidney Stone Cure

Perform this simple procedure for two days: At the first sign of kidney stones or their associated pain, in the morning, on an empty stomach, immediately mix in a jar two ounces of olive oil and two ounces of pure lemon juice; drink it straight down. During the day drink another half cup of lemon juice diluted in two liters (approximately two quarts) of water. Do this for two days. Then on the third day do the following: Prepare twenty ounces (approximately 600 ml) of pure, fresh lemon juice. Drink eight ounces first thing in the morning (water can be taken as a chaser to wash out your mouth). Follow by drinking one ounce of lemon juice diluted in a glass of water every hour for the next twelve hours, making a total intake for that day of twenty ounces of pure lemon juice.

This three-day kidney stone cure can be repeated over and over several times until all the stones are eliminated. Very large stones may take several repetitions of the three-day cleanse and will pass when they are small enough to pass. Most are eliminated in twenty-four hours to three days. It is also recommended you follow a 100 percent alkaline diet with plenty of internal exercises. Adding two to three cups of vegetable juices listed in this section to your diet is also a very effective way to soften renal stones and help this treatment work better.

LIVER AND GALLBLADDER CLEANSING

Elson M. Haas, M.D., founder of the Preventive Medical Center in Marin, California, attests to the power of internal cleansing to heal any number of problems and maintain good health. He says, "Through my twenty-five years in medical practice and health care . . . I have come to believe that the cleansing/detoxification process is the missing link in

Western nutrition and one of the keys to real healing. I have seen hundreds of patients over the years transform regular or persistent illness into health and greatly improved vitality."

After ridding your body of parasites and other disease-causing microorganisms and cleansing the colon and kidneys, you can move on to the liver cleanse. The liver is often called the blood-cleansing organ, as it stores and cleans the blood, especially during sleep. Modern allopathy says the liver's main job is to regulate the level of hormones circulating in the blood and to manufacture bile, which is then stored and concentrated in the gallbladder. The liver actually removes excess bile salts and wastes from the blood, sending them to the gallbladder for storage. The liver could be called the body's chemical factory because if you wanted to build a factory to perform all the chemical functions that the liver does, your factory would cover a hundred-plus acres.

The process of cleansing the tissues in the liver is not to be confused with the liver-gallbladder flush (see page 169), which softens and removes stones from within the liver and gallbladder ducts and is not a tissue cleanse like a liver cleanse is. Liver cleansing is as easy as following the nutritional system outlined in this book, combined with the correct liver-cleansing herbs.

Liver cleansing has a number of benefits:

- Return of normal, healthy metabolism
- Weight reduction, body-shape changes, or in some cases weight gain for those who are underweight
- Reduction in toxins that result in headaches and migraines
- Better focus and clearer thinking
- Improved general feeling of well-being

Liver Herbs

- Milk thistle contains unique chemicals that literally bind to liver cells, coating them. These chemicals protect your liver cells from damage.
- Artichoke leaf has antitoxin effects on the liver while promoting cellular regeneration of damaged tissue.

- Turmeric has powerful antioxidant and anti-inflammatory properties while helping to stop free-radical progression.
- Burdock root is an effective blood cleanser and skin tonic. It also aids in digestion and helps pain associated with arthritis.
- Dandelion root is a liver, kidney, and spleen tonic, strengthening the arteries and providing a rich source of organic iron.
- *Phyllanthus niruri* (*chanca piedra*) is a well-researched liver and kidney herb that shows excellent results. It is also known as stone-breaker for its ability to dissolve gallstones and kidney stones.
- *Picrorhiza kurroa,* also known as *kutki,* one of the oldest medicinal plants in the Nepalese Himalayas, has been shown to be stronger than milk thistle at lower dosages and is an excellent ayurvedic liver herb.
- *Andrographis paniculata,* known in ayurveda as *kalmegh,* meaning "dark cloud," is an ancient herb that's been the focus of a number of recent studies in India and South America, where it grows. It is most effective in serious liver diseases and is also used to treat malaria and viral infections.

Performing a vegetable juice fast while consuming specific juices is also a good way to cleanse the liver without herbal medicine. Juices that aid in liver cleansing include carrot, beets, leafy greens, apples, lemon, and grape. Herbal teas of some of the liver herbs above may also be taken if one is unable to obtain them in herbal tablet or capsule form.

Flushing the Liver and Gallbladder

The history and medical treatment of stones in both the liver and gallbladder and how they affect health date back to Hippocrates. Today, due to stress and diets high in refined carbohydrates and fats, stones in the liver and the gallbladder are common, and the fact is most of us have gallstones and liver stones. Unfortunately, allopathic medicine does not really see this as a problem, nor has there been much research on how stones affect the liver's function on our overall health. Natural medicine, on the other hand, says that it's an underlying cause of many ills. When we learn that the liver performs hundreds of metabolic functions, it makes sense that if it is congested with tiny stones, it's going to cause all kinds of health problems.

Today, people as young as twenty-one have reported having stones so large that their gallbladder has to be surgically removed (fig. 4.2). Many times this drastic measure can be prevented by a simple cleanse that softens the stones naturally, flushing them from the gallbladder into the bowels, to then be excreted from the body. Many traditional cultures still use this method to rid the liver and gallbladder of stones. Having your gallbladder removed surgically should be avoided at all costs as it is vital to digestion, especially the digestion of fats. We do not intend to contradict modern orthodox practices here; rather, we offer you an inexpensive alternative to surgical removal of this vital organ, which is often unnecessary. Liver-gallbladder flushing has also been proven to be beneficial even to those who have had their gallbladders removed by surgery, as the same painful symptoms that caused its removal in the first place often reoccur after the gallbladder is removed. This is because of the presence of intrahepatic stones in the liver, which are extremely common:

- 90 percent of adults have intrahepatic stones (at least three small stones in the liver), but 99 percent of these folks don't know that they have them.
- You can have up to three thousand stones (very small stones like sand, or just a few big stones) in the gallbladder, and up to three thousand in the liver.
- 15 to 30 percent of children age fourteen to eighteen have intrahepatic stones (depending on which country).
- 95 percent of people older than thirty-five have intrahepatic stones and gallstones, but very few of them have any symptoms.
- Most people diagnosed with cancer have intrahepatic stones.

There are no drugs for gallstones in orthodox medicine; hence the surgical removal of the organ is a common practice these days. Therefore, performing a gallbladder cleanse yearly to prevent gallstone formation and the other diseases that are associated with liver stones or gallstones is highly recommended. Gallbladder cleansing also improves general digestion, metabolism of fats, energy levels, and immune function. As the proper digestion of foods is vital for nutrient absorption and energy production, you can see how important a role the gallbladder plays in our overall health.

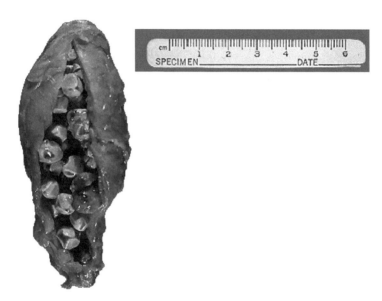

Fig. 4.2. Gallbladder surgically removed. Multiple faceted gallstones are seen in the opened gallbladder pictured here.
(Photo copyright Edward C. Klatt, M.D., University of Utah)

The Liver-Gallstone Flush Protocol

For those with large stones, doing a sudden gallstone flush without proper preparation can result in large stones lodging in the bile ducts, resulting in bile colic, which can be serious. Therefore, to be on the safe side it's necessary to soften the stones before flushing them out. This can be done over a one- to two-week period (depending on the size of the stones) by following an alkaline nutritional program combined with certain foods or herbs that help to dissolve the stones. Drinking two liters (approximately two quarts) of cleavers herb tea daily is one such way of making stones smaller in a short period of time. If you place solid gallstones in a glass of cleavers tea you can observe them completely dissolve in forty-eight hours. The herb *Phyllanthus niruri* may alternatively be used to soften the stones during preparation for the flush if cleavers tea is not available. Another alternative is to drink one liter (approximately one quart) of freshly pressed apple juice and a half liter of pure lemon juice daily for at least one week prior to the liver-gallstone flush, which has been shown to have a similar effect. For those suffering from serious gallstone pain, one drop of pure peppermint oil in a glass of hot water, drunk twice daily, has been shown to reduce painful symptoms. And if you must, go seek emergency medical treatment and take some painkillers or injections to temporarily treat the painful symptoms.

Ingredients:
- 2 liters (approximately 2 quarts) vegetable + apple and lemon juice
- 1 heaping teaspoon of magnesium oxide or 2 heaping teaspoons of magnesium citrate powder (muscle magnesium powder)
- ¼ to ⅓ cup of virgin olive oil or macadamia oil
- ⅔ cup of pure lemon juice
- Peppermint and chamomile tea

Directions:
On the day you flush the liver-gallbladder, take only vegetable juices (including plenty of apple and lemon juice in the mix); several whole apples are allowed during the day until 3 p.m.; treat this like a semifasting day. Then at 3 p.m. take the magnesium powder, which will flush the colon and relax the biliary/hepatic muscle ducts in your liver and gallbladder. After that, only herbal tea is allowed, no more juice. Then immediately before bedtime combine olive or macadamia nut oil with the lemon juice (the combination tastes like oily lemon juice), shake to mix the contents, and drink right down (if you drink slowly you may need to close the jar again and shake because the contents will separate, making it harder to drink). Then go directly to bed with your head up on some pillows and go to sleep on your right side or back. In the

morning or during the next day you will pass stools that will contain liver and gallbladder wastes.

Repeat this procedure once every two weeks, and do four to five flushes for complete cleansing of the bile ducts..

Note: We prefer to use magnesium oxide or citrate instead of magnesium sulfate (Epsom salts), because Epsom salts are very hard on the kidneys, not to mention very difficult to drink. I believe that magnesium oxide/citrate is a far safer alternative and equally effective.

The liver-gallbladder flush is best done after cleansing the colon and kidneys because these eliminatory organs are then more functional in terms of removing the waste products from the liver-gallbladder. Also, note that diabetics can use vegetable juice instead of apple juice to reduce blood sugar spikes, and be sure to carefully check blood sugar levels over the resulting days and weeks after several flushes, as many people report sudden improvements in blood sugar levels. Those with very large stones should first consult a medical practitioner before doing a liver flush.

How It Works and What to Expect

The oil combined with the lemon purges the gallbladder and lubricates the stones, while the magnesium keeps the bowels clear and relaxes the bile ducts, allowing the stones to be released. As the gallbladder is situated horizontally on the right side, lying on your right side on the night of the flush aids in draining the gallbladder of bile and removing the stones.

In the morning upon waking you will need to move your bowels, sometimes urgently, so have easy access to a toilet. Stones will be lodged in the stool and can be retrieved by putting on rubber gloves and breaking up the stool. The stones will float to the top, and you'll be able to pick them out to show off to friends—seriously! Seeing what comes out of your liver and gallbladder is not vital, but for those who want to, it's an amazing sight. The stones are usually a greenish to gray color depending on the mineral salts that bind them, and they can vary in size from a small pea to a large marble. Their texture, ranging from rubbery to quite hard, usually determines how old they are.

How Often Should I Do This Cleanse?

If one has never flushed the liver-gallbladder of stones before, it is recommended that you perform this cleanse once a fortnight, performing four to five flushes to fully cleanse the bile ducts; afterward, once or twice a year is fine.

LUNG CLEANSING

Our lungs are probably the most remarkable life-supporting organs we have. They not only convert the air we breathe into usable oxygen for oxygenating the tissues of the body, they also act as a major eliminatory organ. Through the process of respiration, they remove large amounts of toxins that are a result of the metabolic process. One such waste product is carbon dioxide, so if the lungs are compromised in any way, such as with phlegm, mucus buildup, or poor circulation, leading to poor elasticity, the lungs' detoxification and filtering processes become sluggish and limited. Like constipation of the bowels, lung sluggishness, which is also a type of constipation, can result in health ailments in other organs. Dr. Richard Schulze observes that "the body loses a quart of water every day just by breathing." When the lungs are not functioning correctly, the kidneys work harder, eventually becoming exhausted. From breathing poor air, pollution, or general toxicity of the body, the lungs can become overloaded, at which point you need a lung cleanse.

As oxygen is the number-one nutrient in your body, it seems sensible to regularly maintain and cleanse this amazing organ. It's widely known that one can go months without food and days without water, but without enough oxygen you'll die in minutes; therefore, the importance of the lungs cannot be underestimated, and having them function to their full capacity is vital for every other eliminatory organ. While lung cleansing can obviously improve the function of the lungs, reducing asthma, bronchitis, shortness of breath, and a host of respiratory diseases, I have also found it can help with constipation, depression, fatigue, and even skin complaints.

Herbs for the Lungs

Effective herbal lung formulas contain these three groups of herbs:
1. Antitussives (relieves coughing)
2. Astringents (binding action on mucous membranes)
3. Expectorants (clears out phlegm from the chest)

The following herbs have beneficial effects on the lungs:

- Lobelia is probably one of the most amazing herbs known to Native Americans. Also known as Indian tobacco, lobelia effectively purges mucus from the lungs and surrounding tissues.
- Mullein is rich in iron, magnesium, potassium, sulfur, and vitamins that loosen mucus, strengthen the lungs, and calm inflamed and irritated tissues, controlling coughs.
- Elecampane acts as an expectorant to help those with respiratory disorders, including asthma and bronchitis. It acts as a diuretic and promotes perspiration and elimination.
- Fennel seeds are rich in sulfur and potassium and act as an anti-inflammatory while also soothing mucous membranes.
- Fenugreek seeds soften and dissolve hardened masses of accumulated mucus, expelling toxic waste through the lymphatic system and mucus and phlegm from the lungs.
- Skullcap is not only for the nervous system and for detoxing but is also rich in nutrients; it also synergizes well with other herbs such as fennel and fenugreek, detoxifying the lungs.
- Licorice acts as a cough suppressant, expectorant, and laxative, inhibiting the growth of harmful viruses and acting to stimulate the adrenal glands. It also purges excess fluid from the lungs and throat and body, relieving inflammation.
- *Justicia adhatoda,* known in traditional Indian medicine as *adhatoda,* is ayurveda's most effective lung cleanser, both antibiotic and phlegm reducing; it mixes well with most other herbs and acts to soothe the bronchioles and clean the lungs.

Performing a vegetable juice fast (with smaller amounts of fruit juice) is also a good way you can cleanse the lungs without herbal medicine. Juices that aid especially in lung cleansing include carrot, celery, onion, and grape. Herbal teas that are easily available for cleansing the lungs include fennel, fenugreek, and skullcap. Lung cleansing is best performed after a colon, kidney, and liver cleanse but can be done anytime in an emergency. Because toxins in the bowels and liver supply the blood for the lungs, cleansing the colon and liver can result in a superior health effect for the lungs.

HEART AND ARTERY CLEANSING

Many wonder why we recommend cleaning the other organs first instead of going straight to heart or arterial cleansing if one has heart problems. Many heart conditions of course are caused by diet and lifestyle, but many times they are also caused by poor colon, kidney, and liver health. We often begin cleansing the eliminatory organs first such as the colon and kidneys. This is because if the colon is backed up or the kidneys are not filtering the blood properly and you proceed to detox or flush your liver, you are mostly recirculating your toxins and causing more problems. Many books selling the liver flush or liver cleanse as the cure-all don't even mention this important fact. That is why we recommend cleaning the colon and kidneys before the liver in most cases so that the colon is able to eliminate the toxins via the toilet and the kidneys don't have to strain when filtering the blood while cleansing the liver. After cleansing these organs or during the cleansing process there are specific substances that help to clean the arteries and improve the heartbeat dramatically, both reversing and preventing heart disease.

Cardiocleansing

The heart muscle and the arteries can be cleansed, and doing so helps prevent heart disease and arteriosclerosis. Here are some useful formulas for cleaning your body's blood pump:

Vitamin C, lysine, and proline formulas: Heart Technology makes a proprietary heart formula called Heart Tech for reversing heart disease that was developed by Dr. Linus Pauling. Often called "Linus Pauling therapy" and "orthomolecular nutrition," this therapy deals with the fact that heart and artery disease is caused by a form of chronic, long-term scurvy, wherein the arteries become gradually broken or damaged due to a lack of acerbates and can also become damaged by insulin. The body then uses cholesterol to mend these lesions. It is known that insulin oxidizes cholesterol, causing it to clump together, leading to clots. This therapy strips the arteries of deposits and helps mend the artery lesions. Remember that plaque is found on arterial walls and not in veins, and the difference between the arteries and the veins may explain why this occurs. The arteries must expand and constantly flex to accommodate the rush of blood each time the heart beats and contract between beats, so if the walls become stiff they will begin to crack; the body heals the cracks by filling them in with cholesterol.

Terminalia arjuna (arjuna) and guggul: Both of these ayurvedic herbs have been used for more than two thousand seven hundred years for treating heart disease and are effective in lowering bad cholesterol, reducing angina and heart disease, and cleaning the arteries. In a 2001 study arjuna outperformed vitamin E in a randomized placebo-controlled trial. After only thirty days of supplementation with *T. arjuna,* the test group decreased their average LDL "bad" cholesterol levels by 25.6 percent, with a corresponding 12.7 percent drop in total cholesterol. The groups receiving either the placebo or 400 I.U. of vitamin E had no significant change in either measurement.*

SSKI: This amazing substance (also described earlier in this chapter), a saturated solution of potassium iodide that comes in both liquid and tablet form, not only kills pathogens and protects against radiation

---

*R. Gupta, S. Singhal, A. Goyle, and V. N. Sharma, "Antioxidant and hypocholesterolaemic effects of *Terminalia arjuna* tree-bark powder: A randomised placebo-controlled trial," *Journal of the Association of Physicians India* 49 (2001): 231–35.

poisoning, it also dissolves accumulations of fatty deposits in the arterial system. In an article posted on his website titled "Iodide," Jonathan Wright, M.D., founder and director of the Tahoma Clinic, a holistic clinic in Washington State, describes how when he was a premed student at Harvard University one of his professors, Louis Feiser, made a point of demonstrating to him and to all the other premed students that iodine and iodide make oils, fats, and waxes (cholesterol is actually a wax) more soluble in water. He urged them to remember this fact in their medical practices, as he was sure it wasn't taught in medical school. Dr. Wright recommends six drops of SSKI plus a comprehensive nutritional, dietary, and lifestyle approach for anyone with atherosclerotic clogging.

Megadoses of omega-3 (using flax, perilla, or hemp oil): Many of us are aware of the effects of omega-3 when it comes to thinning the blood and lowering cholesterol, which is why salmon, sardines, and mackerel, as well as fish oils, are promoted as being good for the heart. However, plant sources of omega-3s can be taken in place of eating copious amounts of expensive fish or fish oils, which are often polluted. Usually we recommend a minimum of one tablespoon of flax, perilla, or hemp oil twice daily for those with serious heart and artery diseases.

Oral chelation formulas: EDTA is ethylenediaminetetraacetic acid, an aminopolycarboxylic acid and colorless, water-soluble solid that serves as a chelating agent; it is on the World Health Organization's list of essential medicines and is considered one of the most important medications needed in a basic health system. Using a product with EDTA as one of the main ingredients in a proprietary formula that also contains SSKI, B_6, B_{12}, folate, and high levels of vitamin C and lysine is highly recommended for chelation therapy, along with including omega-3 plant-based fats. It is also recommended you include plenty of kelp and Modified Citrus Pectin (MCP) for maximum chelation efficiency, for both of these have been shown to be excellent in removing mercury and other toxic metals from the blood and tissues. A complete formula should contain ingredients in maximum levels that have been shown to detox heavy metals to clean the arteries while also lowering homocysteine and C-reactive protein levels, which are more important markers for heart disease than cholesterol.

RAW, UNPASTEURIZED APPLE CIDER VINEGAR

Raw, unpasteurized apple cider vinegar may be the best and cheapest detoxifier you can take. Hippocrates, way back in 400 BCE, used apple cider vinegar to heal many of his patients. If you take cider vinegar daily, your allergies will improve, your complexion will have a healthy youthful glow, and you will more easily digest your food, which will give you more overall energy. Similarly, raw coconut-toddy vinegar, described in chapter 3, is an excellent substitute and in many ways even superior to apple cider vinegar because of its higher nutrient content.

Raw vinegars have been used to cure ailments for centuries, not only for specific medical problems, but also to improve one's health, to detoxify the body, and to treat a wide range of diseases related to toxins and acidity. In Asia, vinegar is often called "the best friend of Chinese herbs" because it is frequently used to process herbal preparations. It is also successfully used in modern Chinese medicine. The historical origins of vinegar are not exactly known; it was probably discovered when our ancestors saw that wine exposed to the air turned sour, thereby creating vinegar. It is among the oldest of foods and medicines, well known for its healing properties.

Raw apple cider vinegar or raw coconut vinegar is famous for treating digestive upsets and is also quite effective for flu/cold, allergies, low immunity, infections, skin diseases, high blood pressure, obesity, acid reflux, diabetes, weight loss, and arthritis. It is one of the most successfully used natural remedies today for detoxifying and healing sickness, not only in humans but in natural veterinarian medicine also.

The process of creating this raw apple cider vinegar involves fermenting apple juice to wine or cider, which is then allowed to ferment a second time until the alcohol mixes with oxygen in the air, changing it into acetic acid and water. Apple cider vinegar is often called one of Mother Nature's perfect foods, so it seems fitting that medicinal apple cider vinegar must contain the "mother," a term that refers to the milky sediment at the bottom of the bottle, which should not be confused with commercially made (nonmilky) processed apple cider vinegar, which is only good for taste, pickling, and cleaning. Only vinegar with the "mother" can be used as medicine because it has beneficial minerals (especially potassium), malic and tartaric acids, and enzymes intact.

One of the most vital minerals for detoxifying the body is potassium, and there is no better source than raw apple cider vinegar. Potassium's main function is to promote cell growth and replace dead cells. Lemon juice is also acidic to the taste, like apple cider vinegar, and both digest into an alkaline ash, thereby having a strong alkalizing effect on the body. Raw apple cider vinegar acts as a buffer in the body because the acetic acid reacts with base or acid compounds to form an acetate, thereby rendering them chemically bioavailable for the body's utilization. Apple cider vinegar has been known to destroy microorganisms and viruses while also preventing poisons from reaching the rest of the systems of the body. It has been shown to inhibit the growth of gram-negative bacilli, *Pseudomonas,* and candida. The acid nature of vinegar makes the digestive tract environment unpleasant for germs and fungus. Like traditional fermented food such as Korean kimchi, German sauerkraut, and Japanese natto, apple cider vinegar also acts as a prebiotic, stimulating the proliferation of probiotic bacteria in the colon.

Dosage

Generally, it is recommended you take two tablespoons of raw apple cider vinegar (or raw coconut vinegar) diluted in eight ounces of warm water twice daily. Sip it slowly and enjoy the natural flavor of this natural healing product. Honey or some other natural sweetener can be added, or a slice of ginger for a toddy. In addition to taking it for daily maintenance, for weight loss, and to balance pH, it's especially helpful when there is an acute condition like cold/flu or strep throat.

DRY SKIN BRUSHING

The skin is the largest eliminatory organ in the body, measuring approximately two square meters in most adults. It is a strong yet supple cutaneous membrane that protects us from outside germs and warms or cools us, in addition to detoxifying the body by eliminating toxins through the natural process of sweating. In traditional medicine the skin is regarded as having a close relationship with the lungs; in fact, it is an extension of it because it also breathes, and the condition of the lungs is said to be reflected in the skin, and vice versa. The skin's many functions, from protecting the internal tissues to regulating body temperature, as well as being a major eliminatory organ, means that if it becomes blocked in any way, ill health can and most often does occur. The lymphatic system, much like the superficial layers of the skin, contains a network of capillaries and thin blood vessels while also containing ducts and glandular organs such as the tonsils, appendix, thymus, and spleen. Together these all help to cleanse and maintain the fluids of the body. The lymphatic network also transports fats, proteins, and other substances to the blood system and filters toxins out of the blood capillaries in normal metabolism. So you can see why the skin is such an important system to monitor. In saying this, dry skin brushing is an excellent way to stimulate lymphatic circulation, improving the skin's daily functions.

Dry skin brushing is a very effective traditional way of stimulating peripheral circulation, exfoliating, and improving lymphatic circulation; it works great against cellulite and many other health conditions. I recommend dry skin brushing before bathing be done one or two times a week, always brushing *toward* the heart area. Skin brushing also stimulates the meridians and fascia, in turn affecting the internal organs and glands. Brushes especially formulated for this purpose are made of rigid vegetable fibers and are available at most health-food stores. Dr. Bernard Jensen makes the best brush we have seen yet—it's of excellent quality. There are usually two types available: the body brush has strong, rigid fibers, and the complexion facial brush is much softer.

It's important to note that these brushes should never get wet; they are not to be confused with shower scrubbing brushes, which look similar.

LYMPHATIC DETOXING ON A REBOUNDER

Even NASA agrees that the rebounder, a mini in-home trampoline, is probably one of the easiest, most effective, and beneficial exercises around. In a 1980 study done at the Biomechanical Research Division of the NASA-Ames Research Center, it was found that "for similar levels of heart rate and oxygen consumption, the magnitude of the biomechanical stimuli is greater with jumping on a rebounder trampoline than with running, a finding that might help identify acceleration parameters needed for the design of remedial procedures to avert deconditioning in persons exposed to weightlessness."*

Exercising on a rebounder is kind to the joints of the ankles, knees, and hips, unlike running, and it also has many other benefits that running and cycling do not have. You can do it at the office or at home while listening to music or watching a documentary on TV. Many people might think that as gravity pushes things down, this bouncing action would cause all the lymph to be accumulated in the ankles, causing more swelling, but in fact it's the opposite. Mother Nature has very cleverly created a flap valve system in the lymphatic ducts that allows the circulation of your body fluids to go back up the legs. This requires body movement that resists gravity. Bouncing up and down on a rebounder exercises the muscles by helping them resist the forces of gravity. Unlike a regular trampoline, the aim is not to bounce high and do tricks; the small up-and-down movement creates massive improvements in blood and lymphatic circulation, lung capacity, cardiovascular efficiency, heart circulation, joint health, weight loss, digestion, detoxification, stress reduction, and many other benefits. Besides, it's fun! Start with ten minutes per day and build up gradually to thirty minutes. You can also do interval training with the rebounder by doing two minutes of really vibrant jumping followed by one minute's rest, performing approximately eight cycles.

---

*A. Bhattacharya, E. P. McCutcheon, E. Shvartz, and J. E. Greenleaf, "Body acceleration distribution and O_2 uptake in humans during running and jumping," *Journal of Applied Physiology* 49, no. 5 (1980): 881–87.

EFFECTIVE HYDROTHERAPY AT HOME

There is much to be said for good old-fashioned hot and cold showers. As simple as it sounds, the benefits are many. Stimulating the lymphatic system, activating blood circulation, improving skin health, and detoxifying the body are just some of the benefits of this practice. Dr. Richard Schulze confirms this: "The fastest, strongest and most effective way to increase your blood and lymphatic circulation is the application of hot and cold water." We have seen many of our clients improve their circulation problems and reduce joint stiffness with hot and cold therapy alone.

When finishing a shower with cold water after alternating hot and cold, we develop healthier skin while stimulating the internal organs and meridians. Key acupuncture points all over the body are electrically excited from the changes in temperature on the skin's surface. If you initially cannot deal with doing very hot and cold, try doing warm and cool and work your way up to it. Just as the health of the internal organs (especially the digestive system) can affect the quality of the skin, the stimulation of the skin's surface affects one's internal health.

In a similar way, "icing the spine" involves gently rubbing smooth pieces of ice up the whole spine. This shows any vertebral disharmonies and is a great home remedy for activating the cranial-sacral pump while simultaneously improving local blood circulation to the spine and spinal fluid. Any areas of the skin's surface above the spinal bones that appear red in color show deficient circulation, mostly due to compression. Once the blocked spinal areas are found, appropriate massage techniques, osteopathic treatment, Tao Yin, or yoga therapy can then be used to treat the condition. The spinal column could almost be regarded as an organ because it houses the central nervous system, which controls all our other organs.

URINE THERAPY

A former prime minister of India, the late, respected Morarji Desai, boldly and emphatically declared to the world that he drank urine and practiced urine therapy regularly, and that it was the secret of his longevity and lifelong exuberant health (he died just short of his 100th birthday, in 1995). Although this detoxification therapy is scoffed at by skeptics, of which there are many, for those who have tried it or studied the medicinal properties of urine there is no doubt that this simple therapy has terrific benefits. It's not a surprise that Wikipedia mildly attacks it, not saying that it is dangerous but rather that it doesn't work, with links to pseudoskeptical quack-buster sites as references. Even if you find the thought of urine therapy disgusting, we only ask you to read what we have to say here and do your own research on those who have been healed of cancer and many other diseases using it, and the courageous doctors who use it successfully in their medical practice.

We ourselves have been using urine therapy for most of our lives, as we were first introduced to the external application of urine as children to remedy insect bites and jellyfish stings. We have recommended it successfully in our practices and teachings for decades when performed correctly. In fact, it may just save your life or that of one of your loved ones someday. Urine therapy is an ancient, respected medical practice. In the Vedas it is called Shivambu Kalpa, the "elixir of Shiva," because Shiva was known to be a daily advocate of urine therapy and proclaimed that it was this that gave him his strength and good health. Okay, so some of you might be thinking *Big deal, so it's written in some ancient text.* Well, just take a look at the science behind it.

Urine is a sterile aqueous by-product of the body's amazing filtration system, the kidneys, and is made of approximately 95 percent water, 2.5 percent urea, and 2.5 percent ions, vitamins, enzymes, minerals, bicarbonates, hormones, antibodies, and other trace elements—and absolutely no wastes, so it is a clean, nontoxic medicine. After water, urea is the main component of urine. Urea is synthetically produced on a scale of some one hundred million tons per year worldwide and used in beauty products, tooth-whitening products, medicines and medical skin creams, fertilizers, animal feed, and various plastics and adhesives. Although urea can be toxic at high levels if intravenously injected into the blood, urine therapy does not involve injecting it, nor does it directly enter your bloodstream. Although synthetic urea can cause skin irritations, one's own natural urine does not. Urea is even an FDA-approved medicine used in many medicines today! Due to urea's remarkable and comprehensive antineoplastic (antitumor) properties, it has been extensively studied for its use in cancer treatments and is presently being used in some anticancer drugs. The urea compound drug glycoside is used successfully by the medical establishment in treating both insulin-dependent and noninsulin-dependent diabetes. All this, yet people doubt the power of urine (urea) therapy.

The most common question I hear is, "If urine is so good for you, then why does your body excrete it?" In other words, why does the body excrete valuable nutrients, water, hormones, enzymes, etc., that are critical to its functioning? The kidneys form and excrete urine as a way of removing certain elements in your blood that are simply not needed at that time. Take this for example: After some exercise, you proceed to drink two big glasses of water, and at this point you probably have taken in more water than your body needs. So your kidneys balance the amount of water delivered into your bloodstream by your excessive water consumption, and through urine they excrete whatever amount of water from the blood that is not needed at the time. Although water is a life-sustaining element for your body, it can only deal with so much at any given time, so it gets rid of the excess. The rest of the contents of urine are present because of much the same reason.

Urine is medically called *plasma ultrafiltrate,* a purified part of the blood made by your kidneys, whose primary function is not excretion, but regulation of blood elements. Urine is literally the by-product of blood filtration, not of waste filtration. Blood goes through the liver and is purified, poisons are removed and sent to the intestines to be removed as waste, and eventually this purified blood undergoes a filtering process in the kidneys. Here, excess water, salts, vitamins, minerals, enzymes, antibodies, urea, and other elements that are not needed at the time go on to form urine. The kidneys' function is to keep all the many elements in the blood balanced. It is due to this regulatory process of the kidneys that we can eat or drink more than what our body needs at any particular time.

The taste of urine is different but not disgusting, and it changes depending on what you eat or drink, so it's a different taste every day. Many do not mind the taste, some like it, while others may find it difficult at first; everyone who tries it gets used to it and has no problems in a short period of time.

There are various ways you can introduce urine treatment into your health regimen:

- While you're showering, simply cup your hands and pee into them, then take a good mouthful and swish your mouth thoroughly with it and also have a good gargle. This is great for mouth, teeth, and throat problems and also for general health. If you are immediately ready to try it, try taking a sip and swallow, or if you're not quite ready for that, you can then spit it out and rinse your mouth out with water.

- You can wash and scrub your face thoroughly with it while you are showering. Leave it on your face for several minutes, then shower as normal without any residual smell. This is fantastic for acne and other skin conditions.

- Urinate in a cup and apply it to your face over the sink; leave it for five minutes, and then wash off with water or a natural soap. If you have a skin problem apply it to the problem area in the shower cubical and leave on for five minutes, then wash off with water or leave it on.

- Urinate into a cup, and then pour it into a clean, empty dropper bottle and use it fresh each day as eye drops for eye conditions or as ear drops for ear problems. Do this several times daily. It works wonders for conjunctivitis, sties, ear infections, and many other problems. It also helps to prevent further development of cataracts (as declared by the late Indian prime minister Morarji Desai).

- While in the shower, urinate into a large copper cup, wash and massage your hair for several minutes, then rinse with water for radiant hair, to cure yourself of dandruff, or to prevent hair loss or premature balding.

- For normal internal use, urinate in a cup anytime during the day and take a good sip, gradually building up to several sips. Do this once a day if you are healthy or several times a day in times of mild illness.

- For chronic diseases like cancer and diabetes consume at least one liter (approximately one quart) daily. This of course is to be used in conjunction with a complete medical treatment, not as a single cure. Be sure you are being monitored by your doctor (provided he or she is amenable to this treatment) while also working with a professional health practitioner of urine therapy.

While some people say you should use the midstream morning urine and others say not to, it really doesn't matter. Use it any time, any place, anywhere. Urine has helped in the recovery of many diseases. It is safe for all external applications on the skin, but some internal contra-indications do exist. It is also recommended you improve your diet and remove intoxicants while doing urine therapy. That said, in many cases drug addicts can be helped to reduce and eliminate drugs with urine therapy, especially alcoholics.

Cautions and Contraindications:
- Because prescription drugs are excreted in the urine, if you are taking medications you're going to be recycling them, so you need to be careful with not overdosing on your medications. You may in most cases need to cut your dosage down with the help of your doctor.
- It is also not recommended in the case of a UTI (urinary tract infection). For this problem we recommend taking apple cider vinegar, colloidal silver, and herbal antibiotics like olive leaf extract or an herbal formula from your naturopath or Chinese or ayurvedic doctor. Once your UTI is cured and your urine is not carrying infection, you can use urine therapy safely.
- People with kidney disease should first consult their doctor but can usually still practice it without problems and to great effect by only taking several drops three times daily as a homeopathic dose.
- Do not use urine therapy if you are pregnant.

Fifth Immortal Healer—Lu Tung-Pin
Stop Poisoning Your Body

A person will get well when he is tired of being sick.

Lao-tzu, *Tao Te Ching*

The healing that takes place from eliminating toxins from the body is symbolized by Lu Tung-Pin, who is also called Ancestor Lu. He is perhaps the most familiar of all the Immortals, sometimes considered their leader. His emblems are the magic two-edged sword that dispels evil and gives him the power of invisibility and a horsehair whisk that allows him to fly through the air. He is dressed and honored as a scholar, the hero of marvelous wisdom residing on Stork Peak, although like all the other Immortals he has his eccentricities, in this case that of being a ladies' man, prone to bouts of drunken revelry. He sometimes appears with a tiger. The story goes that Lu Tung-Pin underwent ten trials on his journey to transcending the limitations of his human body. It was in his fourth test that he was charged with looking after sheep in the mountains. A tiger came upon him and his terrified sheep, but Lu Tung-Pin put himself between the tiger and the sheep, and the tiger slunk away, signifying this Immortal's ability to tame the wild forces of nature.

Legend has it that Lu Tung-Pin was born in the eighth century CE. He was a Confucian scholar who converted to Taoism after being initiated into the secrets of internal alchemy by fellow Immortal Chung-Li Chuan.

He can travel thousands of miles in an instant to seek those with kind hearts, especially those who risk their comfort and well-being to help others in great need. Upon discovering such exemplary persons, he uses his supernatural powers to help them transform themselves into Taoist Immortals.

This Immortal represents the element of the Lake or Marsh, which is our drainage of waste from the lower areas. We must remember that if we use poisons they will reside in the lower areas or "ditches" of the body, where they can fester and cause disease. This could very well be called the foundation on which modern medicine stands.

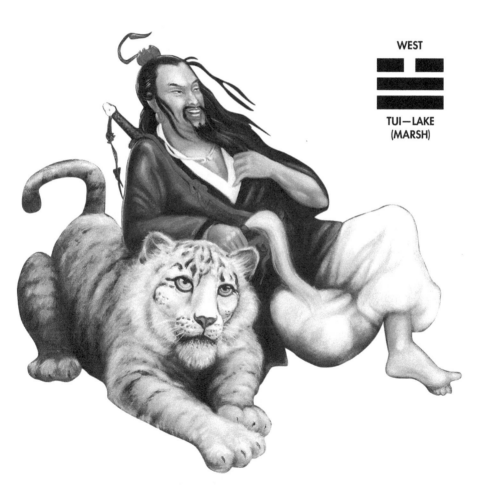

WEST

TUI—LAKE
(MARSH)

Fig. 5.1. Lu Tung-Pin (Lu Dong Bin)

ARE GERMS THE REAL PROBLEM?

The main reason we include this discussion of germs is that there is a common, and incorrect, belief that says that if we are unlucky we will catch some kind of germ and come down with a cold or the flu. The truth of the matter is that nature has provided germs with a purpose, and that purpose is to eliminate wastes from the body. A good example of this is how germs work in the cycle of decomposition of dead plants or animals back into the earth, enriching it with minerals for new life to begin again. Flies do not live inside a clean rubbish bin. Germs have a purpose—to eat waste—so if your body is being regularly infected with germs, then your body is overloaded with wastes or toxins; it's that simple.

Stress, overeating, and eating unnaturally refined foods high in refined sugars and complex carbohydrates overload the system so that it becomes burdened with acid wastes, which the body cannot eliminate fast enough through the eliminatory organs such as the lungs, skin, kidneys, and bowels. This simple scenario is one of the root causes of poor immunity and explains the prevalence of so many infections and immune-system diseases today. Let's look at a few facts to clear up the confusion once and for all.

The "germ theory of disease"—and here we emphasize the word *theory*—proposed by Louis Pasteur in the nineteenth century suggests that diseases arise from infections derivative of airborne germs. This falsely proposes that the human body is sterile (a massive joke today) and that germs attack our innocent bodies as if we were poor victims. Pasteur himself apparently refuted his own theory at the end of his life. Christopher Bird, author of *The Secret Life of Plants* and other books, recounts how "on his deathbed Louis Pasteur . . . declared . . . the microbe is nothing, the terrain is everything." Nevertheless, the germ theory took hold and is still presented as fact by the modern medical establishment, which says that the answer to curing a disease lies in finding the right pills to attack those beastly germs. Is it any wonder that the pharmaceutical industry has praised the germ theory of disease and personified the human being as a demigod instead of teaching the fact that we reap what we sow?

While modern medicine and the pharmaceutical industry have astounded us with advanced pain-killing drugs and amazing surgical techniques, they have been unable to find an answer to the many diseases that exist today and practically all degenerative diseases. In fact, degenerative diseases such as cancer and heart disease are increasing by the hundreds of thousands every year despite all the drugs, diagnostic technology, and laser-equipped surgical procedures. For example, the rate at which diabetes afflicts people even in their youth is alarming. On the same note, despite all the fancy antibiotics and vaccines, infectious diseases are on the increase. To keep up the pace and not look like they don't know what's happening, the medical system gives us new names for all the old bugs, like AIDS, candida, chronic fatigue syndrome, and fibromyalgia, while at the same time we also get promises every year that there will be a magic pill to cure these diseases coming soon.

The Two Opposing Theories of Pasteur and Béchamp

Let's review the two theories of illness that were proposed at the time of the discovery of microbes. They are those of the well-known Louis Pasteur and that of the less well-known Anthony Béchamp, one of France's greatest scientists. One man's theory was based on fact, the other's on pure hypothesis, which, as we have seen, even Pasteur admitted on his deathbed.

Pasteur's theory:

- A disease arises from an attack by external microorganisms.
- All microorganisms are generally to be guarded against.
- The function of microorganisms is consistent.
- The shapes and colors of microorganisms are always the same.
- Each disease is associated with a particular microorganism.
- Microorganisms are the primary cause of disease.
- Disease can "strike" anybody at any time.
- To prevent disease we have to "build defenses."

Béchamp's theory:

- A disease is caused by microorganisms within the cells of the body.
- These intracellular microorganisms' normal function is to build and assist in the metabolic processes of the body.
- The purpose of these organisms' changes is also to assist in the catabolic (disintegration) processes of the host organism.
- Microorganisms are able to alter their shapes or colors to reflect their surrounding environment.
- Every disease is associated with a particular host condition.
- Microorganisms only cause disease when the health of the host organism deteriorates.
- Disease is built by unhealthy conditions within the body.
- To prevent disease, you must first create health.

Pasteur's hypothesis was not a new one. An Italian doctor by the name of Girolamo Fracastoro (ca. 1478–1553) was the first to publish any substantial information on infections and crude microbiology in his 1546 work *De contagionibus et contagiosis morbis, et eorem curatione* (*On Contagion, Contagious Diseases, and Their Cure*). He was the first to divide diseases into three categories: those that infect by instant contact, through intermediate agents, or at a distance through the air. Later, Antonie van Leeuwenhoek (1632–1723), a Dutch tradesman and scientist considered the first genuine microbiologist and dubbed "the Father of Microbiology," found what he termed *animalcula* in saliva through one of the first microscopes, one of his own designs. He described what he saw, and in his drawings included both rod-like and spiral forms. It is thought that the two species he saw are what are today recognized as *Bacillus buccalis maximus* and *Spirillum sputigenum*. Then later, in 1762, an Austrian medical doctor, Marcus Antonius von Plenciz, published a germ theory of infectious diseases. Plenciz stated that there was a special organism by which each infectious disease was produced, that microorganisms were capable of reproduction outside of the body, and that they might be conveyed from place to place via the air we breathe. So there you have it—three centuries or so before Pasteur came up with his amazing discovery, several scientists, even without the use of the more advanced microscopes that Pasteur used to identify bacteria, proposed the same theory that Pasteur proposed.

Yet there were dissenters at the time. Pasteur's contemporary, Béchamp, claimed that germs were part of nature's design for health and not for causing disease. Germs, he said, were nature's scavengers and appeared only when the soil—meaning the body's polluted condition—was conducive to their existence. He asserted that the emphasis should be placed on cleaning the soil instead of attacking the germs. The most famous nurse in the world, Florence Nightingale, agreed. She published an outright attack on Pasteur's theory, nailing it when she said, "Microbes must not be looked upon as separate entities, as they perform a job in the body and have some purpose." She also said, "Wise and humane management of the patient is the best safeguard against infection. The greater part of nursing consists of preserving cleanliness. The specific disease doctrine is the grand refuge of weak, uncultured, unstable minds, such as now rule in the medical profession. There are no specific diseases; there are specific disease conditions."

One theory puts humans as the victims of microbes, while the other more sensibly maintains that the human body will always contain bacteria, and that it is the condition of the terrain of the body's cells that is the key to preventing and treating disease. So the germ theory of Pasteur—or should we say of those who came before him from whom he stole much of his work—is based on misinformation that has led us to the medical crisis that we are in today, in which the conventional approach is to declare all-out war on the body's microflora.

Now that we've cleared up one of the basic assumptions of modern allopathic medicine, let's take a look at the myriad poisons we are exposed to on a daily basis that poison the body's terrain, making us vulnerable to any number of maladies.

THE FACTS ABOUT VACCINES

One of the most contentious subjects in the field of health today, especially since the controversial 2016 documentary *Vaxxed* has come out, is that of vaccines, long assumed to be safe and necessary. Dr. Leonard Horowitz, an internationally recognized authority in the fields of public health, natural medicine, behavioral sciences, and emerging diseases, says of vaccines,

> You lament the additional ramifications of this "license to kill" given to vaccine makers. It dawns on you that this trash legislation not only impacts the millions of young victims of mercury poisoning, but equally guarantees helplessness, if not hopelessness, for those struggling, now and in future years, with myriad cancers attributed to polio vaccine viral contaminations; for Gulf War Syndrome victims made ill by vaccines and drug interactions; for military personnel recently inoculated with anthrax vaccine with up to 85% made ill; for more than a hundred thousand Lyme vaccine injured people; for claimants who cite recent studies that will soon prove early hepatitis B vaccines triggered the international AIDS pandemic; and for the millions of forthcoming smallpox vaccine injured persons who you are told to accept as simply unfortunate casualties of America's new war.*

What are human vaccines made of, how safe are they, and do they really prevent us from getting the illnesses that they supposedly are specifically designed to target? Even though we may not know the answers to these vital questions, many of us do not question the government's efforts to make vaccines compulsory. Strictly speaking, a vaccination is the injection of an impure substance (a virus or poison) into your body based on the assumption that the body will develop antibodies against that disease, in turn aiding in preventing that illness—a great theory that has stood some test of time, but it may be time to let the

---

*www.healingcelebrations.com/essay.htm.

cat out of the bag. Unfortunately, when you study the facts, vaccines can result in serious side effects that often go undetected. For some time now the vaccine myth has been able to stand strong despite all the evidence to the contrary. But nowadays, the moral dilemmas that are created by forced vaccination and the vaccination of schoolchildren without parental consent can no longer be ignored, as we become more aware of the dangers of vaccines.

Without compulsory laws, it would be safe to say that vaccination would not have lasted this long, as since their introduction both the general public and members of the medical profession have questioned their safety. For example, in the autumn of 1901 in Philadelphia there were no fewer than thirty-six cases of tetanus, all following vaccination. After a study of these and fifty-nine other similar cases, a prominent Philadelphia physician and professor, himself once an ardent believer in vaccination, concluded that neither careless dressing of a wound nor infection from a foreign source could account for the cases of lockjaw following vaccination, for, as he pointed out, cases had occurred not only among the ignorant and filthy, but also among those who lived under the most favorable conditions, and even when the utmost precautions had been taken.*

The belief that vaccines are safe and effective is common; after all, it's what doctors and we the public are told by medical governing boards and the drug companies that manufacture these questionable substances. We are brainwashed into believing this by the medical profession, by the media, and by the local drugstore chains and supermarkets that commonly dispense these poisons to the public, such that the public is demanding even stronger and more powerful vaccines to address things like cancer and even obesity.

Way back in the early 1700s, Lady Mary Wortley Montague, English aristocrat, letter writer, and poet, and the wife of the British ambassador at Constantinople, attempted the first vaccinations. She was said to have learned the technique, then called "engrafting," from

---

*Philadelphia County Medical Society session of 1902, vol. 23.

the Turks. After almost a century of human experiments on the British people with a smallpox vaccine that used infectious grafts taken from cowpox, these inoculations, which were at first highly endorsed by the Royal College of Physicians, were eventually condemned by the British Parliament as a criminal offense. Edward Jenner, an English physician who a short time later pioneered the smallpox vaccine and who went on to be regarded as the "Father of Vaccination," later revamped the practice. Due to inconsistent results with vaccines, a formal inquiry led by the Royal Commission and headed by Lord Herschell, the chairman at the time, was to become one of the largest medical research reports in history. Spanning seven years, from 1889 to 1896, with numerous testimonies taken from both health officials and the public, the report left yet another strong question mark on the effectiveness of vaccination, which led to the abandonment of enforced vaccination. Retrospectively, a scientific publication, the *Journal of Pediatrics,* concluded that "the largest historical decrease in morbidity and mortality caused by infectious disease was experienced not with the modern antibiotic and vaccine era, but after the introduction of clean water and effective sewer systems."*

Although vaccines were initially claimed to offer lifelong immunity, there was no scientific proof that they lasted even several weeks, as many people reported contracting smallpox immediately after being vaccinated when the smallpox vaccine was developed. In fact, many public vaccinators such as the English physician and later legislator William Job Collins (1859–1946), who vaccinated thousands over his twenty-five years of work, in the end commented that vaccinations never diminished smallpox, and in fact often produced it. The immunity theory with which vaccination was supported was still a shaky hypothesis. This theory could in no way be compared to the oft-cited cases of Amazonian tribespeople who ingested small amounts of poisons from plants or animals to strengthen themselves, in turn making them immune to the bites and stings of the plants and animals from

---

*"Zinc, diarrhea, and pneumonia" (editorial), *Journal of Pediatrics* 135, no. 6 (1999): 663.

which the poisons were taken—an argument that was used as a rationale for vaccination.

According to a 1980 analysis of historical trends in Switzerland from 1876 to 1977, immunization had little or no effect on the spread of contagious disease.* Researchers noted that there was already a 95 percent decrease in diphtheria death rates even before introduction of the vaccine. Other graphs demonstrate that scarlet fever decreased from 200 deaths per 100,000 in the late 1800s to virtually zero by the 1930s, before drug treatments were introduced. Yet another graph in this study shows typhoid also decreasing, from 50 deaths per 100,000 in 1876 to virtually zero by the 1940s, after which drug treatments were introduced.

It seems clear that shortly after life-threatening contagious diseases began to diminish in the early twentieth century due to improved personal and public hygiene and other lifestyle factors, compulsory vaccinations started—and the purveyors of those vaccines also conveniently began taking the credit for the decrease in infectious diseases. However, when we look at the statistics on vaccines we can see that contagious diseases took a dive well before vaccines were made compulsory. Mortality rates from tuberculosis, diphtheria, scarlet fever, whooping cough, measles, typhoid, polio, puerperal fever, and other diseases all started to fall long before the introduction of either immunization or antibiotics.

Perhaps we are starting to wake up, though. Today, vaccinations are receiving more and more bad publicity in the scientific press, which has noted their link to a number of new types of problems, including autoimmune diseases such as asthma and arthritis, SIDS (sudden infant death syndrome), narcolepsy, leukemia, and many types of cancer. Some say the word *iatrogenesis,* which means "physician-induced illness," describes many of today's new health ailments. Some of these, if not the majority, are clearly due to the overuse of antibiotics or the abuse of prescription drugs. More recent testimonies and studies emerging now

---

*E. Gubéran, "Tendances de la mortalité en Suisse" (Mortality trends in Switzerland), *Schweizerishe medizinische Wochenschrift* 110, no. 15 (1980): 574–83.

are beginning to see vaccines as another deadly culprit. There is much more research needed to confirm whether vaccines really help or hinder; contrary to what you're being told by the mainstream media, there is no clear-cut evidence that validates their widespread compulsory use. Apart from a tetanus or rabies shot, which can save a life in an emergency, we personally do not recommend any vaccines, nor do we personally take them. We urge you to research this subject further if you have any doubts, especially if you have children.

LIST OF INGREDIENTS OF SOME POPULAR VACCINES*

NAME	USES	COMPANY	CONTENTS	MEDIUM
Attenuvax	Measles virus live	Merck & Co.	Neomycin, sorbitol, hydrolyzed gelatin	Chick embryos
Biavax	Rubella and mumps virus live	Merck & Co.	Neomycin, sorbitol, hydrolyzed gelatin	Human diploid cells (from human aborted fetal tissue)
Flu Shield	Influenza trivalent, types A & B	Wyeth-Ayerst	Gentamicin sulfate, formaldehyde, polysorbate 80, tri(N)butyl phosphate, thimerosal	Chick embryos
Havrix	Hepatitis A	SmithKline Beecham	Formalin, aluminum hydroxide, phenoxyethanol (antifreeze), polysorbate 20, residual MRC5 proteins	Human diploid cells (from human aborted fetal tissue)
IPOL	Inactivated polio	Connaught Labs	3 types of polio virus, formaldehyde, phenoxyethanol (antifreeze), neomycin, streptomycin, polymyxin B	VERO cells, a continuous line of monkey kidney cells

*According to the *Physicians' Desk Reference* 1997.

Fearmongering over "Stealth" Viruses

H1N1 virus, swine flu, SARS, anthrax, smallpox, new killer flus, and the common cold are all anaerobic diseases. The bacterial and viral transmission vectors of these illnesses are also anaerobic. Anaerobic means that they cannot exist in oxygen-rich environments; therefore, by definition none of these illnesses can exist if our tissues and organs maintain sufficient levels of oxygen when these pathogens first invade the body. There are a variety of ways to keep the body strong and healthy by introducing oxygen into the body, the subject of chapter 1. Medical forms of ozone and oxygen therapy are one way to more active oxygen. Home supplementation with other forms of active oxygen, such as H_2O_2 and the oxygen products I described in the beginning of this book are another effective way of boosting the body's oxygen levels. Also, colloidal silver, as explained in chapter 4, boosts oxygen levels in the body. Chapter 8 describes the Beck Protocol, yet another way to protect yourself from stealth viruses.

Here are the facts on viruses:

- In 2001, more than 36,000 people (young and old) died of the common flu in the United States. Almost all had compromised immune systems, either through poor diet or other lifestyle factors. Another possible source of their poor immunity is linked to drug side effects and vaccine-induced toxicity and autoimmunity.
- There has been almost no mention of widespread mortality caused by the flu in previous years, and the SARS virus to date has killed no one in the United States.
- Herbs such as *Andrographis,* olive leaf, and *Lomatium* (desert parsley) have a good record of curing viral epidemics fast, and articles about them have been published in the scientific literature for several years now, which is something government authorities or your doctor might be unaware of or might have forgotten to mention to you.

If you take two people, one who has been diagnosed with SARS and the other some regular pneumonia or flu, you would not be able to tell the difference between the two ailments. Many people may not be aware that influenza and pneumonia are major contributors to the many deaths and hospitalizations among the elderly today. Influenza and pneumonia are the leading cause of death from infectious disease in Canada. In fact, in 1996 there were 7,627 deaths from pneumonia and influenza in Canada alone. Researchers have admitted that with even the most sensitive tests, they can only find evidence of the SARS virus in 40 percent of these cases. Rather than being an actual public health emergency, "severe acute respiratory syndrome," or SARS, could better be called a "sickening and repulsive scam." According to the World Health Organization, SARS inflicted a death rate of less than 4 percent. In Hong Kong, this alleged "worst medical disaster," as described by the mainstream media, in reality killed only ten people out of 316 known cases. But since this only takes into account those ill enough to seek medical help, the actual ratio of deaths to infections is certainly far less. In contrast, the 1918–1919 flu pandemic killed approximately one-third of the 60 million people afflicted. Even in light of the facts, many people still buy into the fearmongering hype, rushing off to get vaccinated without properly educating themselves on the long-term side effects of vaccines or the many available natural medicines that can cure these illnesses.

THE BIG BUSINESS OF PHARMACEUTICAL DRUGS

Charles Vincent, professor of psychology at University College London, whose research focuses on the causes of harm to patients, the consequences for patients and staff, and the methods of improving the safety of health care, says,

> Medical error is the third most frequent cause of death in Britain after cancer and heart disease, killing up to 40,000 people a year— four times more die from this cause than all other types of accidents.

Provisional research figures on hospital mistakes show that a further 280,000 people suffer from non-fatal drug prescribing errors, overdoses and infections. The victims spend an average of six extra days recovering in hospital, at an annual cost of £730 million for England alone.

Few of us are aware of the laws the World Health Organization installed in 1963 in the United States, Europe, and Australia regarding health supplements, called the Codex Alimentarius, whose purpose, as stated by the WHO, is "to develop harmonized international food standards, which protect consumer health and promote fair practices in food trade." Nothing could be further from the truth. The restrictions imposed on the availability of health supplements as a result of this law mean that soon you will have your right to choose how to protect your health taken away from you. In fact, many of the health supplements you take today may go on a prescription basis (thereby controlled by Big Pharma), while some of your favorite supplements may become totally unavailable. Most of us are unaware that such restrictions are being pushed by governments with the assistance of multinational pharmaceutical companies, and we go about our daily lives unaware that our health freedoms and rights are being stolen from us. Many believe these new restrictive bills on health supplements will increase people's reliance on pharmaceutical drug companies by eliminating alternative options or either making those options impossible to obtain or forcing you to get a prescription from an allopathic doctor who has no training in twenty-first-century nutritional medicine. A German doctor, Matthias Rath, the first director of cardiovascular research at the Linus Pauling Institute in Palo Alto, California, provides a concise summary of the current state of ethics of the pharmaceutical industry:

Throughout the twentieth century, the pharmaceutical industry has been constructed by investors, the goal being to replace effective but nonpatentable natural remedies with mostly ineffective but patentable and highly profitable pharmaceutical drugs. The very nature of the pharmaceutical industry is to make money from ongoing diseases.

Like other industries, the pharmaceutical industry tries to expand their market—that is, to maintain ongoing diseases and to find new diseases for their drugs. Prevention and cure of diseases damages the pharmaceutical business and the eradication of common diseases threatens its very existence. Therefore, the pharmaceutical industry fights the eradication of any disease at all costs. The pharmaceutical industry itself is the main obstacle, why today's most widespread diseases are further expanding, including heart attacks, strokes, cancer, high blood pressure, diabetes, osteoporosis, and many others. Pharmaceutical drugs are not intended to cure diseases. According to health insurers, over 24,000 pharmaceutical drugs are currently marketed and prescribed without any proven therapeutic value.*

Dr. Rath adds that "millions of people and patients around the world are defrauded twice: a major portion of their income is used up to finance the exploding profits of the pharmaceutical industry. In return, they are offered a medicine that does not even cure."

According to the *Journal of the American Medical Association* (April 15, 1998), the known dangerous side effects of pharmaceutical drugs have become the fourth leading cause of death after heart attack, cancer, and stroke.

Many people today put blind faith in allopathic medicine's drugs and the companies that manufacture these inorganic chemicals that we call "medicine." Let me briefly explain the process of pharmaceutical testing and approval, and why over 100,000 people die each year in the United States from FDA-approved drugs. When you read this, you'll understand why it's no wonder that natural supplements are becoming harder and harder to obtain, even when virtually no deaths occur from nutritional or herbal supplementation compared to that of pharmaceutical drugs.

Drugs today are tested over short periods of time, and on limited numbers of people (almost always men, not women), so the long-term safety and side effects are relatively unknown. The drug companies

---

AOK Magazine, April 1998.

generally design their own studies, in turn controlling all the raw data. Often when results are unfavorable, drug manufacturers can sometimes prevent these findings from even coming to light. After quick trials that often seem unregulated in terms of length, the new drugs are released to the public for us to consume. It is here in the population where the true testing takes place, and it is we the consumers who are the guinea pigs. If the drug sells well and has minimal side effects or deaths, it passes; if numerous side effects or deaths occur it is taken off the market and nothing more is said; no further investigations, so that Kim Kardashian and Brangelina can dominate the news headlines again.

Most of the new pharmaceutical drugs developed today are for generating profits for drug companies and their shareholders; they offer very few new treatments and no actual cures. According to recent research, only 15 percent of drugs approved by the FDA between 1989 and 2000 had any significant clinical advantage over existing drugs. What's more, many drug manufacturers do not even consider developing drugs for rare or incurable diseases because they wouldn't offer financial rewards to shareholders. Moreover, it seems that drug companies today have a stronger influence over the U.S. Food and Drug Administration than at any previous time.

The Prescription Drug Takeover

In 2001, the editors of the world's most prestigious medical journal, the *New England Journal of Medicine,* changed their policy, allowing them the right to refuse publication of studies sponsored by pharmaceutical companies, which actually constitute the majority of published studies. This decision was made because most companies were found to be extensively influencing the results of drug trials. Unfortunately for us, it only took until June 2002, a few months later, for this and other medical journals to relax this commendable policy—not because the trials became more truthful, but because it got worse. Medical journals were finding it increasingly difficult to find *any* drug studies to publish in their journal pages that did not have close financial ties to the drug companies that sponsored them. Marion Moss, a former investigator for the Texas attorney general's office, says that "during the eight years when I was an investigator . . . I had numerous occasions to work with the FDA on cases involving potential health fraud. I repeatedly saw cases against large corporations go unchallenged. Instead, the agency chose to pursue cases involving alternative health-care providers."*

In 2006, the United States alone spent an estimated $5,000 per person per year on health care, which is more than any other nation in the world, yet we are far from being the healthiest country; in fact, we're way down at number 25 in world standards. As prescription drugs are the fastest-rising part of our health care expenses, the amount that Americans spend on drugs has increased by 15 percent a year for the past few years, which is five times the rate of inflation. Despite all this, we're seeing no correlation with improved health. It is becoming clearer that drugs are neither curbing disease rates nor effectively treating them. In fact, from these openly available drug statistics it's safe to say that the drug companies are poisoning us. Even the respected *New England Journal of Medicine* (February 7, 1991) concludes that "about 90 percent of the patients who visit doctors have conditions that will either improve on their own or that are out of reach of modern medicine's ability to solve."

Today many people have become emotionally and physically weak, eager to give their power to heal themselves over to "authorities" and not even question the medical system. Many people do not realize that prescription drugs were initially designed as a last resort, in dire cases when herbs and other natural medicines didn't work. In such cases chemical drugs would only be administered to buy time until the real cause of an illness could be established and the natural treatment could be administered. In times past, all healing was achieved from plant sources much more successfully than the drugs of today. Synergistic blends of herbs for detoxification purposes and appropriate rest during illness were common right up until prescription drugs arrived on the scene. It seems quite clear that as people became more familiar with going to the doctor's office for their pills and then immediately returning to work,

---

*www.alkalizeforhealth.net/about.htm.

prescription drugs became increasingly common. The once-heralded natural cure has now become a thing of the past, to the point where most orthodox medical people regard natural therapies as pure snake oil. How corrupt and ignorant our society has become! In addition to all the various horrible side effects of drugs, they are also very acidic and deplete the body of nutritional stores, causing further deficiencies. Prescription drugs such as diuretics, antacids, antibiotics, and even oral contraceptives are all known to cause nutritional depletion, which then cause a host of other diseases. While Americans spend more on antacids each year than on health supplements, the restrictions of health supplements are ever increasing.

CHEMOTHERAPY

Author and journalist Barry Lynes, author of *The Healing of Cancer,* quotes Allen Levin, M.D., as saying, "Most cancer patients in this country die of chemotherapy. Chemotherapy does not eliminate breast, colon, or lung cancers. This fact has been documented for over a decade, yet doctors still use chemotherapy for these tumors." This should come as no surprise. Presently in the UK, 200,000 people are diagnosed every year with cancer, and of those diagnosed, 152,500 of them die. In the United States this rate is even higher. As these deaths are recorded as cancer deaths, the statistics easily cover up how many deaths are really being caused by using radiation, chemotherapy, and surgical techniques in an attempt to cure cancer. If one is diagnosed with cancer and decides on the allopathic route, then this means radiation and chemotherapy, which involves a cocktail of toxic pharmaceutical drugs, all of which have possibly more health dangers than the cancer itself and are perhaps even more unpleasant than any cancer.

Chemotherapy uses toxic forms of radiation in an attempt to destroy cancer cells. At the same time, because it is not specific to the cancer site, it also destroys your entire immune system. On that note it is estimated that 67 percent of people die using the prevailing cancer protocol as a result of opportunistic infections that are in turn the direct result of immune system failure. This is due to the aggressive, toxic nature of radiation and chemotherapy. Dr. Walter Last, N.D., in an article published in a 1998 issue of *The Ecologist* (volume 28, no. 2), says that "after analyzing cancer survival statistics for several decades, Dr. Hardin Jones, professor at the University of California, concluded, 'Patients are as well, if not better off, untreated.'"

Even though chemotherapy and allopathic cancer protocols demonstrate appalling results, with little solid medical evidence that chemotherapy can even prolong life, we never cease to be amazed when patients continue the prescribed treatment right up to their deaths. There seems to be a lot of ignorance due to some hidden influence of allopathic medicine boards, and this is resulting in horrendous suffering. If there is virtually no scientific evidence demonstrating the effectiveness of chemotherapy on any large scale, and there is so much information proving its ineffectiveness, then why are so many people willing to undergo such a devastating treatment? Not even the doctors themselves would follow this protocol:

> Scientists based at McGill Cancer Center sent a questionnaire to 118 lung cancer doctors to determine what degree of faith these practicing cancer physicians placed in their own therapies they administered. They were asked to imagine that they had cancer, and were asked which of six current trials they would choose? Only 79 doctors responded, of which 64 would not consent to be in any trial containing Cisplatin, one of the common chemotherapy drugs they were trialing, (currently achieving worldwide sales of about $110,000,000 a year). Fifty-eight doctors of the 79 found that all the trials in question were unacceptable due to the ineffectiveness of chemotherapy and its unacceptably high degree of toxicity.*

One cancer patient described the nightmare treatment: "This highly toxic fluid was being injected into my veins. The nurse who was

---

*Phillip Day, *Cancer: Why We Are Still Dying to Know the Truth* (Credence Publications, 2000).

administering it was wearing protective gloves because it would burn her skin if just a tiny drip came into contact with it. I couldn't help asking myself that if such precautions were needed to be taken on the outside, what is it doing to me on the inside? From 7 p.m. that evening I vomited solidly for two and a half days."*

Most people do not realize that allopathic cancer treatment involves *no* natural treatments, nor does the medical establishment invest any of their profits into research on natural protocols to address cancer. You are poked, diced, cut, poisoned, and radiated till your immune system shuts down and your hair falls out, and in most cases you die, or by some rare miracle your cancer gets scared into remission. We would much prefer to die with some dignity or search every corner of the globe for people who have healed themselves of cancer successfully, without such chemical torture, and begin to apply those techniques. Maybe it is the slim hope of a cure that people persevere on this horrendous route.

When I talk to cancer patients undergoing chemotherapy and to my own clients about their relatives who have decided to use this method instead of changing their diet, cleansing their body, and eradicating the causes of cancer, they all report to have an uncomfortable inner feeling about chemo but feel compelled to undergo it anyway on advice of their doctor. It is as if every time they see their oncologist, a stronger opinion is planted in their subconscious minds. This could be the result of a strong submissive attitude combined with all those magical diplomas on the wall of the doctor's clinic. It could be because of the way people are diagnosed in allopathic medicine, and how a prognosis is forced on them—like a robot receiving instructions from its master. Some clients explain how their relatives heard the news and what followed from their doctor's mouth after they were initially diagnosed. Such comments as, "The cancer that you have, Bill, is a very rare type of lymphatic cancer, the type that creeps up on you gradually and then metastasizes all over your body very quickly. This is why we need to get started on the chemotherapy treatment

---

*www.cancertutor.com.

immediately or you will die in three months." British journalist John Diamond recounts his personal ordeal with cancer in his best-selling book *Because Cowards Get Cancer Too:*

> What if those denying alternatives were right? What if the truth was that no life had ever been saved by radiotherapy and that there was every chance that my cancer would be made worse by it being irradiated? What if the truth as pronounced by a couple of books was that the main effect of cancer surgery was to release stray cancer cells into the body, allowing them to set up home elsewhere. . . . I turned to the medical books for solace and got none.*

Diamond initially began his chemotherapy as a staunch supporter of modern orthodox medical methods. Then, after suffering tragically during his treatment, having his voice box cut out and losing his ability to speak (he was a broadcaster by profession), and then losing his ability to taste before he finally died, he expressed a note of doubt in his last writings, proving that even he, a staunch supporter of the modern medical establishment, was beginning to wonder. Diamond died in March 2001 at the age of forty-seven, joining so many celebrities before him, such as Linda McCartney and George Harrison, plus 150,000 or more British citizens who perish each year after being diagnosed with some form of cancer and undergoing chemotherapy.

Ralph Moss, in his book *Questioning Chemotherapy,* says, "Chemotherapy usually doesn't cure cancer or extend life, and it really does not improve the quality of the life either. Doctors frequently make this claim, though. To most it is just common sense that a drug that makes you throw up and lose your hair and wrecks your immune system is not improving your quality of life." To understand the FDA's definition of the term "effective treatment" demonstrates a bigger picture in the story on cancer treatment success in allopathic medicine. The FDA states that a treatment producing 50 percent or greater reduction in tumor size for twenty-eight days is an "effective treatment." However,

---

*John Diamond, *Because Cowards Get Cancer Too* (Vermilion Press, 1999).

in the majority of cases there is absolutely no correlation between the shrinking of tumors in the first twenty-eight days and the cure of the cancer in the long run, and any extension of life for that matter. So many times when patients or family members hear the doctor say, "This has been an effective treatment," everyone breathes a sigh of relief, thinking that it means a cure is just around the corner, or a lengthening of life at the very least. What this really means is a temporary tumor size reduction only.

In the UK alone, £2.8 billion a year is spent in the valorous attempt to cure cancer using toxic radiation and inorganic chemical drugs. That's approximately £6,800,000 a day; in the United States this amount is ten times higher, at approximately $100 billion annually. With this in mind it is important to note that Bristol Myers, which incidentally owns patents on twelve of the nearly forty FDA-approved chemotherapy drugs, has their president, past president, chairman of the board, and several of their directors also holding board positions at the influential Memorial Sloan Kettering Cancer Center. With this, we leave you to your own conclusions as to what is really happening in "Cancer, Inc." Understand this the next time someone comes knocking on your door asking for more money for cancer research; the hard-earned money you donate is being spent on the further development of ineffective drugs and toxic treatments, while none of it being spent on treating the true cause of cancer with natural methods.

Dr. James Watson won a Nobel Prize in 1962 for determining the shape of DNA. During the 1970s he served for two years on the National Cancer Advisory Board. In 1975, he was asked about the national cancer program. He declared, "The American public has been sold a nasty bill of goods about cancer." Many doctors I have spoken with personally regarding this matter believe there is a tremendous conflict inside the minds of most oncologists and other medical practitioners. While the majority of doctors may be honest, sensitive, caring persons, you're in a tight situation when you've been trained for so many years in medical school with such a high level of knowledge of these poisons, radiation, and deadly drugs. It must be difficult for oncologists when they know deep down inside that the tools you have to work with against cancer are extremely limited and quite toxic. There is added pressure when seeing what happens to other doctors who attempt to go against the grain and begin treating cancer with so-called alternative techniques like oxygen therapy, sodium bicarbonate therapy, naturopathy, and herbal or nutritional medicine. Suddenly you are subjected to armed raids by medical police departments and the loss of your license to practice medicine, smeared for the rest of your life by your colleagues and mentors or perhaps even the whole allopathic medical profession.

There is a saying that goes like this: "Develop an effective cancer treatment = Go to jail." If you have cancer yourself and you are in your doctor's office, we encourage you to ask if he would undergo the same treatment that he is prescribing for you if he himself had this cancer, or would he prescribe it for his own family members if they had cancer. You may be surprised that many doctors would shudder, not answer this question directly, and instead repeatedly reinforce your critical situation or your current prognosis or simply change the subject by using a lot of technical medical jargon.

A study that set out to accurately assess the actual benefit by chemotherapy in the treatment of adults with the most common types of cancer, showed that it provided almost no benefit.* The paper did attract some attention in Australia, the native country of the paper's authors, yet was completely ignored around the world. Their paper, a meta-analysis, analyzed the results of all the randomized, controlled clinical trials (RCTs) performed in Australia and the United States that reported a statistically significant increase in five-year survival rates due to the use of chemotherapy in adult malignancies. Survival data were drawn from the Australian cancer registries and the U.S. National Cancer Institute's Surveillance Epidemiology and End Results (SEER) registry, spanning the period January, 1990, until January, 2004. Overall the study concluded that chemotherapy con-

---

*G. Morgan, R. Ward, and M. Barton, "The contribution of cytotoxic chemotherapy to 5-year survival in adult malignancies," *Clinical Oncology* 16, no. 8 (2004): 549-60. See www.icnr.com/articles/ischemotherapyeffective.html for an article summarizing the results of the study.

tributes just over 2 percent to improved survival in cancer patients. There were a few exceptions, such as in cases of acute lymphocytic leukemia, Hodgkin's disease, nonseminomatous testicular cancer, choriocarcinoma, Wilm's tumor, and retinoblastoma, which do show some positive response to chemotherapy. But the study points out that these types of cancer account for only 2 to 4 percent of all cancers, leaving some 96 to 98 percent of other cancers, for which chemotherapy remains hugely ineffective. Despite this landmark study and further mounting evidence of chemotherapy's lack of effectiveness in prolonging survival, oncologists continue to present chemotherapy as a rational and promising approach to cancer treatment.

DENTAL POISONING

There is abundant scientific evidence to prove that the mercury in dental amalgam fillings is not safe; over time amalgam suppresses the immune system considerably and affects brain function. Patrick Stortebecker, former associate professor of neurology at the Karolinska Institutet, Sweden's top medical school, says that "the average amalgam filling will release up to half of its mercury content over a ten-year period (50 percent corrosion rate). It will therefore release between 68 and 130 micrograms per day, per filling."

Mercury amalgam restorative material generally contains 50 percent mercury in a complex mixture of copper, tin, silver, and zinc. It has been well documented that this mixture continually emits mercury vapor, which is dramatically increased by chewing, eating, brushing, and drinking hot liquids. Mercury has been shown to have damaging effects on the kidneys, central nervous system, and cardiovascular system; it has been implicated in gingival tattoos and may be a culprit in Alzheimer's disease, chronic fatigue syndrome, and MS. While mercury amalgams are detrimental to the patient, mercury vapors are also an occupational hazard for dental practitioners as well, not to mention the environmental impact of mercury. One study concluded that "dental amalgams, or fillings containing mercury, account for 3.7 tons of mercury discharge from dental offices each year. Mercury waste results when old mercury fillings are replaced with new ones. Mercury and dental fillings are flushed into chairside drains and enter the wastewater system, making their way into the environment through discharges in rivers and lakes, incineration, or land application of sewage sludge."*

In recent years, Norway, Sweden, Denmark, Russia, and Japan have enacted laws banning the use of amalgam, while Canada recommends limiting its use. Very recently the European Union (EU) totally banned the use of amalgam for children under the age of fifteen and for pregnant and breastfeeding women, a ruling that includes twenty-eight countries with a population totaling half a billion people. Moreover, the United Nations finalized a treaty in 2013 that includes important provisions to reduce and eliminate mercury pollution, one of them being a requirement for countries to phase down the use of dental amalgam. Charles Brown of Consumers for Dental Choice and the World Alliance for Mercury-Free Dentistry notes that "countries that have phased out amalgam recognize that mercury-free dental fillings are readily available, affordable and effective." In response to the mercury treaty provisions he explains, "This pushes the reset button on dentistry. Now the rest of the world can benefit from the experience of those countries."†

Unfortunately, the United States has not yet benefited from the leadership of European countries. While Maine, California, Connecticut, and Vermont have enacted legislation that requires that informed consent brochures be given to patients in a dental office before getting any teeth filled, the American Dental Association has said for the past 150 years that the mercury in amalgam is safe and does not leak. Other organizations of the medical establishment, including the Mayo Clinic, the American Academy of Pediatrics, the U.S. Environmental Protection Agency, the esteemed *New England*

---

*R. F. Erdlich, S. K. Rhoads, H. S. Cantrell, S. M. Azavedo, A. T. Newkirk, "Banning mercury amalgam," www.fda.gov/downloads/Adviso...e/DentalProductsPanel/UCM236379.pdf.

†Dr. Mercola, "New U.N. Treaty on Mercury Requires Countries to Phase Down Dental Amalgam." http://articles.mercola.com/sites/articles/archive/2013/02/05/mercury-un-treaty-abolishes-amalgam.aspx.

Journal of Medicine, and the American Cancer Society have also declared that amalgam fillings are safe, despite the overwhelming scientific evidence to the contrary on dental amalgam's links to a host of serious ailments and numerous scientific studies that support the fact that the mercury in amalgam is toxic. It seems that the FDA approved mercury fillings under a grandfather clause. Like asbestos, which at one time was claimed to be very safe for insulation and other industrial and building uses (or for that matter, like DDT, which was widely used as a pesticide in the United States in the 1940s and 1950s; glyphosate, a commonly used herbicide; and a host of other toxic substances that have gotten the government's official seal of approval), we are told that amalgam is perfectly safe.

What many of us do not realize is that there is still a large percentage of the population walking around with amalgam inside their mouths while it continues to leach small quantities (more than enough to destroy one's health) of mercury into their systems. Some dentists are now advertising amalgam removal with the discreet suggestion that it is dangerous and should be removed. Some more open-minded dentists are actually offering research evidence in the form of brochures that detail the dangers of dental amalgam and how important it is to be removed and replaced; some brave dentists are even making documentary videos that can be seen on YouTube warning people about the dangers of amalgam. One such dentist, Richard Fischer, says, "I do not feel comfortable using a substance designated by the EPA to be a waste disposal hazard. I can't throw it in the trash, bury it in the ground, or put it in a landfill, but they say it is okay to put it in people's mouths. That does not make sense."

Dr. Hulda Clark demonstrates in her book *The Cure for All Cancers* that amalgam removal has a close link with successful cancer recovery as well as many other immune-related conditions. Dr. Clark states that the removal of dental amalgam fillings (and also dead teeth from root canals) is a core factor in beating cancer and many other diseases because the mercury inside amalgam filling suppresses the immune system so much that complete recovery from serious illness becomes impossible without such an important procedure. She also claims that the mercury in amalgam attracts particularly dangerous microorganisms such as the human intestinal fluke, which has been shown to have a direct link with nearly all types of serious cancers.

If you have any dental amalgam tooth fillings, we highly recommended that you get them replaced as soon as possible, as the chances are fairly high that they are leaching mercury into your body every day. After removing your fillings and replacing them with a sealed composite resin, perform a complete heavy-metal, organ, and parasite detoxification program as described in the previous chapter.

Root Canal Controversy

In his book *Root Canal Cover-Up,* George E. Meinig, D.D.S., says, "Today, both patients and physicians have been 'brainwashed' to think that infections are less serious because we now have antibiotics. Well, yes and no. In the case of root-filled teeth, the no-longer-living tooth lacks a blood supply to its interior, so circulating antibiotics don't faze the bacteria living there because they can't get at them."

The teeth, as an important structure of the body, have a tremendous impact on one's overall health. The hidden dangers root canal procedures can pose to your health have been researched thoroughly, almost without any public awareness, for several decades. Once such researcher, Dr. Weston Price, began looking at this issue as far back as 1900, and he was at the forefront of establishing the link between root canals and disease. From 1900 to 1925, Dr. Price led a sixty-man team of researchers whose findings have been suppressed until now. With the help of his team he discovered that a whole host of systemic illnesses could result from latent infections lingering inside filled root canals. He went as far as to say that the millions of bacterial colonies that become entrenched inside the structure of teeth after root canals cause the largest number of diseases ever traced to a single cause.

What did Dr. Price observe to bring him to believe that root canals can cause arthritis and many other chronic degenerative diseases? He witnessed what is called the *focal infection theory* and presented it to the American Dental Association, for whom he served as its first research director. This theory states that bacteria in root-filled teeth can easily spread (metastasize) to other tissues and organs in the body. These microscopic organisms, which are usually harmless inside the mouth, begin to lurk in a complex maze of tubules before migrating into the interior of the tooth, where they colonize and spread. Although this theory is regarded as fact today, in 1925 the world's leading dental authorities as well as the American Dental Association failed to acknowledge this, claiming that antibiotics after root-canal therapy would prevent any latent infections. Even after the roots are removed during a root-canal procedure, the tooth remains, with a maze of tubules that were once rich in fluids and nutrients from its root. This is where the anaerobic bacteria live, mutate, and hide, away from antibiotics, only to then migrate into surrounding tissue before entering the bloodstream and then circulating throughout the body. The strength of your immune system is a major factor in how far these microorganisms can spread. If it is strong, the bacteria will not be able to get into your body, but if your immune system is weakened, they can really party hardy.

In many documented cases Dr. Price repeatedly found that after removing infected teeth, patients' health ailments would suddenly begin to improve. One experiment that astounded him occurred when he removed a seemingly healthy root-filled tooth from a woman suffering from arthritis and planted it under the skin of a healthy rabbit. After forty-eight hours he discovered the rabbit exhibiting signs of severe arthritis, while the woman was feeling much better. He performed similar procedures with many patients suffering from different illnesses, wherein the rabbits always contracted the specific illnesses that the patient had suffered from. Teeth that even looked good on an X-ray were storehouses for bacteria waiting to hatch into the bloodstream. Dr. Price was then further astounded when he discovered that the waste toxins produced from the mutated bacteria could be more dangerous than the actual bacteria.

Today holistic dentistry is a relatively small field, but this is changing fast as more and more people become aware of the important link between a healthy mouth and a healthy body. Choosing a dentist, like choosing a medical doctor, is more important than you think. One such dentist,

Victor Zeines, the author of the book *Healthy Mouth, Healthy Body,* is the founder of the Institute of Natural Dentistry, where he educates and trains other dentists in innovative, groundbreaking dental programs that offer more of a total wellness program rather than just focusing on filling holes. Dr. Zeines states that "conventional dental care can often cause more harm than good, because its treatments include mercury fillings, root canals, and fluoride treatments that fail to reduce cavities effectively and are linked to cancer, heart disease, toxic poisoning, and autoimmune illnesses such as asthma and arthritis." An effective way to prevent tooth decay and other dental problems is with an alkaline diet, as outlined in the nutritional program in chapter 3, combined with regular flossing and brushing and dental checkups. During Dr. Price's lifetime he traveled to many parts of the world studying different cultures and found only a few small pockets where people did not have cavities or dental disease. These cultures lived on diets of fresh, unprocessed, unrefined whole foods—just like the program outlined in this book. Even without the availability of toothbrushes, fancy toothpastes, or dental floss, these few cultures were almost 100 percent cavity-free.

"FOODS" THAT KILL

The Food and Nutrition Science Alliance reports that 52 percent of calories in the American diet come from fats and sugars alone. These are truly substances that kill. I do not use this description lightly; these foods—if you could call them foods—don't just have poor nutritional value (most are highly processed or refined); they also deplete the body of nutrients, in turn destroying your health. The following are some of the major "nonfoods" or "fake foods" commonly consumed in today's diet: sometimes the cure for your disease can simply involve not ingesting the things that are poisoning you.

Refined Wheat and Gluten Products

Do you remember making papier-mâché at school? The glue was made of wheat flour and water. Flour and water form glue. White (wheat) flour is an unnatural, processed, refined product that is not only starved of nutrients, it also depletes the body of nutrients. Most commercial breads, pastries, and baked flour products are made from this health-depleting, nutritionally starved flour that is processed, refined, and commonly bleached to appear more white and attractive. Whole wheat flour is not much better and still overly processed. "Whole-grain" stone-milled unprocessed flour does have some nutritional value and can be okay in small amounts but is still a poor food for most of us.

Wheat is best avoided by most folks as it is highly mucous-forming and high in gluten (food glue), which can block nutrient absorption into the body through the intestines. As most bread today is made from highly processed wheat flour that is devoid of fiber and nutrients and full of gluten, cut it way down or cut it out completely. If you eat gluten, make sure you are eating the whole grain itself and not the processed flour; eat only whole grains such as rye or spelt breads or pasta, available from health-food stores and in some supermarkets. As wheat slows the metabolism considerably for most blood types, completely cutting out wheat products and replacing one's carbohydrate intake with low-glycemic, complex, gluten-free whole grains can have a great benefit on weight loss and the immune system immediately. If you are suffering from any autoimmune condition I urge you to avoid gluten completely. There are many alternative grains that are gluten-free and make great-tasting breads and pastas. Some gluten-free grains are brown rice, buckwheat, quinoa, amaranth, and millet. Sprouted grain breads that use biodynamic organic wheat, rye, and spelt (such as Ezekiel) are tolerated by those who tolerate small amounts of gluten as they are raw and organic, but listen to your body when consuming these traditional organic breads and consume in moderation.

Processed, Refined, Trans-Fat Oils

What most of us do not realize is that oils are literally the blood essences of plants. As plants do not have blood as such, they contain oil, which has a variety of very healing essential nutrients for humans. When oil is extracted from the plant source, whether it be from a sunflower seed, almond, soybean, or an olive fruit, it becomes completely unstable and begins to oxidize as soon as it is out of its original environment. Chemical reactions occur, and these can be cancer forming.

Most commercial vegetable oils are extracted using a high-heat processing method combined with chemical solvents because it is cheaper. Long ago, the ancient Egyptians discovered that processed and heated oil quickly becomes rancid from oxidation, which creates what are known as *trans fats*. Trans fats attack liver and brain cells, contributing to autism, ADHD, and several other learning problems, as well as contributing to cancer and heart disease. Margarines and other vegetable-oil spreads are loaded with trans fats, which are highly dangerous to your health. The high temperature that vegetable oils are subjected to during manufacturing causes the oil to break their hydrogen bonds, creating a strong chemical reaction; this turns vegetable oils into a dangerous health hazard that can harden and block arteries, and instead of lowering cholesterol they increase it.

If the vegetable oil you buy does not specifically state "cold-pressed," do not consume it. As 95 percent of the vegetable oils sold commercially in modern supermarkets are processed, it is essential to exercise consumer awareness when it comes to purchasing vegetable oils. Often we see a TV personality telling us that we should eat those supposedly cholesterol-free processed vegetable oil spreads that look like butter but aren't, instead of the real thing, butter. Unfortunately, most of us are uneducated in modern nutrition, just like the doctors who recommend these harmful butter substitutes. So we buy these carcinogenic products, thinking we are doing ourselves a favor because, as advertised, it is "better than butter." Nothing could be further from the truth. Here we have a typical example of big business preying on the public's and many doctors' lack of general nutritional knowledge. Heat-treated oils and hydrogenated oils such as those found in vegetable-oil spreads made to look like butter are very indigestible and indirectly raise cholesterol levels. This is why people in countries such as France and Switzerland, who prefer real butter over fake butter, have much lower levels of cholesterol than their American and British friends, who eat large amounts of the processed vegetable oil and artificial butter and margarine—one reason these countries rank high in terms of cholesterol ratings. Remember that when poly- and mono-unsaturated oil is heated, it goes rancid, becoming highly indigestible and therefore quite dangerous. These vegetable oil spreads are made by cooking the oils at high temperatures, making them solidify, and then adding a coloring agent to make the result turn yellow so it *looks* like butter, and you buy it.

What does slip unnoticed into many people's shopping carts are the premade salad dressings (most of which contain canola oil, even the "organic" variety), packet sauces, and packet pastas. These products are so damaging to the heart and arteries because they contain unstable, rancid, trans fats that have been heated at extremely high temperatures and can cause cancer and many other diseases. To eat these is to pay the price in terms of your health, as the body cannot and does not digest these unnatural, processed, man-made fats. Get into the habit of reading labels and strictly avoid anything with vegetable oils (unless cold-pressed) and canola oil.

Pasteurized Dairy Products

In her book *The Cure for All Diseases,* Dr. Hulda Clark says, "People need to realize that pasteurization is not sterilization. All milk products go off if left in the fridge for too long, showing that bacteria and microorganisms are contained within them."

Cow's milk is designed for baby cows, not humans. While that may seem obvious, many people have been brainwashed into thinking that cow's milk is some sort of health food. Today's cow's milk is highly processed and pasteurized (heat-treated), which destroys raw milk's natural enzymes, causing incomplete digestion of the sugar and fats in milk. Even worse, we see most supermarkets selling UHT (ultrahigh-temperature processed) milk, which is often sold unrefrigerated. Even more disturbing is the fact that more than 80 percent of the organic milk sold in the United States is UHT-pasteurized. The official U.S. government definition of an ultrapasteurized dairy product stipulates "such product shall have been thermally processed at or above

280 degrees Fahrenheit for at least two seconds," either before or after packaging, to produce a product that has an extended shelf life.

Processed cow's milk, especially UHT milk, is devoid of natural enzymes, so it is very difficult to digest. Getting your hands on unprocessed fresh, raw cow's milk is virtually impossible, as it is banned from being sold to the public on the basis that it supposedly is not safe for human consumption. I find this amazing, as we drank enzyme-filled raw milk until relatively recently. Pasteurization allows big companies to lengthen the shelf life of milk for months, allowing more control over the market and the farmers.

One of the biggest lies of corporate marketing over the last century was saying that milk is a great source of calcium. It never was and never will be. Any educated twenty-first-century nutritional doctor will tell you that for every 100 grams of calcium found in milk, there is approximately 90 grams of phosphorus. Phosphorus bonds to calcium and literally blocks the absorption of calcium into the bones or even depletes it from your body. This is why the Japanese, who consume the lowest levels of cow's milk products in the world, have the lowest levels of osteoporosis and the strongest bones, and countries like the United States and Great Britain, which consume the largest amounts of dairy products, have the highest rates of osteoporosis in the world. Milk does nothing to prevent osteoporosis, as these cultural pictures demonstrate.

If you prefer to get your nutritional advice from a person who is well paid to tell you to drink milk in a TV ad, then go ahead. Otherwise, get the facts from someone not working for the dairy industry. I still find doctors who have virtually no education in nutrition giving out nutritional advice that says that milk is good for your bones. If you want to know about drugs, disease diagnosis, or surgery, go to your doctor for sure; but if you want accurate information on nutritional facts, think about talking to a professional naturopath. Do not be fooled into thinking your body needs cow's milk for health. You have no more need for cow's milk than you do for dog's milk or elephant's milk. Healthier alternatives to cow's milk include vegetarian sources such as rice and almond milk. And good sources of calcium that are low in phosphorous include sesame seed butter (tahini), nuts, and green leafy vegetables.

Sugar

Processed sugar is by far one of the most dangerous nonfoods widely consumed today, and a major killer. What we are talking about here is processed, refined white sugar and its other names, sucrose, fructose, and glucose. Brown sugar is actually white sugar with molasses spun back into it for color and is not much better for you. White sugar is a totally unnatural product, contrary to what you may be told on TV. White sugar does not contain a single nutrient required by the body, only refined, empty calories. It thus causes mineral imbalances and often contributes to arthritis, migraine headaches, mental disorders, depression, diabetes, and other degenerative diseases. Much of the glucose in products is synthetically made by treating cornstarch with hydrochloric acid. After extensive processing, there are many by-products that are made from sugarcane. Processed sugar and its many forms are devoid of nutrients and in fact deplete nutrients from the body. Raw cane sugar, which is only found at some health-food stores, is used traditionally in Asian cooking and does have some nutritional value and can be taken safely in small amounts.

Soft Drinks

The word *soda* derives from the word *sodium* and is so named because these beverages are sodium rich and potassium depleted. High levels of sodium in the body are directly related to cancer, according to German-born physician Dr. Max Gerson (1881–1959), founder of the Gerson Institute clinics in Tijuana, Mexico, and in Hungary, and a specialist in cancer causes and alternative treatments. As our bodies are designed for a potassium-to-sodium ratio of 4:1, foods rich in sodium such as animal products, processed foods, and soda drinks raise it to 2:1, a level commonly found in people with cancer. Sodas are also highly acidic and have a pH as low as 2.5 (with the pH of 7 being neutral), so you can see how dangerous these chemical beverages can be for your health. The bubbles in spring or ionized water are pure oxygen, but the bubbles in soft drinks are carbon dioxide, which then forms carbonic acid, a toxic by-product of the body. One can of a soft drink contains on average eight to ten teaspoons of highly processed sugar. It also contains other highly refined chemicals that are extremely dangerous to your health. Most also contain caffeine, which overstimulates the adrenal glands, producing yet more overacidity of the body and especially the stomach. Sodas also contain many artificial flavors and colors that impede proper liver function and have been shown to contribute to serious illnesses. The unusually high levels of phosphorus found in sodas pull calcium from the bones, causing osteoporosis and other mineral imbalances.

Diet sodas are especially dangerous because they contain artificial sweeteners. There is no evidence to prove that saccharin, a popular artificial sweetener, is safe in even small quantities. Saccharin derives its name from the word *saccharine,* meaning "sugary." The word is used figuratively, often in a derogative sense, to describe something unpleasantly overpolite or overly sweet. Saccharin is a by-product of bitumen from coal tar and is thus extremely dangerous. Aspartame, another common artificial sweetener found in diet soda, is a neurotoxin that has been shown to cross the blood-brain barrier, causing brain cancer and blindness in laboratory tests. Many people choose diet sodas because they are promoted as a diet alternative having no calories, but these "lite" sodas actually cause more weight gain than normal "heavy" sodas because of the chemicals in the artificial sweeteners. Although they may contain no calories, they indirectly affect and slow down the metabolic organs such as the liver and thyroid. They do not contain calories as they advertise, which is true, but they slow the metabolism, causing more weight gain in the long run.

Common Salt

Table salt and other common processed salts sold in grocery stores are not natural as many people think, nor do they occur in nature or in natural foods. Common table salt is a man-made chemical poison. Sodium chloride does occur in nature in combination with other trace mineral salts in the ocean from which it is derived. Consuming processed table salt and regular processed sea salt in any quantity causes mineral imbalances that lead to problems with the kidneys, blood pressure, and hardening of the heart and arteries and fluid retention. Replacing processed table salt with unprocessed Celtic sea salt, a true medicine that is available at health-food stores, is highly recommended and imperative for good health.

MSG

Commonly known as the "Chinese restaurant syndrome," the symptoms of MSG poisoning are many. MSG has been around since the early 1900s, but that does not make it safe. Today its consumption is at a record high, and it is commonly found in products like packaged soups, sauces, flavored snacks, chips, nuts, condiments, processed meats, and in most fast foods. It has serious links to diabetes, weight gain, asthma, neurological damage, learning disorders, endocrine dysfunctions, allergies, and more. MSGTruth.org is a very informative database created by former food-processing engineer and scientist Carol Hoernlein that has plenty of helpful information. Carol earned her degrees in food science and bioresource (agricultural) engineering at Rutgers University and worked in the research and development departments at the largest global food companies as a food scientist and food-process development engineer. She has also appeared in many well-known documentaries, such as *The Beautiful Truth* (2009). Go through your whole kitchen and start reading all product labels and throw out anything with this poison in it. Start reading all labels of products you are buying and look for an ingredient labeled "E621," or its full name, *monosodium glutamate*. Better still, throw out anything with any *E* numbers listed in the ingredients.

Coffee

Caffeine, contrary to many people's beliefs, is a poison. When concentrated, one drop injected into small rabbits produces instant death from heart failure. Instant coffee is highly acid forming and poisonous to your liver and digestive system. This is why it is often prohibited in patients suffering from ulcers. Coffee has a negative influence on the immune system and the nervous system because it creates sympathetic dominance (i.e., the fight-or-flight response), which is why it is so heavily promoted in the workplace, because it keeps you overstimulated and "on edge," ready for emergencies. Taoist health wisdom strongly recommends avoiding coffee, especially instant coffee, which is highly processed and harmful to one's health. Coffee may also inhibit B_{12} and other vital nutrients and minerals in your gut, drain the adrenal glands and kidneys, and interfere with GABA transmissions in your brain. Taoists view coffee as a "chi drainer," meaning that in the long term it takes more energy from your vital organs than it gives.

Consuming fresh, unprocessed, organic coffee that has been decaffeinated by means of water processing in small quantities can, for some people, result in minimal to no health problems and in some cases more energy, provided that only one cup is consumed daily. This organic form of decaffeinated coffee still contains small amounts of caffeine, and you can become more sensitive to it when consuming less, which is a good thing. In a healthy person one cup per day would be the maximum. If one is experiencing any health problems, avoid it altogether. Replace it with tea, especially green tea or oolong tea (both contain smaller amounts of caffeine), which have been shown in medical studies to prevent cancer, reduce obesity, and increase health because of their antioxidant properties.

Food Sprays and Pesticides

Going organic was once seen by many as being only for hippies, but these days it is a positively sensible idea. Today there are so many reasons that we need to begin heading back to our organic origins. Not so long ago, in the early 1900s, all food produce was organic, cancer and heart disease were not so common, and people did not have serious allergies like they do today. When you walked into a grocery store a sign did not advertise the food as organic or pesticide-free because everything was organic and pesticide-free in every store. Synthetic agrochemical pesticides had simply not yet been invented. Technically speaking, all plant food is organic, as it is based on carbon; however, since World War II, the word organic has been applied to food that has not been grown with synthetic chemicals, including pesticides and herbicides. With the advent of chemical-based agriculture, however, giant food companies have taken over the food supply, and with these toxic chemicals they're able to produce food faster and at a lower cost (read: higher profits) and are also able to keep supply above demand.

Organically grown produce, on the other hand, is not covered in a cocktail of poisonous chemicals. The average conventionally grown apple can contain up to twenty to thirty artificial poisons on its skin, even after you rinse it. Not only does chemically grown food contain toxic chemicals, it's less nutritious and tasty. Organic produce contains up to 50 percent more vitamins, minerals, enzymes, and other micronutrients than intensively farmed produce does, although this higher level depends on the mineral content of the soil it's grown in. Eating organic food is also a sure way to know that you are not eating any GMOs, since they have been introduced into the food chain by giant chemical companies. In fact, some of these companies are the same companies that invented chemical warfare. According to the Organic Consumers Association, "Supported by a $1.5 million grant from the U.S. Department of Defense, research at the Salk Institute has identified a gene that may link certain pesticides and chemical weapons to a number of neurological disorders, including the Gulf War syndrome and attention deficit/hyperactivity disorder (ADHD).*

Another reason to go organic is that the food is much more nutritious:

> Over a 2-year period, organically and conventionally grown apples, potatoes, pears, wheat, and sweet corn were purchased in the western suburbs of Chicago and analyzed for mineral content. Four to 15 samples were taken for each food group. On a per-weight

---

*Environment News Service, "More Evidence—Pesticides Cause Brain Damage," March 17, 2003, Organic Consumers Association, www.organicconsumers.org/old _articles/foodsafety/gulfwar040903.php.

basis, average levels of essential minerals were much higher in the organically grown than in the conventionally grown food. The organically grown food averaged 63% higher in calcium, 78% higher in chromium, 73% higher in iron, 118% higher in magnesium, 178% higher in molybdenum, 91% higher in phosphorus, and 125% higher in potassium and 60% higher in zinc. The organically raised food averaged 29% lower in mercury than the conventionally raised food.*

If you eat dairy or meat products, going organic has never been more essential to safeguard your and your family's health. Conventionally raised dairy cows and other farm animals are fed a dangerous cocktail of antibiotics, hormones, antiparasite drugs, and many other synthetic medicines on a daily basis, whether they have an illness or not. These drugs are passed directly on to the consumer when he or she is eating the dairy or meat products. Many of these chemicals are carcinogenic and contribute to a host of ailments. Animals that eat organic food or are grass-fed, on the other hand, show stronger immune systems. Be aware, meat eaters, that approximately 99 percent of nonorganic factory-farmed animals in the United Kingdom are fed GM soy; these figures are similar in other developed nations like the United States. Notably, there has never been a reported case of foot and mouth disease in organic, grass-fed cattle in the UK to date. Besides the fact that organic produce tastes a whole lot better than nonorganic, as the fruit and vegetables are full of juice and flavor, it's worth considering that organic food may not necessarily be more expensive than intensively farmed, chemically sprayed foods, as we tend to pay for these conventionally grown foods in the long run if you consider that we spend billions of dollars every year cleaning up the mess that pesticide use makes in the environment.

---

*"Organic food is more nutritious than conventional food," *Journal of Applied Nutrition* 45 (1993): 35–39; article cited by Organic Consumers Association, www.organicconsumers .org/old_articles/Organic/organicstudy.php.

HOUSEHOLD AND
PERSONAL-CARE PRODUCT CHEMICALS

Dr. Morton Walker, the author of ninety-one consumer books and over five thousand journal articles on natural and nontoxic methods of healing, says that "each person living in Western industrialized countries today is known to be at least a thousand times more polluted with toxic metals and/or heavy metals than anyone who lived when Christ walked the earth." No doubt many of these substances are to be found right in your own home. Are you aware that most household cleaning, personal-care, and beauty products contain dangerous chemical solvents and other petrochemicals that are carcinogenic and that also suppress the immune system? The website www.projectcensored.org reports that "in 1997 the number #2 censored story was cancer caused by cosmetics and personal care products."

It seems many of the by-products of the petroleum industry are being used in food and personal-care products as cheap foaming agents and preservatives. While it is impossible to list all the chemicals presently being used in food and personal-care products today, this information is easily available. Most of these synthetic chemicals show major carcinogenic properties and immune-suppressing effects. According to Dr. Hulda Clark, who has written extensively on cancer as well as solvent- and parasite-related illnesses, certain parasites have affinities for certain solvents. For example, benzene, a petroleum by-product used in personal-care products and some processed foods, has a close relationship with the human intestinal fluke. According to Dr. Clark, all those who test positive for the human intestinal fluke have high levels of this solvent inside them.

It is impossible to list all the chemicals that are used in our everyday products, and most of us don't read the labels on every product and research the ingredients, so how can we be assured that we are not buying products containing dangerous solvents and other chemicals? Thanks to an Australian company, there is now a simple pocket manual called *The Chemical Maze* that thoroughly details the major chemicals in commercial foods and personal-care products, including those misleading E-plus-a-number abbreviations that hide many toxic substances. This compact pocket manual gives you more power, allowing you to make safer choices on the products you purchase. This vital information is a major threat to chemical giants who produce these products—products that contain suspect petroleum-based chemical by-products that go by mysterious number abbreviations and are commonly found in personal-care and nutritional supplements. What you will discover is that these dangerous chemicals are basically in all the household and personal-care products found in the average supermarket. Thankfully, there are a few companies committed to selling organic, biodegradable, chemical-free household cleaning and personal-care products in health-food stores and online. Unfortunately for us consumers, it's difficult for these companies to enter the mainstream supermarket chains, as they risk opposition from large chemical corporations that control the market and corner the large chains with a better financial deal. And beware of "greenwashing." This term refers to when companies use tricky packaging and labeling, advertising a few ingredients on their cover label as "natural," even though the product is not certified organic or even natural. Make sure to look for registered organic certification.

Remember that the skin is the largest organ in the body, with the capacity to absorb anything placed on it. Soaps, shampoos, creams, and perfumes placed on the skin or near your mouth are absorbed into your bloodsteam immediately. One unusual but sensible way to determine if your personal-care products are safe is to ask, "Would I drink or eat the products that I'm placing on my body?" If the answer is no, then it is highly likely that the product you are using is harmful and contains dangerous toxic or carcinogenic chemicals. If it is not safe to eat or drink, do not put it on your body. In my clinical practice I see numerous conditions, including fatigue, autoimmune diseases, and poor immunity that are related to overexposure to toxic personal-care products. Not only do I ask my patients when they come to see me to bring in all the supplements and drugs they are currently taking, I also ask them to bring in all their personal-care products. Most bring in large bags or small suitcases full of toxic, chemical-laden personal-care products such as underarm spays, toothpastes (which go inside the mouth), and moisturizing creams. When I take the time to sit down with them and read the ingredients and cross-reference them with chemical reference books such as *The Chemical Maze,* they are shocked and begin to associate their health condition not only with their diet and lifestyle, but also with these toxic chemical-based products that are directly applied to the skin or the inside of the mouth.

Remembering that anything you place on your skin will be immediately absorbed into your body, begin to be aware of these petrochemical-based, cancer-causing agents. Talcum, for example, is a mineral called tremolite, which is a form of asbestos, but many of us just slap it on, thinking it's safe. But would you eat this? A 1998 study published in the *American Journal of Epidemiology* concluded that applying talcum to the body can increase a woman's chances of developing ovarian cancer.*

Start by reading the labels of the products you are using now and see if any of there are any dangerous chemicals or mysterious numbered ingredients in them. If there are, stop using them immediately and begin using the steps outlined in chapter 4 on cleansing. I highly recommend you do some research on the amount of industrial chemicals that enter your body daily via household and personal-care products. One study shows that women absorb up to five pounds of damaging chemicals a year from beauty products alone, all of which are slowly or sometimes quickly killing them.†

Parabens

Butylparaben, ethylparaben, isobutylparaben, isopropylparaben, methylparaben, propylparaben—these are just a few of the names that refer to

---

*L. S. Cook, M. L. Kamb, and N. S. Weiss, "Perineal powder exposure and the risk of ovarian cancer," *American Journal of Epidemiology* 145, no. 5 (1997): 459–65.
†Fiona MacRae, "Women Absorb Up to 5 lbs. of damaging chemicals a year thanks to beauty products," www.dailymail.co.uk/health/article-462997/Women-absorb-5lbs-damaging-chemicals-year-thanks-beauty-products.html.

parabens, common preservatives that have been linked to breast cancer. They are all used to prevent bacteria in personal-care products but once upon a time organic essential oils did this job and did it much better. A 2012 study indicated that 99 percent of breast cancers showed high concentrations of these parabens.*

Isopropyl and Wood Alcohols

These are colorless, volatile, flammable liquids. This toxic solvent is denaturant (a poisonous substance that changes another substance's natural qualities). Isopropyl alcohol is found in hair-coloring products, body rubs, hand lotions, aftershave lotions, fragrances, and many other cosmetics. This petroleum-derived substance is also used in antifreeze. According to *A Consumer's Dictionary of Cosmetic Ingredients,* inhalation or ingestion of isopropyl and wood alcohol vapors may cause headaches, flushing, dizziness, mental depression, nausea, vomiting, narcosis, and coma.

Mineral and Petroleum-Based Oils

Baby oil, that innocently marketed product we're all familiar with, is 100 percent mineral oil, which is derived from crude oil. And this commonly used petroleum ingredient coats the skin just like the plastic wrap you put over your food. The skin's natural immune barrier is compromised and so is its ability to breathe; so too is its ability to absorb the natural moisture factor (moisture and nutrition). As your skin is an eliminatory organ, the skin's ability to release toxins and breathe is impeded by this "plastic wrap," which can promote acne and other skin conditions, including the premature aging effect. And to think that mothers put it on their newborns. . . .

---

*L. Barr, G. Metaxas, C. A. Harbach, L. A. Savoy, and P. D. Darbre, "Measurement of paraben concentrations in human breast tissue at serial locations across the breast from axilla to sternum," *Journal of Applied Toxicology* 32, no. 3 (2012): 219–32.

Polyethylene Glycol (PEG)

This chemical is used in antifreeze, in cleaners that dissolve oil and grease, and to stabilize and thicken products. Because of their effectiveness, PEGs are often used in caustic spray-on oven cleaners and in many personal-care products, even toothpaste. PEGs do strip the natural moisture factor, leaving the immune system vulnerable. There is actually no difference between the PEG used in industrial products and that used in your personal-care products. It is used in industry to break down protein and cellular structure, so it easily moves through your skin when it's found in most forms of makeup, hair products, lotions, aftershaves, deodorants, mouthwashes, and toothpaste. Because of its ability to quickly penetrate the skin, the EPA requires workers to wear protective gloves, clothing, and goggles when working with PEG. The material's safety data sheets warn against skin contact, as PEG has systemic consequences, such as brain, liver, and kidney abnormalities.

Sodium Laurel Sulfate and Sodium Laureth Sulfate (SLS and SLES)

Used as detergents and surfactants, these two closely related compounds are found in car-wash soaps, garage floor cleaners, and engine degreasers. Yet both SLS and SLES are used more widely as one of the major ingredients in cosmetics, toothpaste, hair conditioner, and about 90 percent of all shampoos and products that foam. Mark Fearer, in an article titled "Dangerous Beauty," says, "In tests, animals that were exposed to SLS experienced eye damage, along with depression, labored breathing, diarrhea, severe skin irritation, and corrosion and death."

According to the American College of Toxicology, both SLS and SLES can cause malformation in children's eyes. Other research has indicated SLS may be damaging to the immune system. Skin layers may separate and inflame due to its protein-denaturing properties. It is possibly the most dangerous of all ingredients in your personal-care products. Research has shown that SLS when combined with other chemicals can be transformed into nitrosamines, a potent class of carcinogens that cause the body to absorb nitrates at higher levels than when eating nitrate-contaminated food (and it has been found that SLS stays in the body for up to five days). Other studies have indicated that SLS easily penetrates the skin and enters and maintains residual levels in the heart, the liver, the lungs, and the brain. This poses serious questions regarding its potential health threat as it is a common ingredient in shampoos, cleansers, and toothpaste. If your toothpaste does not list the ingredients, it is highly likely to contain these two dangerous chemicals.

Coloring Agents

Products labeled FD&C or D&C followed by a number are coloring agents known to cause skin irritation and sensitivity. Many are also believed to be carcinogenic. Many color pigments cause skin sensitivity and irritation, and the absorption of certain colors can cause depletion of oxygen in the body and even death according to *A Consumer's Dictionary of Cosmetic Ingredients*. As most of these artificial chemicals are derived from coal tar, there is a great deal of controversy about their use. Additionally, the majority of animal studies have shown them to be carcinogenic.*

Synthetic Fragrances

Synthetic (nonessential oil) fragrance is present in most deodorants, shampoos, sunscreens, and skin- and body-care products, baby products, and in all nonorganic laundry and dishwashing products, so please buy organic products only. All of the compounds in fragrances today are synthetic, and most are carcinogenic or otherwise toxic. Fragrance listed on a label can indicate the presence of hundreds of separate ingredients, and all of them are man-made and synthetic. Symptoms reported to the FDA have included headaches, dizziness, rashes, skin discoloration, violent coughing, vomiting, and allergic skin irritations.

---

*For more information on toxic coloring agents see http://articles.mercola.com/sites /articles/archive/2011/02/24/are-you-or-your-family-eating-toxic-food-dyes.aspx.

Clinical observation has shown that exposure to synthetic fragrances can affect the central nervous system, causing depression, hyperactivity, irritability, inability to cope, and other behavioral changes. These are just a few of the industrial chemicals that enter your body if you use commercial personal-care products daily. Again, I recommend referring to the pocket guide to chemicals, *The Chemical Maze,* by Bill Statham as a simple guide for your family.

There are many countries now producing excellent certified organic personal-care and beauty products. Personally we have found that the strictest standards for organic labeling are found in Australia, with products of excellent quality and integrity. A company called Synthesis Organics, www.synthesisorganics.com, manufactures with the highest standards, and their products contain Taoist energy-imbued waters and oils. These are the best-quality products that we have personally tested.

Sunblocks

The increasing rates of skin cancer have placed the use of sunblock creams right up there with taking vitamins in terms of "healthy" habits. Yet despite all the slapping on of sunblocks, 50 percent of all cancers in the United States in 2002 were skin cancers, of which nearly 10,000 cases were fatal. In the 1960s your risk of skin cancer was 1 in 600, but today this has jumped to 1 in 60—and this is despite the massive increase in the popular use of sun-protection agents. It seems as if we're being told the sun is bad for you, that it causes cancer, but that's simply not true! Vitamin D (synthesized from sun exposure), which is deficient in many people today, has actually been shown to prevent cancer. During my medical studies in college I was introduced to a theory presented by one of my professors: that the use of sun protection creams combined with using sunglasses are two prime reasons that skin cancer ranks as the most common type of cancer today. Initially when people hear a statement like this they think it sounds ridiculous because of all the brainwashing we've been subjected to on the importance of using chemical sunblocks and protecting ourselves from the sun, but when we look at the facts, this professor's theory makes a whole lot of sense.

Commercially made sunblock creams are made from industrial petrochemical by-products. While they do help minimize your chances of getting burned, they contain an array of carcinogenic petrochemicals. As the skin is the largest organ in the body, anything that is placed on it is absorbed into your body. These chemicals can quickly be absorbed into the epidermal layers of the skin and react with the DNA of your cells, and also go into the bloodstream, clogging up the liver. Furthermore, although sunblocks limit you from getting burned by the sun, they do not protect you from the damaging UVA rays that actually cause skin cancer. By far the best way to reduce sunburn is by wearing clothing and limiting your exposure to the sun to the morning and the afternoon, avoiding exposure to the sun at midday, when the highest number of damaging rays are present.

A fascinating health fact is that broccoli extract is better than common sunscreen for preventing skin cancer. A recent study conducted by a team of researchers at the Johns Hopkins University School of Medicine found that the chemicals in broccoli, including sulforaphane, glutathione, S-transferase, and superoxide dismutase, when applied to the skin, can neutralize the DNA-damaging molecules that are created in the skin by the mix of oxygen and sunlight. They can also temper the inflammatory reactions that can turn precancerous cells into life-threatening tumors.[*]

According to Dr. Sharon Moalem, a British researcher, regular use of sunglasses most surely increases our risk of skin cancer. This is because the amount of melanin, the brown pigment produced by your skin that protects you from sunburn damages, is primarily regulated by the eye's perception of UV light. When you wear sunglasses it easily tricks the body into thinking it is shady and the body stops producing the optimal levels of melanin, making you more susceptible to being injured by the sun. As well, if you walk around all day in your swimsuit and nothing else but your sunglasses, you are more likely to get burned, increasing your skin cancer risks.

---

[*]Rick Weiss, "Broccoli Extract Could Help Head Off Skin Cancer," *Washington Post,* Tuesday, October 23, 2007.

Omega-3 Deficiency and Skin Cancer

There is strong evidence that the sudden increase over the last century in omega-6 fats (from common vegetable oils) and deficiencies of omega-3s (from flax, perilla, hemp, and fish) disrupts the omega-6:3 ratio, causing cancer, especially skin cancer. In 1993, the Department of Social and Preventive Medicine of the University of Queensland Medical School, Australia, published a study finding a 40 percent reduction in melanoma among those who ate fish regularly. In June 2001, the prestigious National Academy of Sciences published a comprehensive review titled "Omega 3 but not omega 6 fatty acids inhibit AP-1 activity and cell transformation in JB6 cells," showing that the omega-6:3 ratio was the key to preventing skin cancer development.

There are many natural, nontoxic ways to protect yourself from the sun's damaging midday infrared rays, such as not sunbathing between 11 a.m. and 3 p.m. Also, use only natural sun creams available from health-food stores that contain no petrochemical by-products or carcinogenic chemicals. Use aloe vera gel always after sunbathing to cool your skin and prevent burning. Do not be a consumer dummy; avoid getting sucked into the corporate marketing lies that sunlight is dangerous and bad for you and that you need to slather yourself in a dangerous cocktail of cancer-causing chemicals to protect yourself. Get educated about basic nutritional facts, such as getting your omega-6:3 ratios correct.

Healthy Alternatives

We see many clients whom we advise to stop using commercial personal-care and household cleaning products immediately and replace them with organic plant-based products from the health-food store or use homemade products. They usually just agree and then go home and do nothing about it. Most of them seem to think that this kind of advice is too extreme and that we are crazy or we are getting a cut from the local health-food store. Unfortunately, many of these people who doubt me have a terribly hard time getting well. Most blame me, the health practitioner, or the one before me. Some blame their job, relationship, or even the herbs or medicines that just are not enough. The fact is their body is laden with cancer-causing, immune-suppressing chemicals because of their lack of awareness of how dangerous they really are, combined with their persistence (even after being told) in using them. The thinking seems to be that if they are so dangerous, why would they be allowed to be sold?

We live in a corporate-dominated world where money is more powerful than doing the right thing. I strongly suggest replacing your chemical products with plant-based products immediately, and be especially aware of marketing tricks in which companies use terms like *natural, nature organics,* or *naturally sourced* on their bottles. Most of these products are full of bad ingredients with a little plant extract included for advertising purposes. The only way to be safe is to read the label of ingredients and then use the pocket chemical guide *The Chemical Maze.*

There are many recipes available online for making your own cleaning products, perfumes, shampoos, and skin creams, but if you do not have the time to make your own, your local health-food store stocks them. Most health-food stores sell traditional olive or coconut oil soaps and natural, chemical-free cosmetics. Most commercial soaps dry your skin anyway, so you are compelled to also buy the same company's (or its subsidiary's) skin cream, which in turn poisons you. Toothpaste is a big one in disguise, because most people do not understand that anything they put inside the mouth is quickly absorbed into the gums and down the back of the throat. Every time you brush your teeth with those fancy-colored, hot-flavored toothpastes you see advertised, you get partially poisoned. Simple ingredients like lemon juice, baking soda, vinegar, and hydrogen peroxide are all you need for household and personal cleaning. These few simple ingredients replace hundreds of toxic products.

THE FACTS ON FLUORIDE

Even the book that doctors have on their own desk for drug referencing contains information stating that fluoride is dangerous. The *Physicians' Desk Reference* states: "There are reportedly more than 11 million Americans with diabetes. Since many diabetics drink more liquids than other people, these 11 million Americans probably should not drink fluoridated water, because in doing so, they will receive an excessive dose of fluoride. Kidney disease, by definition, lowers the efficiency of the kidneys, which is your main route of fluoride elimination. So those people with kidney disease also shouldn't drink fluoridated water."

The first occurrence in history of fluoridated drinking water occurred in Nazi concentration camps. Nazi scientists had little concern about fluoride's supposed beneficial effect on the prisoners' teeth; instead, the alleged reason for mass-medicating water with sodium fluoride was to sterilize humans and dull their senses, turning the people in the concentration camps into calm submissiveness. The Nazis dreamed of a world dominated and controlled by Nazi philosophy; therefore, the German chemists worked out an ingenious plan to control the masses. The original plan was to control and reduce the population with mass medication of drinking-water supplies by producing sterility in women and chemical intoxication. It just so happens that sodium fluoride, the same inorganic chemical that is added to some of today's cities' and towns' water supplies, was the ideal chemical for the Nazis' purpose of population control. Nazi chemists clearly proved that repeated doses of fluoridated water will in time reduce one's power to resist domination, by poisoning and narcotizing certain areas of the brain. Basically, fluoride makes you more submissive to those who govern and control you. Furthermore, it may not even prevent dental caries, the rationale for its use in toothpaste and in drinking water:

> The use of professional dental applications of fluoride may not be providing any benefit to children, even though they are widely used and generally accepted to reduce the rate of tooth decay. This study evaluated the association between this practice and the number of cavities.

The data from over 15,000 children and for treatment provided by over 1,500 different dentists were analyzed. The researchers followed up with the children for a period averaging over 5 years. No differences in tooth decay rates were seen for "baby" or permanent teeth.[*]

According to a German study published in 2000 in the journal *Community Dentistry and Oral Epidemiology,* a number of towns and cities in the former East German Republic stopped the artificial fluoridation of their water. Though they braced themselves for a corresponding rise in dental cavities, incredibly, the dental decay rates actually went down. Although this outcome would seem contrary to commonly held beliefs on fluoridation, cavity rates are still coming down throughout Germany, regardless as to whether water is fluoridated or not. Researchers studied more than 15,000 children in the formerly fluoridated German towns of Spremberg and Zittau. Children had been examined repeatedly over the past twenty years. Cavity levels in twelve-year-old children significantly decreased during the years 1993 through 1996. These results provide even more support for the contention that caries prevalence may continue to fall after the reduction of fluoride concentration in the water supply.[†]

Even in minute quantities, as in toothpastes, sodium fluoride is a deadly poison, affecting the brain and nervous system. Sodium fluoride water solutions are used in some European countries for the cheapest and most effective rat killers known to chemists: it is colorless, odorless, and tasteless, and there is no antidote to this poison that brings about instant and complete extermination of the rodents.

Understand that sodium fluoride is an entirely different chemical compound from the element fluorine or organic calcium fluorophosphates, which occur naturally in our water supply and are needed to

---

[*]S. A. Eklund, J. L. Pittman, and K. E. Heller, "Professionally applied topical fluoride and restorative care in insured children," *Journal of Public Health Dentistry* 60, no. 1 (2000): 33–38.

[†]W. Künzel, T. Fischer, R. Lorenz, and S. Brühmann, "Decline of caries prevalence after the cessation of water fluoridation in the former East Germany," *Community Dentistry and Oral Epidemiology* 28, no. 5 (2000): 382–89.

build and strengthen bones and teeth. This organic calcium fluorophosphate, which is derived from a whole food nutritious diet, is actually an edible organic salt. Why then would government doctors and scientists, with the overwhelming evidence of the effect that the inorganic chemical sodium fluoride has on health problems, persuade politicians to fluoridate our public water supplies? There are many theories about the rationale for this insane practice, including that put forward by chemist Emanuel Bronner, a nephew of Albert Einstein who had been a prisoner of Nazi Germany during World War II, and who went on to gain fame as the inventor of Dr. Bronner's soap:

> It appears that the citizens of Massachusetts are among the "next" on the agenda of the water prisoners. There is a sinister network of subversive agents, Godless "intellectual" parasites, working in our country today whose ramifications grow more extensive, more successful and more alarming each new year and whose true objective is to demoralize, paralyze, and destroy our great Republic—from within if they can, according to their plan—for their own possession.*

Those countries that have banned fluoride in the water supply are Sweden, Norway, Denmark, Germany, Italy, Belgium, Austria, France, and the Netherlands. Despite these bans on water fluoridation, the United States continues in its efforts to achieve the goal of fluoridating every community water supply within its borders. Allopathically trained dentists are familiar with the American Dental Association's promotion of fluoride. In fact, this is probably where you were told that fluoride is good for you, despite fluoride's toxicity and the numerous studies that reveal increased tooth decay after fluoride use, not decreased, and the fact that cities where fluoride is used show increased rates of cancer caused by unscheduled DNA synthesis and mutagenic effects on the body's cells.

A past president of the American Medical Association, Dr. Charles

---

*From a letter published in the *Catholic Mirror,* Springfield, Mass., January 1952.

Heyd, has said, "Do not drink fluoridated water. . . . Fluoride is a corrosive poison which will produce harm on a long-term basis." According to studies by Dr. Gerard Judd, a chemist on the Manhattan project, where he worked with fluoride, and later authored *Good Teeth, Birth to Death,* the United States sees a 22 percent increase in decay every sixteen years with fluoride use.

There are three basic compounds commonly used for fluoridating drinking water supplies in the United States: sodium fluoride, sodium silicofluoride, and hydrofluorosilicic acid. Having sodium fluoride in our water is one thing, but sodium hydrofluorosilicic acid is one of the most reactive chemical species known to man, with the ability to eat through metal and plastic pipes and corrode many materials, including stainless steel, while also dissolving rubber tires and melting concrete. This is just one of the many chemicals added to your water supplies to supposedly produce healthy teeth.

The allopathic-oriented American Dental Association states that fluoride is safe, as do the politicians and companies that make these chemicals, but there is no hard evidence to back up this claim—in fact, quite the opposite, as shown in almost all studies. George Meinig, a founder of the American Academy of Endodontics, says, "You have been led to believe the fluorine makes teeth harder. The fact is it actually makes teeth softer."*

Studies show that fluoride does the following:

- Inactivates sixty-two enzymes
- Increases the aging process
- Increases the incidence of cancer and tumor growth
- Disrupts the immune system
- Causes genetic damage
- Interrupts DNA repair and enzyme activity[†]

---

*"The Fluoride Controversy," http://articles.mercola.com/sites/articles/archive/2008/01/02/fluoride-controversy.aspx.

[†]Studies cited in "The Fluoride Controversy," http://articles.mercola.com/sites/articles/archive/2008/01/02/fluoride-controversy.aspx.

We do not believe that the public is aware of the long-term dangers of fluoridated water or anything with fluoride in it, such as toothpaste, and in fact that most of the population is ignorant of the facts. This may be because people assume that governments are looking out for our best interests, but this sort of attitude has put us in the health crisis we are in today. Let's step out of the cloud we've been in and start talking to our local government officials about ending the poisoning of our communities.

The good news is that there are simple ways you can remove sodium fluoride from your body and pituitary gland, which is where it tends to accumulate. Substances such as SSKI iodide; foods rich in iodine like seaweeds; selenium and foods rich in selenium such as Brazil nuts; boron and foods rich in boron like beans, almonds, prunes, dates, and raisins; and the herbs turmeric and tamarind have all been shown to be beneficial for removing the accumulation of fluoride.

Sixth Immortal Healer—Li Tieh-Kuai

Internal Exercises and Structural Balance

The sages awaken through self-cultivation;
Deep, profound, their practices require great effort.
Fulfilling vows illumines the Heavens.
Breathing nourishes youthfulness.

FROM *THE JADE EMPEROR'S MIND SEAL CLASSIC*
TRANSLATED BY STUART ALVE OLSON

The healing of internal exercise and structural balance is symbolized by Li Tieh-Kuai. Li was born during the second-century CE Han Dynasty and is sometimes depicted in Chinese art as a dirty old beggar with an unkempt beard and dirty face, walking with the aid of a large iron crutch. Li lived in the mountains for forty years, where he devoted himself to practicing meditation. Legend has it that Li earned his epithet Iron Crutch Li as a result of an incident on his path to attaining immortality. It seems that Li was once handsome and fit and had mastered the Tao to the point where he could go for weeks without food or water, so deep was his meditation. Word of his accomplishments eventually reached the sage Lao-tzu, the sage who authored the Tao Te Ching, who decided to mentor him.

> Eventually, Laozi [Lao-tzu] taught Li how to make a voyage of the spirit—separating his soul from his body in order to travel to the celestial realms. After this final lesson, the Old Master invited his pupil to visit him in the heavenly abode of the immortals and gods. Duly excited by this possibility, Li Tieguai began to prepare for his journey, instructing his most prized student in how to care for his material body while he was away. As a contingency, he further advised the young man that his body should be immediately cremated if he did not return within seven days. Unfortunately, while Li Tieguai's spirit was off among the celestial spheres, his pupil received some troubling news: His beloved mother had taken ill. Though he was consumed by anxiety over his mother's health, the young apprentice remained conscious of his duty to his master and continued his vigil over Li's lifeless body. However, on the evening of the sixth day, this stress proved to be too taxing. The student, sure that his master had forever departed the material realm, quickly burned his body and rushed home to tend to his mother. Soon after, Li's soul returned to our plane, only to find that his fine-featured body had been reduced to a pile of ashes. Fearful that he should be extinguished, Li quickly entered the first available material form that he could find—the body of a recently expired beggar-man.*

Initially repulsed by this unattractive body due to ego clinging, Li finally accepted it when his teacher convinced him that with it he would realize the irrelevance of the physical body and thereby gain immortality.

This Taoist Immortal represents the element of fire, the symbol of action, warmth, circulation, and activity, as well as representing the phoenix rising from the ashes. Taoists have long maintained that if we

---

*"Li Tieguay," *New World Encyclopedia*.

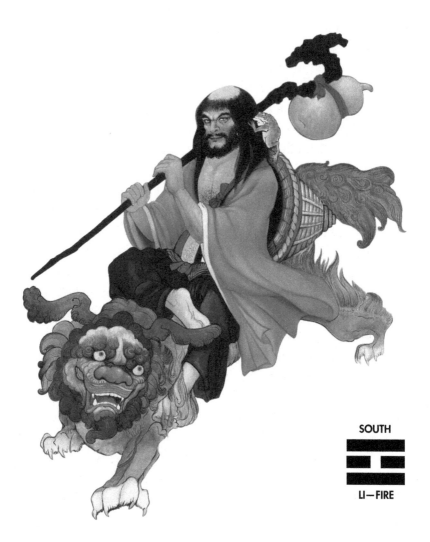

SOUTH

LI—FIRE

Fig. 6.1. Li Tieh-Kuai (Li Tie Guai)

do the correct exercises, especially the internal ones, our body will need less food and gather its chi from the cosmos.

What the ancient Egyptians were referring to in the proverb "Exercise is the daughter of health" was internal exercise rather than external exercise. Many of us do not even realize that there is actually a difference between the two. Activities like swimming, running, cycling, aerobics, and working out at the gym are all external exercises. External exercises work on the physical body, on the muscles and joints. While they do affect the internal organs by increasing circulation, they do not work on balancing the subtle energetic, magnetic, or bioelectric fields within the human body. For this, internal exercises such as yoga, Tai Chi, and Chi Kung are taught in traditional medical systems to balance the subtle energy fields of the body and thereby improve the internal health of the organs and energy pathways of the body, mind, and spirit. Internal exercises must be combined with external exercises if one is to achieve true health.

We are constantly hearing stories of professional athletes such as runners and swimmers falling ill and even dying of serious illnesses like stroke and pneumonia at very young ages. These top athletes may have had external fitness but they did not have internal health. Going to the gym and having a physical fitness regimen does not give you health. True health originates internally and radiates outward. The exercises taught in the ancient systems of yoga and Chi Kung are proven health practices that emphasize both internal and external fitness. By the same token, traveling to India or China and studying with a yoga master or guru, or having many books on spirituality will not give you internal health and fitness; daily practice of just a few simple exercises that can be learned very easily will, however. That said, it is highly recommended that for maximum effectiveness of an internal exercise practice, you should seek a qualified teacher who can work with your personal needs.

When we perform external exercises, our body produces a larger amount of waste products along with more free radicals. When exercise is done incorrectly and when one does not take nutritional supplements while exercising to combat the side effects of exercise, illnesses can result, especially those of the immune and nervous systems. Exercising without nutritional supplementation is like trying to run a car without oil; it will eventually burn out your engine. It is a big fallacy that external exercises are a replacement for healthy eating and internal exercises. It is an even bigger fallacy that exercise brings a youthful body and long life, as those who do a lot of exercise in their younger years, such as marathon runners, have also been shown to have shorter life spans. Lactic acid, a by-product of muscle metabolism, is usually cleaned up by the lymphatic system during and after exercise, but if the body produces high enough levels it can literally melt muscle tissue and fry your immune and nervous systems. Today's sports headlines are packed with stories about top athletes dropping dead either on or off the sports arena for this very reason. This preventable scenario is mainly due to increased acid levels in the body that comes about because of a combination of strenuous exercise without proper supplementation and a poor diet.

Consuming "energy bars" and "energy drinks" that proliferate nowadays is not the answer to gaining back energy lost through exercise. Many people in the United States and Canada are aware of the story of Brian Maxwell, a Canadian athlete, track coach, entrepreneur, and philanthropist, and the originator of the PowerBar. Maxwell was an excellent athlete and marathon runner (external exercise) who was part of the Canadian Olympic team that boycotted the 1980 Moscow games. Sadly, despite all the exercise in the world, he died in 2004 of a heart attack at the age of fifty-one. Maxwell's million-dollar company produces "energy" bars whose main ingredient is high-fructose corn syrup, a type of processed, GMO sugar, as well as "milk protein," another kind of sugar that comes from pasteurized cow's milk. Both these ingredients raise insulin levels, considerably damaging the arteries and the heart itself, forming the right conditions for a heart attack. In the 1970s it was commonly thought among many in the medical profession that if you ran a marathon you would never get heart disease, but Maxwell certainly proved that not to be the case.

We are increasingly hearing about professional athletes dying on football fields and basketball courts. Athletes, professional and non-professional, are beginning to see the dangers of taking synthetically produced nutritional supplements and eating high-carbohydrate diets and are beginning to head back to the original organic whole-food nutritional supplements and low-carb diets. We are slowly beginning to understand that when we exercise on a regular basis we literally burn up several times more nutrients compared to just sitting around. It's like when you're driving and if you're too hard on the gas pedal, you'll have poor mileage; similarly, those who exercise need to understand that what you burn up during exercise must be replaced or illness will result, and you cannot get what you need from processed food supplements and isolated vitamins and minerals.

Just as important are the fuels we burn during exercise. Waste products (just like car exhaust) need to be eliminated from the body at optimal levels. If there is a problem with the exhaust of a car, the car will pollute; similarly, if the eliminatory organs of the body are not excreting the acid waste products that are produced from exercise at fast enough levels, the body will pollute in its own wastes. These days many athletes are doing more cross-training and incorporating yoga and Tai Chi into their regimen to balance the side effects of too much external exercise. External exercises such as running create acidity in the body and burn large amounts of vital nutrients from the tissues, while internal exercises such as yoga, Tai Chi, and Chi Kung can actually conserve nutrients while helping to alkalize the tissues of the body. This is because the exercise techniques involved in these internal disciplines balance the systems of the body while also energizing them.

EXERCISE AS A FORM OF MEDICINE

In a consumer report survey in India of approximately 46,000 people, most found that exercise was just as effective as prescription drugs for handling health problems such as arthritis, back pain, and prostrate problems. In fact, for health ailments such as allergies, depression, and insomnia it scored better than any medications, even natural ones. The Food and Nutrition Science Alliance meanwhile has reported that "poor diet and lack of exercise are related to just as many cancer cases as smoking."

The effects that internal exercises such as Tai Chi have on health have been extensively studied of late. A meta-analysis of forty-seven studies from English and Chinese databases done at Tufts Medical Center concluded that Tai Chi practice brought considerable improvements in balance and strength, respiratory function, flexibility, immune function, and a reduction in pain from arthritis and muscular tension.* Another study carried out in 2002 on elderly women concluded that there were significant improvements in balance, functional mobility, and fear of falling after just two thirty-minute Tai Chi classes a week over the twelve-week period of the study.† Expert panels, convened by organizations such as the Centers for Disease Control and Prevention (CDC), the American College of Sports Medicine (ACSM), and the American Heart Association (AHA), along with the 1996 U.S. Surgeon General's Report on Physical Activity and Health, have all reinforced scientific evidence that links regular exercise to various measures of cardiovascular health.‡

It is impossible for us to demonstrate in this book the hundreds of internal exercises that we know to be helpful for curing disease or for one to regain optimal health and maintain it. Because such an in-depth review is beyond the scope of this book, we will focus on the exercises that we personally have found to be the most effective and simplest to perform. For some of you these exercises are not new; in that case, we only wish to remind you of their importance and that they need to be incorporated into even an advanced program of health exercises. For those who are experiencing them for the first time, they are here for you to begin your journey with internal exercise and to encourage you to explore more of the internal exercise systems that are available, such as yoga and Chi Kung.

INNER SMILE AND SIX HEALING SOUNDS (INTERNAL ALCHEMY EXERCISE)

Taoist sages discovered that consciousness is rooted not only in the brain, but is found in every cell and every organ of the body. By

---

*C. Wang, J. P. Collet, and J. Lau, "The effect of Tai Chi on health outcomes in patients with chronic conditions: A systematic review," *Archives of Internal Medicine* 164, no. 5 (2004): 493–501.

†H. M. Taggart, "Effects of Tai Chi exercise on balance, functional mobility, and fear of falling among older women," *Applied Nursing Research* 15, no. 4 (2002): 235–42.

‡Jonathan Myers, "Exercise and cardiovascular health," *Circulation* 107, no. 1 (2003). https://doi.org/10.1161/01.CIR.0000048890.59383.8D.

literally smiling into the organs, thanking them for the work they do, we can reawaken the intelligence of the body. The Inner Smile meditation is often combined with the sacred Six Healing Sounds meditation and is a simple and enjoyable practice for all ages, especially children. Traditionally regarded in China as an inner alchemy Chi Kung exercise, it seems to have originated among ancient Taoists, who were both philosophers and medical doctors. Just as we need good nutrition to nourish our physical body, we also need to nourish our emotional and spiritual bodies. The Inner Smile offers an excellent way to cultivate and activate the healing energies that are always around us. Using color and sound to activate and reenergize the body at a cellular level, this exercise is similar to many modern meditation techniques, yet surprisingly more powerful.

The Taoist masters have long held that each of the six main organs have an associated color and sound vibration. As more recently scientists have discovered that what actually makes sounds and colors different is their vibratory rate, this may well explain how this internal exercise works. From personal experience, whether you believe this or not, the Inner Smile and Six Healing Sounds exercises really get results on the physical, emotional, and spiritual levels. Some people may find that at first using your mind's eye to visualize your internal anatomy is slightly difficult, but with regular practice it gets quite easy, even for those who struggle with creative visualization. Because your organs are actually in the place where you visualize them and do vibrate to the colors and sound vibrations mentioned here, many will find this exercise much easier than, for example, visualizing a forest or some nice garden, images often used in modern creative visualization techniques. Visualization of something that does exist and is so close and personal, in this case actually inside you, is more natural and free-flowing.

Inner Smile Meditation Combined with the Six Healing Sounds

We recommend spending at least three minutes on each elemental organ, and make the healing sound at least three to six times on each organ, drawing each sound out for several seconds when voicing it.

☯ Prior Relaxation

Sit comfortably with a straight spine, either in a chair or sitting cross-legged on the floor; the most important thing is that your spine is erect and your neck is fully extended to allow the full flow of blood and energy up to your brain.

1. Close your eyes, and begin to draw your attention inward. Listen to your breathing for several minutes as you inhale and exhale in a relaxed fashion.
2. Begin then to smile, but rather than smiling outward as you usually do in life, begin to smile back in, toward yourself. With your eyes closed and using your mind's eye (the third eye), visualize smiling back into yourself, as into a mirror. See your inner smile smiling back toward and into your body (fig. 6.2). We will begin by smiling into the lungs.

☯ Metal Element (Lungs' Sound)

The lungs are the center for energy cultivation and vital chi in the body. They regulate the opening and closing of the pores and also skin health.

1. See the left and right lungs in the chest cavity; they extend down to touch the liver and the spleen (fig. 6.3). Many of us use only the upper half of the lungs when breathing, being unaware of how far they actually extend down into the body.
2. The healing color of the lungs is pure white, like the color of snow. Send this color into both lungs, seeing them being covered in the color white. Begin to visualize this color cleaning the lungs gently and smoothly. Eliminate any browns or blacks that occur when visualizing the lungs.

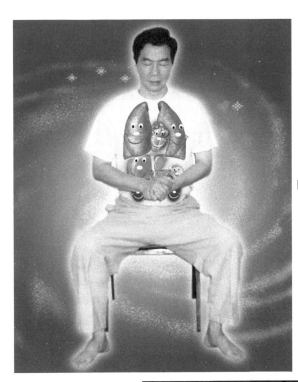

Fig. 6.2. Smile down into
your vital organs.

Fig. 6.3. Make the
sound sss-s-s-s-s-s,
the sound of a snake,
with your tongue
behind your bottom
teeth.

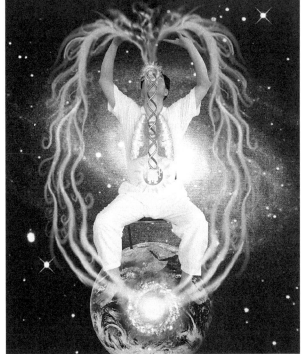

3. Once cleaned with the color white, raise your arms in front of you and rotate the palms to face upward, letting the eyes follow them, while you make the sound sss-s-s-s-s-s, the sound of a snake, with your tongue behind your bottom teeth.

◎ Water Element (Kidneys' Sound)

Feel the kidneys working, each day filtering all the body's wastes and regulating blood pressure and the acid-alkaline balance and many other duties that the kidneys perform each day for us.

1. Smile down into the kidneys, which are in the upper part of your lower back, one on each side of your spine (fig. 6.4).
2. Visualize the color dark blue inside and around both kidneys. Using your imagination, clean the kidneys with the color blue, leaving no area unpainted with this color.
3. Once complete, lean forward with your hands clasped around your knees and make the sound choo-oo-oo-oo. Try shaping your lips like you are blowing out a candle. Send this sound deep into the kidneys, as if you are talking to them. Then move on to the liver.

◎ Wood Element (Liver's Sound)

The liver is a workhorse and needs regular attention in the form of positive energy and inner love.

1. Visualize the liver, located under the right rib cage, and smile into it (fig. 6.5). See it cleaning your blood, producing bile, and regulating your metabolism.
2. Visualize the color green, as in the color of grass, and see the liver being covered in this color. Use an imaginary paintbrush, if you like, to color it until it is completely green.
3. Once completed, clasp your hands over your head, palms up, and press your palms upward (pressing slightly more with the right

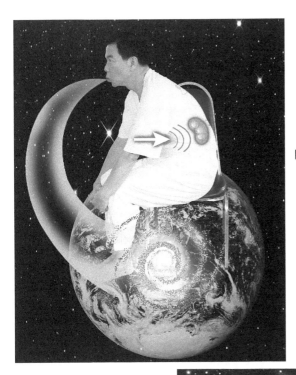

Fig. 6.4. Make the sound choo-oo-oo-oo, and try shaping your lips like you are blowing out a candle.

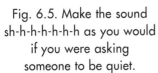

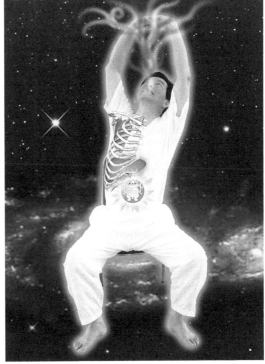

Fig. 6.5. Make the sound sh-h-h-h-h-h-h as you would if you were asking someone to be quiet.

palm) while you make the sound sh-h-h-h-h-h-h as you would if you were asking someone to be quiet. Then move to the heart.

☯ Fire Element (Heart's Sound)

The heart is the only muscle in your body that works twenty-four hours a day, even when you are sleeping or unconscious. It never rests and is fully functional to the day you die.

1. See the heart resting in the cavity of the lungs slightly left of center in the chest (fig. 6.6).
2. Smile down into the heart, and begin to visualize the color red, the color of clean blood. See the heart bathing in the color red and being cleaned and nourished by this color.
3. Once complete, assume the same position as you did for the liver with your palms pressing upward above your head (but this time push harder with your left palm), and direct the heart's sound haw-w-w-w-w-w, into the heart. The sound is like a deep, relaxing moan that originates from the chest rather than from the throat. Then move on to the spleen and pancreas.

☯ Earth Element (Spleen's/Pancreas's Sound)

The spleen, pancreas, and stomach are related to digestion and assimilation in traditional medicine and to the element of earth, hence they are responsible for taking nutrients from food and creating the energy that supplies the other organs.

1. See the spleen, pancreas, and stomach lying in the midsection of the torso toward the left-hand side under the ribs (fig. 6.7).
2. The healing color for these organs is yellow. Visualize the color yellow like the color of a sunflower, and begin to see these organs covered in this color.
3. Once these organs are cleansed in the color yellow, place the fingers of both hands just below the sternum on the left side, press

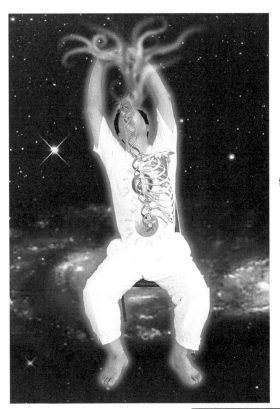

Fig. 6.6. Make and direct the sound haw-w-w-w-w-w, like a deep, relaxing moan that originates from the chest rather than from the throat, into the heart.

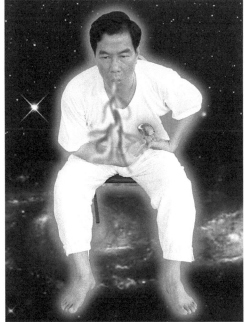

Fig. 6.7. Make the sound who-o-o-o-o-o, originating in the throat and send it down into the spleen and pancreas.

in with your fingers, and lean forward while making the sound who-o-o-o-o-o. The sound originates in the throat. Send it down into the spleen and pancreas. Then move to the lungs.

◉ Triple Warmer (Triple Warmer's Sound)

The triple warmer is considered an organ in traditional Chinese medicine, but without a physical form, as it takes the form of all the organs inside the body. Its function is to regulate the relationship between all other organs and regulate body temperature and the relationship with our internal and external environments.

1. Lie down on your back and close your eyes to work on your triple warmer (fig. 6.8). When you are sensing your triple warmer, try to visualize all the colors of your organs one at a time and then simultaneously. Visualize blue in the kidneys, green in the liver, red in the heart, yellow in the spleen, and white in the lungs.

2. Once you can see all the colors inside your body, exhale and make the sound hee-e-e-e-e-e, sending it to all the organs and then to your whole body.

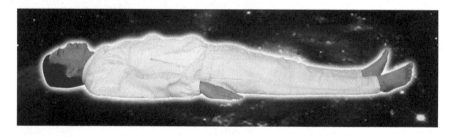

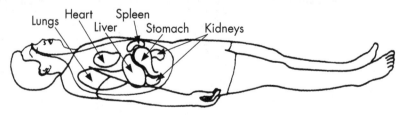

Fig. 6.8. Make the sound hee-e-e-e-e-e, sending it to all the organs and then to your whole body.

The Six Healing Sounds, combined with the Inner Smile Meditation, as described above, is best practiced before bedtime, as it helps to cool down overheated organs, providing restful sleep. Some people enjoy it during the afternoon to invigorate themselves if they're feeling tired or if they still have many things to do before the day's end.

PRANAYAMA, BREATH CONTROL

The word *pranayama* is generally translated as "breath control," but as with most English translations from ancient languages like Sanskrit, it does not convey the full meaning of the word. If we break down the word *pranayama* we find the word *prana,* which is known by the Chinese Taoist term *chi* and the Japanese term *ki.* Often translated as "life force energy" or "vital force," prana is the primordial force that directs the flow of energy of the universe. When one learns to effectively tap into this form of subtle energy and direct it through the nadis, or energy meridians, one can greatly benefit one's health. The second half of the word *pranayama,* the word *yama,* means "control" or "to direct," but many believe that the real word here that conveys the message is actually *ayama,* which suggests a vastly greater explanation of the purpose of pranayama, as it literally means "expansion" or "to extend." What all this means is that the true essence of pranayama lies in our ability to extend and direct our life-force energy beyond the dimension of the physical body and into the other four *koshas,* or bodies.

Yogic philosophy acknowledges the existence of five pranic bodies, or koshas, that encompass the entire human dimension, including their influence on disease. So you can see how great an effect the simple yet profound breathing exercises here can have, not just on your physical body, but also on your mental and emotional well-being.

The five subtle bodies (koshas) affected by pranayama are:

1. The ananamaya kosha: the material/physical body
2. The manomaya kosha: the mental/emotional body
3. The pranamaya kosha: the electrical/energy body

4. The vijnanamaya kosha: the psychic/astral body
5. The anandamaya kosha: the enlightened/transcendental body

While pranayama has a positive influence on all dimensions of the human body, it is primarily focused on the pranayama kosha, the energy body; this kosha can be subdivided into five different pranas, or energies, which correlate with the five elements and the five physical chakras or nerve plexuses within the central nervous system:

1. Vayana: Stored in the base chakra, this prana relates to the earth element and the nerve plexus within the perineum. Its ability is to act as a storehouse for the other pranas.
2. Apana: Located within the navel chakra, this prana relates to the water element and the sacral nerve plexus. Its purpose is to provide energy for the kidneys, colon, anus, and reproductive organs.
3. Samana: This prana is found in the solar plexus chakra and is associated with the fire element. It affects and controls our digestion, assimilation, and adrenal glands and regulates the metabolism.
4. Prana: Found in the heart center, this prana correlates to the heart chakra, the element of air (metal), and the heart nerve plexus of the upper spine. This prana regulates respiration and speech.
5. Udana: Located within the throat chakra, this prana corresponds to the ether/wood element and has a governing effect on the areas of the body above the neck and the five senses.

While it is not compulsory to understand completely the five koshas (bodies) and the five pranas (life-force energies) to benefit from these pranayama exercises, knowing something about them can assist you in understanding the vast healing capabilities of the body and how one has a great opportunity to tap into them for the clear purpose of cultivating them and utilizing them for self-healing.

Kapalabhati, Breath of Fire

Swami Vishnudevananda (1927–1993), founder of the International Sivananda Yoga Vedanta centers and ashrams, who established the world-famous Sivananda yoga teacher-training course, one of the first yoga teacher-training programs in the West, confirmed the vital importance of pranayama—yogic breath control—to one's overall health: "Pranayama is the link between the mental and physical disciplines. While the action is physical, the effect is to make the mind calm, lucid, and steady."

The Sanskrit word *kapalabhati* translates as "skull shining," and it is also commonly known as the "breath of fire" because it invigorates and raises the body's heat; it is also known as "frontal brain cleansing" because it improves your complexion by increasing circulation to the brain, skull, and face. The speed at which this exercise is done will differ from beginner to advanced practitioner, so it is best to start slowly and steadily and begin to gain speed as one gains inner confidence. One of the purposes of this ancient exercise is to rid the body of excess carbon dioxide that builds up in the blood from incomplete, lazy breathing. As it invigorates, it is best done early in the day and not before bedtime.

Although Kapalabhati is classified as a pranayama exercise in yoga, it is also included as a part of the six yogic purification and cleansing exercises known in the Vedas as the *shatkarmas*. *Shat* means "six," and *karma* means "action" or "process." Pranayama is generally defined as a form of breath control, as it is stated in many classic ayurvedic texts that when one controls the breath, one can also control the movement of energy (prana or chi). The practice of pranayama enables one to effectively activate and regulate the *pranayama kosha* (life-force energy body) that controls every chemical reaction in the body.

The two pranayama aspects of Kapalabhati are (1) *pooraka* (inhalation); and (2) *rechaka* (exhalation).

Kapalabhati Pranayama

Sit in a comfortable position, in a straight-backed chair or cross-legged on the floor on a mat or cushion, or stand comfortably with a straight back. Most important is that the spine is very straight so that the central column and nervous system is not compromised in any way. This and all pranayama exercises are done breathing through the nostrils unless otherwise specified.

1. When in a comfortable position, take three slow, deep breaths in and out through the nose.
2. Just as you are ready to exhale the third out-breath, begin the exercise by forcing the abdominal muscles to contract, which naturally forces the breath out of the nostrils in a short spurt, like one is squeezing the remaining air from a balloon.
3. Immediately after forcefully exhaling like this, in a short spurt, relax the abdominal muscles, which will naturally allow the diaphragm to descend back into its natural abdominal cavity, causing a passive, effortless inhalation. Then repeat step 2, force-contracting the abdominal muscles to push the air out of the nostrils.

Repeat this cycle continuously, approximately every second for thirty seconds (or breaths), and then relax and repeat from the beginning, starting with step number 1 and going through the whole cycle of thirty breaths. Do three cycles of thirty breaths each.

Note: The contraction of the abdominal muscles causes the diaphragm to move up in the thoracic cavity, pushing the air out of the lungs more completely than a normal breath does. This allows complete exhalation of carbon dioxide, which in turn allows for maximum oxygen absorption into the bloodstream inside the alveoli of the lung tissue.

☯ Benefits

In ayurvedic medicine, Kapalabhati is said to purify and balance both the *ida* and *pingala* nadis, or meridians, that circulate up the spinal column; these two nadis are actually represented in the modern medical symbol as the caduceus, a snake spiraled around a central column.

It also helps relieve tiredness and sluggishness while cleansing the lungs of toxins, in turn helping asthmatics and other respiratory diseases. This exercise also strengthens the digestive system and calms the nervous system.

Nadi Shodhana, Alternate Nostril Breathing

The Hatha Yoga Pradipika (chapter 2, verse 2) is clear about the benefits of pranayama, and specifically a form called *nadi shodhana,* an exercise involving alternate nostril breathing, sometimes called "channel clearing breath," and breath retention: "When the breath wanders, the mind is also unsteady. But when the breath is still, so the mind and the yogi live long. Therefore one should retain the breath."

Nadi means "channel"; *shodhana* means "purifying" or "clearing." This practice helps clear out blocked energy channels in the body, which in turn relaxes and calms the mind. Traditionally, nadi shodhana includes breath retention, fixed-ratio breathing, and the repetition of certain "seed" mantras; for beginning pranayama students, it's best to focus only on the inhales and exhales.

Nadi Shodhana Pranayama

Preparation

Sit in a comfortable position with the spine as straight as possible. Preferably this technique is practiced in a cross-legged position (use a cushion under your sit bones to support your spine in an upright position); if sitting cross-legged is not possible, you can sit erect in a straight-back chair. As with all pranayama, make sure the spine is straight and lengthened all the way to the top of the head by stretching the back of the neck muscles upward.

1. With both hands resting in your lap, place your left hand in the Chin mudra (thumb and index finger gently touching each other)

and the right hand in the Vishnu mudra (thumb and ring finger touching (while index and middle finger are tucked under toward the palm).

2. Bring the hand in Vishnu mudra up to the face; separate the thumb and ring finger slightly so that you can be ready to use these fingers to alternately block the right and left nostril respectively.

❂ Actual Breathing Practice

1. Block the right nostril gently with the right thumb, leaving the palm facing upward in a receiving gesture and leaving the ring finger and little finger resting lightly on the left nostril but not blocking it, and breathe in fully through the left nostril for the count of four (fig. 6.9A).
2. Once full inhalation has occurred block both nostrils and hold the breath for the count of twelve (fig. 6.9B).*
3. Then after the count of twelve, unblock the right nostril by letting the thumb off, and exhale gradually and fully to the count of eight.
4. Immediately after the exhalation, inhale once again to the count of four, but this time through the right nostril, keeping the left nostril blocked with your ring finger and little finger (fig. 6.9C).
5. Once again, after a count of four, block both nostrils, holding the breath steady for twelve counts.
6. Release the left nostril, and exhale gradually to the count of eight.

This is one full round of Nadi Shodhana. Repeat the cycle five times if you are new to this practice, and after several weeks work your way up to ten full rounds.

---

*Note that there are several versions of Nadi Shodhana; some do not include lengthy breath retention between inhalation and exhalation.

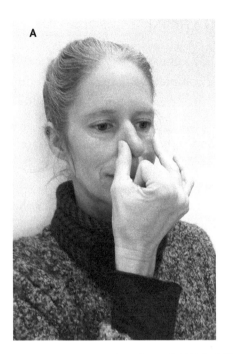

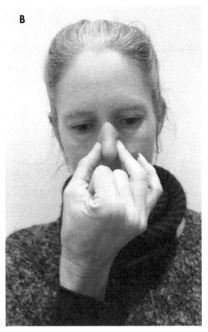

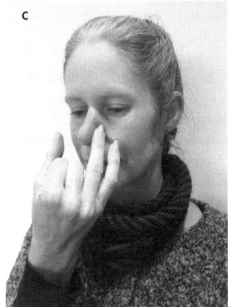

Fig. 6.9. Nadi Shodhana,
alternate nostril breathing

SUN SALUTATION

Swami Santayana Saraswati (1874–1937) praised the yogic practice of Sun Salutation, *Surya Namaskar,* as "a complete *sadhana* [spiritual discipline] in itself, for it includes asana, pranayama, mantra, and meditation techniques."

Surya means "sun" in Sanskrit, and *namaskar* means "to salute." Besides being a practice found in Indian yoga, this exercise also has links to ancient Egyptian yoga (Sema), where it symbolizes the cycle of birth and death. Ra is the Egyptian sun god, and his birth in the morning from our eastern sky symbolizes the birth of a soul into the world of time and space and the ego-personality. It is said that the sun never becomes bored of doing the same thing over and over, rising and setting; it never abandons its duty, nor does it offer excuses as to why it is not possible for it to perform its important duty. Similarly, as we get up each day and perform our mundane tasks such as brushing our teeth, taking a shower, eating and drinking, we need to also exert a certain amount of energy to perform our physical and spiritual practices on a daily basis, avoiding lame excuses such as "I did it yesterday" or "I couldn't be bothered today." Just because you ate or washed yesterday, do you take a break today? Of course not! Be vigilant and consistent like the sun; daily practice is required by all of us.

Although this exercise comes from the Indian hatha yoga tradition, modern Taoists are open to all practices and learning. As many of Master Chia's books have focused on the Chinese Chi Kung exercises, we feel that including the Sun Salutation here reminds us that all forms of spiritual practice have their place in the Taoist pursuit of supreme health and longevity. Spiritually we need to strive to be like the sun (Ra), performing our duties unceasingly until it becomes effortless.

The Sun Salutation involves twelve flowing movements and spinal positions, each with a different effect on the organs, glands, muscles, and joints. When performed in the proper sequence, doing Sun Salutations can invigorate and strengthen the entire body, and they are an excellent warm-up before performing more advanced postures.

The benefits of the Sun Salutation are many:

- Lengthens and straightens the spinal column
- Increases blood supply to the spinal and cranial nerves
- Strengthens and relaxes the whole spine
- Activates the cranial-sacral pump
- Regulates breathing
- Increases mental focus
- Regains lost flexibility
- Increases circulation to the lower limbs
- Prevents back pain and scoliosis

Sun Salutation

To begin, stand tall with the feet slightly apart, toes pointing straight forward, hands by the sides.

Position 1. Inhale and exhale, bringing your palms together at the chest in prayer position; center your body and bring your focus to your heart center (fig. 6.10).

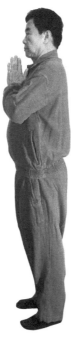

Fig. 6.10. Position 1

Position 2. On a deep inhalation, sweep your arms out and up over your head, stretching the arms up high and slightly backward over the head; focus on lengthening the spine more than on bending so far back (fig. 6.11).

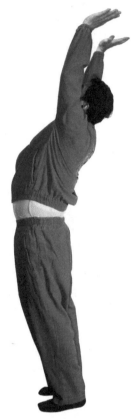

Fig. 6.11. Position 2

Position 3. On an exhalation, bend forward, hinging from the hips; put your hands on the floor (or as close to the floor as you can) next to your feet, and flat on the floor if possible. Make sure that your fingers are in line with your toes and relax your neck, letting your head hang, and then slowly straighten the knees as much as you can (fig. 6.12).

Position 4. On an inhalation, stretch your right foot back as far possible; you may need to rise up on your fingertips to do this. Put your right knee on the floor with the top of the foot flat on the floor; stretch the back of your neck, arching and lengthening the spine (fig. 6.13).

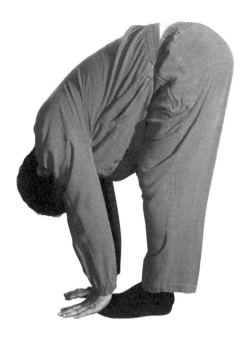

Fig. 6.12. Position 3

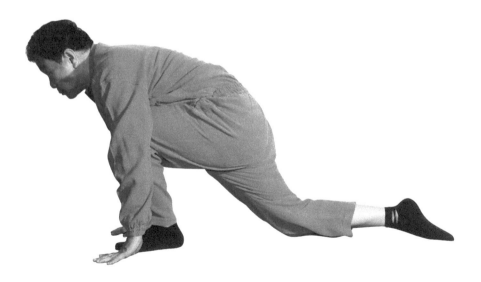

Fig. 6.13. Position 4

Position 5. Retaining the inhalation from the last move, hold the breath, lift your right knee off the floor, and bring the left leg back the same as the right, toes on the floor and flexed, heels pushing straight back. In this position with both legs back, form a straight, flat plank—the push-up position (fig. 6.14).

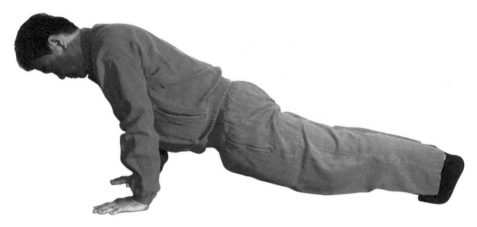

Fig. 6.14. Position 5

Position 6. On an exhalation, slowly lower your knees to the floor, then lower the chest to the floor, your breastbone between your hands; put your forehead down to touch or nearly touch the floor. The buttocks will be slightly raised off the ground when done correctly (fig. 6.15).

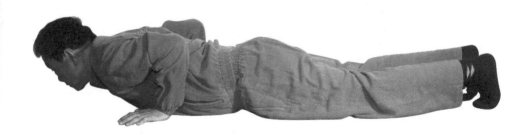

Fig. 6.15. Position 6

Position 7. On an inhalation, lengthen and straighten the spine while simultaneously arching up and back; your legs and hips remain touching the ground (fig. 6.16).

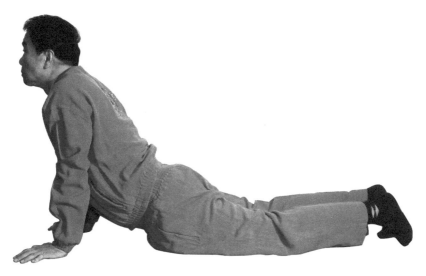

Fig. 6.16. Position 7

Position 8. On an exhalation, begin raising your hips, dropping your head between the arms, relaxing your neck; stretch the back of the legs toward the floor (fig. 6.17) in downward dog position. Don't worry if your heels don't touch the floor.

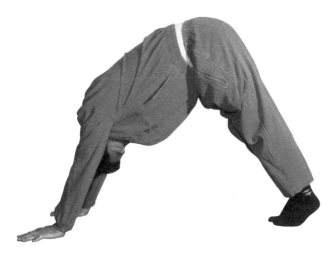

Fig. 6.17. Position 8

Position 9. On an inhalation, bring your right foot forward in line with and between your hands. Your left knee touches the floor as you stretch your left instep against the floor; lengthen your spine and extend your neck by stretching the back of your head out (fig. 6.18).

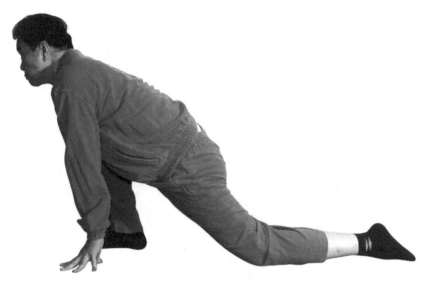

Fig. 6.18. Position 9 (same as position 4 but on the other side)

Position 10. Exhale, stepping the left leg forward to meet the right, keeping your hips as high as possible and your sit bones lifted (fig. 6.19).

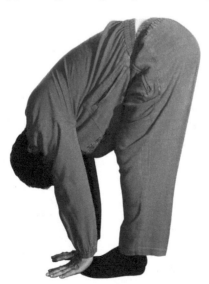

Fig. 6.19. Position 10
(same as position 3)

Position 11. Inhale and stretch back up like when you started out, bringing your arms overhead, arching slightly back (but avoid pushing the hips forward). Stretch the spine lengthwise as well as slightly backward (fig. 6.20).

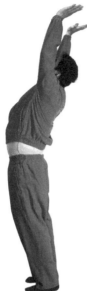

Fig. 6.20. Position 11
(same as position 2)

Position 12. Exhale, bringing the palms together at the chest in prayer position (fig. 6.21).

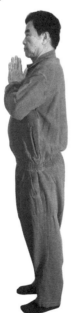

Fig. 6.21. Position 12
(same as position 1)

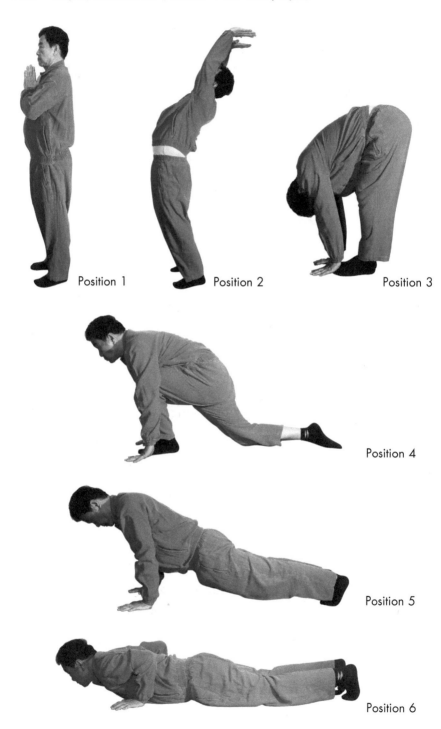

Position 1

Position 2

Position 3

Position 4

Position 5

Position 6

Fig. 6.22. Sun Salutation (positions 1–6)

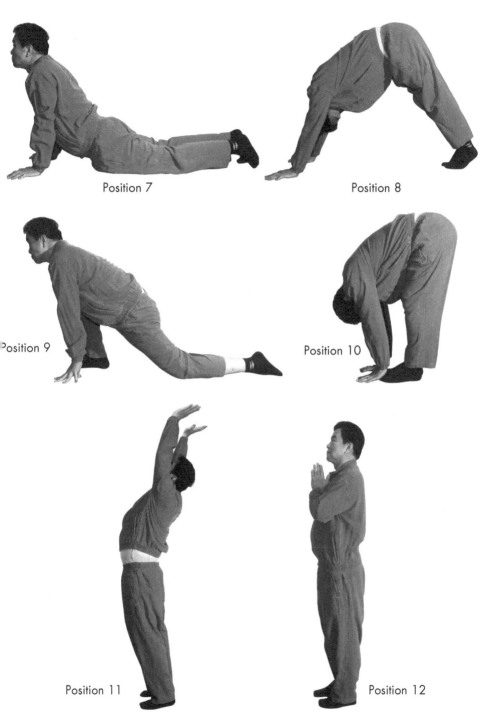

Position 7

Position 8

Position 9

Position 10

Position 11

Position 12

Fig. 6.23. Sun Salutation (positions 7–12)

SECRET CHINESE WEIGHT-LOSS EXERCISE

Ancient Chinese Taoists were famous for their ability to simplify health issues and get to the root of many health complaints by performing simple yet powerful exercises such as those seen in Chi Kung, Tai Chi Chuan, and Falun Dafa (Kung). One such exercise, which was taught to me by an old Chinese doctor I met in Thailand, is simply translated as the "weight-reduction exercise." While this exercise shows remarkable results for increasing metabolism and burning calories, it can also work the other way around for those suffering from a lack of appetite and excessive weight loss. Many of those who first look at this exercise without actually doing it are astounded that it could possibly do anything, as the exercise itself does not involve any real major movements—no running, jumping, stretching, swimming, hurdling, or biking, but rather a steady pose (asana) in two positions that when performed correctly activates the major meridians associated with digestive fire and metabolism. While the exercise itself looks easy, it does demand focus, strength, balance, and quite a bit of determination. When performed for just five minutes each day, this exercise can burn more calories than many aerobic workouts, and without expensive equipment or fancy workout clothes.

 ## Weight-Loss Exercise

To begin, stand with the spine completely straight and feet apart, slightly wider than shoulder width.

1. Bend the knees enough so that you feel as if you are riding a horse. This is called the *horse stance* in Chi Kung. Stretch your arms out in front of you, parallel to the floor, palms facing down (fig. 6.24A).
2. Keeping your pelvis tucked under and not poking the buttocks out, gently come up on the balls of your feet near the toes while moving your body weight slightly forward to balance (fig. 6.24B).
3. Maintain a firm balance for at least one whole second, and then softly return back to the original stance.

Repeat this up-and-back movement for five minutes each day after doing your Sun Salutations.

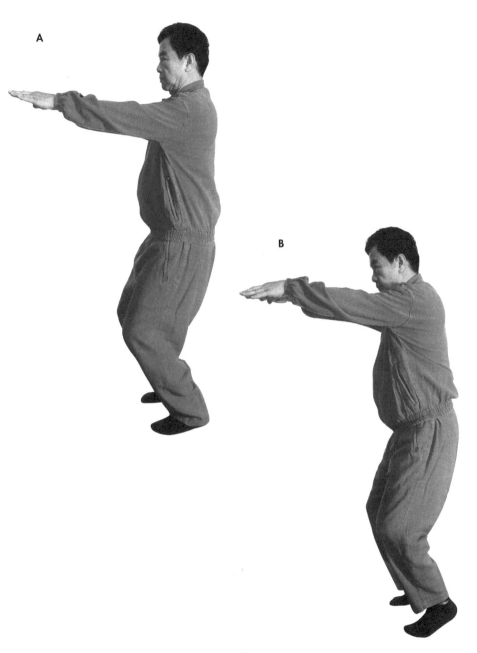

Fig. 6.24. Weight-Loss Exercise

THE FIVE TIBETAN RITES

Way back in 1939, Peter Kelder published *The Five Tibetan Rites of Rejuvenation*. The Five Tibetan Rites, as they are known, possibly predate many modern yoga asanas by at least seven hundred years; therefore, many people believe they could not have derived from either Tibetan or Indian forms of yoga, but rather from some other ancient Indo-Tibetan culture. It has also been suggested that these rites are related to Kum Nye, a form of Tibetan spiritual exercise similar to Tai Chi and Chi Kung. According to Kelder, the first time they appeared outside of Tibet was during the English occupation of India, when an English army officer took refuge in a Tibetan monastery and saw them being performed. After performing the exercises with the monks for some time he went on to experience such incredible longevity that it appeared to be an age reversal of sorts. After he brought the Five Tibetans, as they are called, back to the West and shared them with Kelder, the exercises (or *rites* as they are more accurately called) began to circulate among health and longevity enthusiasts, and their popularity continues to this very day. That said, what is important is not the origin of these exercises, but rather their immense benefits when one commits to spending fifteen minutes a day performing them.

Although the Five Tibetans can be performed by anyone, anyone with spinal injuries is advised to first consult his or her health care practitioner before beginning. I personally have seen those with spinal abnormalities and even spinal curvature diseases receive great benefits from performing these exercises daily. It is not necessary to perform more than twenty-one of each of the five exercises daily, which is said to be enough. The breathing must be continuous and deep. There is no need to hold the posture, but rather use the in- and out-breath to dictate the speed at which the two positions of each exercise are done.

The Five Tibetans are one of the oldest and most proven ways to improve posture, strength, muscle tone, energy level, and general well-being. Those who learn and perform them daily testify as to their simplicity and the benefits to both mind and body.

The Five Tibetan Rites

The Five Tibetan Rites are simple to perform according to your level of strength and flexibility, as you can begin performing only several of each of the Five Rites and then gradually, over a period of several weeks, work your way up to twenty-one repetitions.

Rite 1

Stand tall with arms outstretched, and slowly turn (approximately three seconds duration for each circle) in a clockwise direction while pivoting on one foot (fig. 6.25). Do twenty-one rounds, and then stand with your hands at your sides and breathe deeply; relax for one minute before moving on to the next rite. In the beginning you might experience a slight dizziness, so take your time building up to twenty-one turns. To avoid dizziness it helps to "spot" like a ballet dancer when doing this exercise; that is, hold your gaze fixed on one spot and spin the head around to that same spot as you turn in circles.

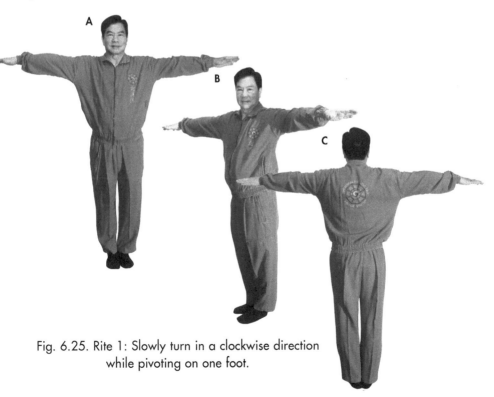

Fig. 6.25. Rite 1: Slowly turn in a clockwise direction while pivoting on one foot.

⟳ *Rite 2*

Lie flat on your back on a mat. If needed, support your lower back by tucking the thumb sides of your hands under your lower back; otherwise place them firmly by your sides, palms down (fig. 6.26A). Take a deep breath in, and then on an exhalation bring your legs into an upright position, lifting your head and bringing your chin into your chest while leaving your upper back flat on the mat (fig. 6.26B). Breathe in while lowering your legs and your head and returning to your starting position. Repeat up to twenty-one times.

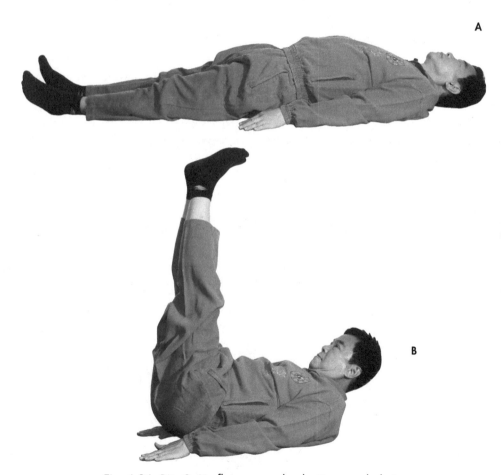

Fig. 6.26. Rite 2: Lie flat on your back. On an exhalation, bring your legs into an upright position as you lift your head, bringing your chin in toward your chest.

❀ Rite 3

Kneel on a mat with your toes flexed and tucked under your feet, and support your lower back with your palms resting against your thighs, placing your chin on your chest (fig. 6.27A). Take a deep breath in, and then on the out-breath bend backward as far as you comfortably can while keeping your hips stationary (fig. 6.27B). Return to the starting position on an inhalation. Repeat up to twenty-one times.

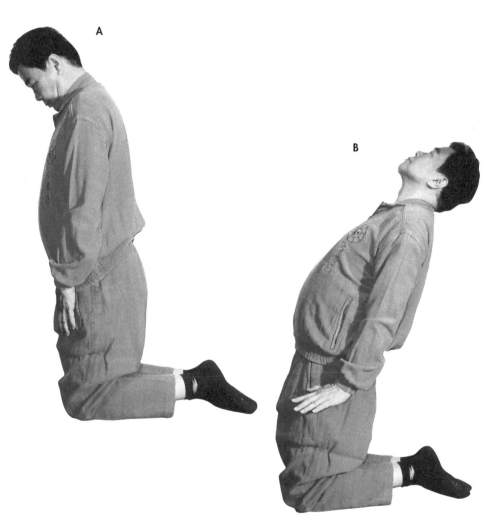

A

B

Fig. 6.27. Rite 3: Kneeling, move your chin down toward your chest, and on the out-breath bend backward.

🜂 Rite 4

Sit on a mat with your legs straight; move your chin down toward your chest, and place your hands on the floor beside your hips, fingers pointing toward your feet (fig. 6.28A). Take a deep breath in, and on an exhalation use your upper-body strength and legs to push your hips up so that your body is in a tablelike position, with knees bent at a right angle (fig. 6.28B). On an inhalation, return to your starting position. Repeat up to twenty-one times.

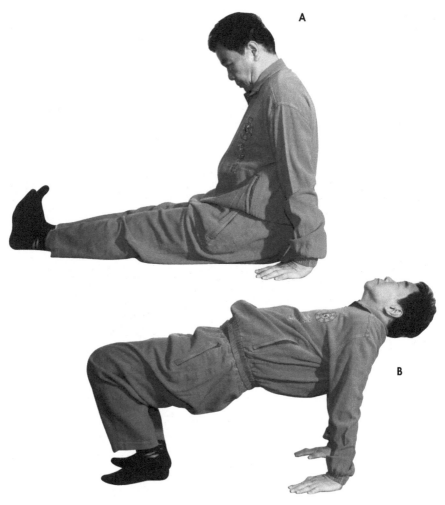

Fig. 6.28. Rite 4: Sit with legs straight, chin to chest. On an exhalation push yourself upright into a tablelike position, knees bent at a right angle.

🌀 *Rite 5*

In a push-up position but with the spine lifted and bent slightly backward, support your whole body off the ground with only your hands and flexed toes touching the mat (fig. 6.29A). Keep your hands directly below your shoulders. Take a deep breath in, and push your bottom up in the air, keeping your legs and spine straight, forming a triangle shape somewhat like the downward dog pose in yoga (fig. 6.29B). Exhale, and repeat up to twenty-one times.

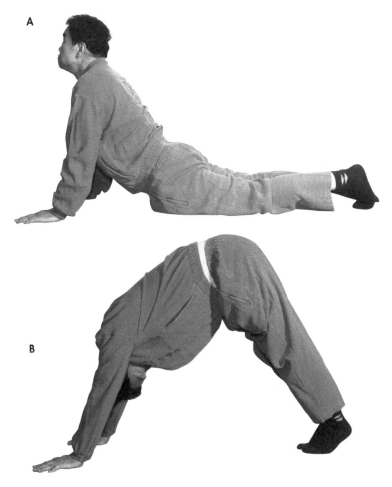

Fig. 6.29. Rite 5: Pushing up, bend your spine backward, and then breathe in, forming a triangle shape (similar to downward dog pose in yoga).

CORRECTING YOUR POSTURE

Many people are aware that when they slouch or maintain poor posture at a computer, typing becomes slower and more difficult. Ask any professional piano player about the importance of good posture when playing and they'll tell you it's almost as important as your talent. A 1994 study concluded that "the significant influence of posture on health is not addressed by most physicians. . . . Posture affects and moderates every physiologic function from breathing to hormonal production. Spinal pain, headache, mood, blood pressure, pulse, and lung capacity are among the functions most easily influenced by posture."*

In the 1800s it was not uncommon for women to suffer from myriad health problems as a result of the fashion of wearing tight whalebone corsets. Going back much further, the ancient Greek physician Hippocrates observed the link between specific postures and health ailments. He discovered that children who developed poor posture in the upper back above the diaphragm tended to suffer from deformed chests, hoarseness of the voice, lung diseases, and breathlessness later on in life, while children who developed this deformity below the diaphragm developed lower bowel diseases, kidney disorders, and poor circulation to the lower extremities when older.

Over a hundred years ago a professional actor and singer from Australia by the name of Frederick Matthias Alexander uncovered and explained the link between posture and concentration and how this affects our physical and emotional health. The Alexander technique, whose principles were developed in the 1890s, is based on what Alexander called "primary control," whereby the head is lifted gently upward from the body, allowing the back to follow. The Alexander technique is based on the idea that our posture holds a vital key to the free flow of energy through our body's electrical circuits and meridian pathways. When our posture is incorrect, the energy flows more slowly or is weaker, in turn causing problems with motor skills and thought

---

*J. Lennon, C. N. Sheeley, R. K. Cady, W. Matta, R. Cox, and W. F. Simpson, "Postural and respiratory modulation of autonomic function, pain, and health," *American Journal of Pain Management* 4 (1994): 36–39.

processes, which in turn affect our optimal performance no matter what we're doing. Alexander's mantra was, "Let my neck be free so that my head moves forward and up, in such a way that my spine lengthens and my back widens, and my knees release forwards."

Poor posture can be caused by a lack of body awareness, as most people don't really understand the importance of maintaining correct posture, especially when they're alone and not out in public or when performing routine activities. Curvature of the upper spine (kyphosis) causes a counterbalancing arching of your lower spine (lordosis), which pushes the abdomen forward and causes the chest to cave in. This type of incorrect posture places pressure on so many different nerves and muscles that it can result in restlessness, irritability, digestive disturbances, and depression.

One of the keys to making good posture easy and comfortable is to understand the importance of the neck. The muscles in the head and neck affect all the other muscles in the body via the cranial nerve reflexes and other acupuncture reflexes. When adjusting the posture of the neck muscles, by stretching and lengthening the cervical spine (neck spine) and bringing the chin inward and not down, you can affect the posture of the entire spinal column. Lifting the crown (the top of the head) toward the sky in turn lengthens the back of the neck and brings the chin slightly inward. This simple action encourages the lower back to lengthen and straighten via reflex nerves.

You can experiment with this yourself: try sitting in a cross-legged meditative position with a nice straight spine and without bending the back, just tilt the head forward slightly. Within a few seconds you'll feel your lower back also slouching. There are many reasons this happens; one is due to the strong connection between the cranial and sacral nerves and their muscles and how each can affect the other. Rather than focusing entirely on keeping your back straight and lengthening the spine when performing physical activities or when sitting at a desk, focus instead on your neck and the position of the cranium. Another exercise you can do to understand how your body balances itself is to lean against a wall with your right side. Once you're leaning against the wall with your right side and right ear up fairly close to the wall, lift your left leg. You may find you can't because your body can't shift to the right to balance itself.

There are many reasons we develop poor posture, from emotional trauma to physical injuries and accidents. One obvious but vastly overlooked reason that so many of us have incorrect posture is that our head is approximately the same size and weight as a bowling ball. Besides this, it rests on top of a very small, movable support column, and the neck muscles are anatomically not strong enough to support such a heavy structure. When we look at other muscles that support weight-bearing structures, they are much stronger. So physically, when your head moves forward in front of the shoulders, the compressive forces are transferred to your spine, muscles, and ligaments. This causes gravity to pull the head down farther to the ground, while the body resists the force of nature using the muscles attached to the head and neck, causing muscle strain and pain. It is estimated that for every inch the head moves forward, an additional fifteen to thirty pounds of tension is placed on the muscles of the neck.

How to Correct Your Posture

Stand in front of a full-length mirror in your underwear with no shoes on. Stand as you normally would, and then check yourself. Try doing this sideways while noticing the subtle curvature of your spine. It is normal to have a mild inward curve behind your neck and lower back, but not too much. Take a look at your chin, making sure that it is not pushed too far forward, which is a common mistake. Think *as tall as possible,* and try to imagine that a cord is attached to the crown of your head, lifting it upward. Avoid leaning on one leg more than on the other when standing in one place for any period of time, which causes the hips to become misaligned. Stand on both legs with equal weight, with hips slightly thrust forward. Men especially need to avoid putting their wallet in their back pocket and then sitting down in a chair or car seat, a common cause of many back ailments. I highly recommend an ergonomic chair that promotes better posture. Use the chair's height adjustment feature so you're not looking down, which makes the chin drop, in turn causing the lower spine to do the same.

Our bodies are designed to avoid pain and to gain pleasure. If any movements cause pain in the body, it remembers this and attempts to move in another way. Retraining your body's posture may be uncomfortable at first, and it may feel more natural to have the poor posture you're used to, but persistent daily correction will in time pay off, resulting in correct posture and improved health. Practicing the Sun Salutation and the Five Tibetans also helps to lengthen the spine and promote better posture, while also bringing more focus and concentration.

THE HEALTH DANGERS OF TOO MUCH SITTING

Dr. James Levine of the Mayo Clinic has said, "Sitting is more dangerous than smoking, and kills more people than HIV and is more treacherous than parachuting. We are sitting ourselves to death." Today we sit more than at any other time in history due to lengthy time at the computer or driving vehicles, and it is causing humans massive amounts of health problems. Right now you're probably sitting or lying down while reading this book, but the more you stay put the more your body becomes agitated and the blood and lymph circulation stagnates. It is true that sitting for periods, especially in correct mediation posture, or lying in relaxation yoga poses on a firm surface can induce relaxation and aid in recovery from stress, especially when you're focused on your breathing. But the greater reality is that the human body is built to move and has over three hundred sixty joints.

When you sit for periods of time at work, at home, or driving a vehicle the muscles and bones in your back, especially in your lower back, receive excessive wear and tear. Your ability to take a deep breath is compromised and your diaphragm is restricted. Your chest cavity is not able to expand fully in a seated position; thus, you receive less oxygen into your lungs, blood, and brain.* If you look at small children

---

*For more information see https://www.youtube.com/watch?v=wUEl8KrMz14; and http://www.huffingtonpost.com/the-active-times/sitting-is-the-new-smokin_b _5890006.html.

after they begin to walk they naturally don't sit very much; rather, they prefer to squat, especially when performing activities like building sand-castles or playing with Legos.

Taoists say that excessive sitting damages the spleen and stomach and their associated energy meridians, which govern the holding of things in their correct places. When this "holding" is depleted it causes prolapses and swelling. The very act of sitting squashes and compresses the spine and spinal nerves, causing numbness and swelling, and weakens the vital energy force. On a scientific level sitting for long periods also decreases the amount of a protein called lipoprotein lipase, a special enzyme that breaks downs fat in the blood vessels and brain, causing your brain to become sluggish. Yet when we sit for computer work we are most often in great need of good brain activity. Recent scientific studies have also linked sitting for too long to certain types of cancers, diabetes, kidney disease, and even heart disease and have documented the fact that inactivity causes millions of deaths per year worldwide.

This is why many modern workspaces are now installing desks that raise up so office workers can also stand for periods during the day and continue working at the computer. While this is helpful we must also perform internal exercises that combat the side effects of sitting for long periods. While sitting is the problem, standing is not the best and only solution. These two simple Taoist exercises can help to compensate for the damages of excessive sitting time.

 ## Exercises to Combat Excessive Sitting

Every thirty to sixty minutes, take a three- to five-minute break and try these two Taoist internal exercises.

For both exercises, stand with your feet apart at one and one-half times shoulder width, with your feet pointing directly forward, knees slightly bent, and your tail bone tucked gently under. Your neck and spine should be long with the chin slightly pulling toward the back of your brain.

✪ Exercise 1

As you inhale, gently try to push both your inner ankle bones and your heels toward each other without moving your feet. Continue to squeeze them toward each other as you complete your inhalation and relax them as you exhale. Take long, slow deep breaths with a particular focus on long, relaxed exhalations.

Do you begin to feel what happens to your lower back and buttocks muscles? If you are doing this correctly you will feel a gentle tightening in them and also in the muscles of your anus, and as you relax they will relax further. Practice this inhalation and exhalation while squeezing the muscles and then relaxing them for twenty slow breaths.

✪ Exercise 2

You can do this either against a wall or freestanding, whatever feels best for you.

1. Beginning in the same original standing position, stretch both arms out straight to the sides, level with your heart, palms and fingers facing up to the sky with a slight distance between each finger, just enough to fit a chopstick between them.
2. Then, as you inhale, simply begin to squat down as far as you feel comfortable and maintain your balance as your bring your hands together in prayer position at the heart center.
3. On the exhale, begin to rise up again, releasing the hands and stretching them out to the sides level with your heart again.

Remember to inhale as you go down and exhale as you push up. Perform twenty breath cycles deep and slow, again focusing on coming up slowly with long exhalations. As you practice this regularly you will begin to squat lower and lower and become more confident.

After the twenty cycles make fists with your hands and rub your kidneys in a circular fashion as you lift and bounce your heels on the ground. At the same time make the kidneys' healing sound, choo-oo-oo-oo, as taught in the Six Healing Sounds section.

Simple Abdominal-Diaphragm Lock (Uddiyana Bandha)

In both Taoist and Indian systems of yoga, locking exercises (*bandhas*) are Internal Alchemy yogic locks that when exercised allow energy (chi) to flow through certain areas of the body after they have been locked and then released. This is similar to building up pressure in a garden hose by blocking the flow of water and then releasing it. Just as the water from the hose flows with more force after it has been blocked, temporarily blocking and then releasing energy in your body allows the energy to flow more freely throughout the superficial meridians and also through the deep internal meridians, which are known as *nadis* in India. Exercising the bandhas involves breath retention for several seconds while simultaneously making a contraction in a particular part of the body. The abdominal-diaphragm lock known in India as *uddiyana bandha* (lifting of the diaphragm) involves taking a deep breath in through the nose, filling the belly and expanding the rib cage, and then breathing out completely, emptying your lungs and compressing your diaphragm, while sucking in your abdominal area and pulling your internal organs upward as much as you can.

Hold this position for several seconds while adjusting your posture in the hips, spine, and neck as best you can during the breath retention. Then take a deep breath in again, filling your abdominal cavity as you relax. Do this several times per day while sitting at a computer or at work. It can also traditionally be done while standing up and bending forward slightly. The sitting format allows you to incorporate the practice easily into your workspace environment to help you relax and to improve your digestion, which is affected from sitting for long periods. This practice will also help organ circulation and bring oxygen to the brain for concentration at work.

FACIAL FEEDBACK

Just changing the facial muscles by your own willpower can release chemical endorphins and neuropeptides that are stronger than any known antidepressant drug. Many medical practitioners are unaware of the power of manipulating the physical parts of the body to bring about chemical, electrical, and emotional changes. The Taoists wrote about it two thousand years ago, but only now is modern medicine giving it a name: *facial feedback*. The facial feedback hypothesis says that our facial movements have a strong influence on our actual emotional experience. For example, a person who is forced to smile during a social event will actually come to find the event more of an enjoyable experience. Charles Darwin was one of the first to popularize the theory that physiological changes caused by emotions have a direct impact on, rather than being the consequence of, that emotion. American philosopher and physician William James also proposed that, contrary to common belief, awareness of bodily changes activated by a stimulus is the emotion itself. This hypothesis was further supported by an oft-cited 1988 study that proves that people's facial activity influences their affective responses.[*]

Scientists have more recently discovered an inseparable link between our facial expressions and the tiny chemical messengers called *neuropeptides*. When we smile, tiny chemicals are released into the bloodstream from our hormonal glands. These chemicals are responsible for feelings such as relaxation, peacefulness, and happiness. Even if you are feeling depressed or angry, forcefully using your face muscles to smile for several minutes can release massive amounts of chemical messengers that trigger peace and tranquility. This may explain why such exercises as the Inner Smile can heal many physical ailments while also balancing the emotional and mental bodies. Try this: the next time you're feeling angry, depressed, or anxious, sit and smile forcefully for several minutes even though you really don't feel like it. At first it may feel unnatural,

---

[*]F. Strack, L. L. Martin, and S. Stepper, "Inhibiting and facilitating conditions of the human smile: A nonobtrusive test of the facial feedback hypothesis," *Journal of Personality and Social Psychology* 54, no 5 (1988): 768–77.

and you will need to really force yourself to do it because you do not feel like it. After five minutes, evaluate how you feel. Using facial movements like these can release chemical endorphins that affect our mood almost immediately.

RELIEF FROM DENTAL STRESS

Many laypeople, even dentists, have never heard of "dental dysfunction syndrome" and how it can cause dental stress or how serious this missing diagnosis really is. It's estimated that millions of Americans suffer from myriad problems, including high blood pressure, heart problems, Parkinson's disease, multiple sclerosis, and mental illness, due to this little known jaw ailment. One could probably say that dental stress is a gray area in conventional dentistry, though it is commonly treated by holistic dentists. Most people wouldn't think of going to a dentist if they were suffering from headaches, migraines, constipation, or chronic fatigue syndrome because that's what doctors are for, right? But there are many reasons that dentists can do more for you than a doctor in some cases. When your skull bones and the muscles that control your jaw—the masseter and temporal muscles—don't align with each other, serious problems can result. This misalignment causes the jaw muscles to compensate heavily, leaving the muscles distorted with tension. You may say, "This sounds obvious, so what does this do to the rest of the body?" Well, what really happens next is that this tension in the jaw can spread to affect surrounding muscles in the head and neck, in turn traveling to other muscles around the body. As all the meridians in the body have a connection running through the teeth and gums, this can unbalance your complete meridian network, resulting in organ dysfunction.

If you could imagine sitting on a seat that had a tack on it, to avoid pain from the tack sticking you in your rear end you could possibly lift up one side. That may sound easy, but when you hold this posture for any period of time, all the other muscles in the body are affected, and the whole body becomes very stressed. The trouble with dental stress is that you cannot get up and sit in another chair; this tension is with you 24/7. After the tension gets to a certain level, it crushes the temporomandibular joint (TMJ), affecting several cranial nerves, including the vagus nerve. When you note that 40 percent of the nerves that run to the brain go through the temporomandibular joint, it's understandable that headaches and migraines are just some of the serious health ailments a TMJ disorder can cause. Your motor and sensory skills can also be affected, causing nervousness, anxiety, palpitations, and depression. This impairment can also affect the cranial-sacral pump, which is responsible for moving the cerebrospinal fluid to the brain and central nervous system, which generally effects the movement of nutrition to the brain and spinal nerves, causing a host of mental and physical health problems.

There are many causes of dental stress, ranging from accidents in childhood to orthodontic procedures. As our bones are still soft when we're growing, even slight impacts from a parent hitting a child or certain orthodontic procedures can trigger it. Yes, it's true: many orthodontic procedures that involve straightening the teeth can actually cause dental stress. In adults this can also be caused by dental procedures or incorrectly made dentures. Finding out if you have dental stress can be as easy as observing the tongue for marks, or looking for tension in the face muscles. Another way is by bringing your teeth together flat and trying to swallow consistently five times in a row without slowing down. If you have difficulty swallowing and have to take a break after two swallows, it can be a sign of dental stress.

Treatment for dental stress involves going to a holistic dentist or one with experience in these practices and having a dental splint inserted onto your molars, raising them as small as the thickness of a hair, which can help immediately in many cases. It is possible to have jaw dysfunction for several years before problems such as dental stress or nerve compression begin, so it pays to consult a holistic dentist.

VAGUS NERVE STIMULATION (VNS)

There are actually twelve pairs of cranial nerves in the brain, and the vagus nerve is known as the tenth one, sometimes called *cranial nerve X*. The word *vagus* means "wanderer" and is related to the word *vagabond* because it wanders to nearly every part of the body, affecting every organ it touches. The vagus nerve's importance in health has been known to osteopathy and chiropractic and has been popularized in books written by Dr. Theodore A. Baroody. Allopathic medicine is also discovering the importance of this nerve. Vagus nerve stimulation (VNS) using a pacemaker-like device implanted in the chest is a treatment used since 1997 to control seizures in those who suffer from epilepsy, and it has recently been approved for treating drug-resistant cases of clinical depression. VNS may also be achieved by maneuvers such as holding the breath for a few seconds or dipping the face in cold water. The vagus nerve can affect virtually every organ or gland in the body, causing pain, numbness, and acid production if misaligned or pinched by the spinal column.

The vagus nerve is the only cranial nerve that travels beyond the head and neck to other organs, as far as the colon. The nerve originates from the medulla oblongata and then goes into the neck, chest, and abdomen. The vagus is unique in that it contains both motor and sensory fibers. The vagus nerve fibers are parasympathetic nerves, except the throat branch nerves, which go to the larynx and pharynx. The heart, lungs, spleen, liver, stomach, intestines, and kidneys are all supplied with motor fibers from the vagus nerve. The nerve's main functions are to regulate taste, aortic pressure, and heart rate, and stimulate digestive organs and functions. As the vagus nerve affects the vocal cords, pressure on this nerve can cause speech impairment and even loss of speech. Severe pressure on the nerve can even result in death due to its effect on the heart and digestive organs. Many cases of gastroparesis, a condition where the stomach takes too long to empty its contents, are in fact caused by pressure on this nerve. Instead of taking pills for your stomach bloating, heartburn, and other stomach problems, which only address symptoms, manipulation of the spine and cranium or acupuncture can be used to take pressure off this nerve. As your general practitioner is not trained or educated in chiropractic, osteopathy, acupuncture, or cranial-sacral therapy, it's no wonder so many people are taking pills for pain that is caused by vagus nerve pressure.

The vagus nerve controls the movement of food through the digestive tract, so if it is damaged or pinched, the muscles of the stomach and intestines don't work fully, and the movement of food is slowed or even halted. Diabetes also can damage the vagus nerve if blood sugar levels remain high over long periods. The high blood sugar levels "burn" the vagus nerve by producing chemical changes in nerves, damaging the blood vessels that carry oxygen and nutrients to them. This nerve also has a close link to many heart problems. During rest, the vagus nerve sends "slow down" messages to the heart. When you are active or stressed, the sympathetic nerve sends "speed up" signals to the heart by releasing adrenaline, which makes the heart beat faster and work harder. The vagus nerve protects the heart from too much adrenaline, which causes high blood pressure and heart disease. So you can see that you cannot have a healthy heart without a healthy vagus nerve. Current research is investigating the link between vagus nerve stimulation and brain damage regeneration; it is believed that vagus nerve stimulation may accelerate brain recovery from such things as head injuries and strokes.

Many of the acupuncture points used in auricular (ear) acupuncture stimulate the vagus nerve, in turn numbing other major nerves in the body partially or completely, allowing tooth extraction and in some cases surgery to be done without anesthesia. The use of acupuncture anesthesia (which affects the vagus nerve) in surgery in place of pharmaceutical anesthetics results many times in patients being able to walk out of most surgeries the same day as the operation, returning home for a more comfortable recovery because of not having to recover from anesthesia. This practice alone could save the health care industry a lot of money by substantially cutting the length of hospital stays following surgery.

Practices such as osteopathy, acupuncture, cranial-sacral therapy, yoga, and several other therapies can help address and structurally align the body, which can take pressure off the vagus nerve. There have been many positive reports in acupuncture and osteopathic studies with lingering illnesses such as migraines, stomach pain, heartburn, reflux, and overacidity of the digestive tract being improved immediately after as little as one session due to adjustments of the spinal column and cranium. This in turn releases pressure on the vagus nerve. No drugs or herbs can do this job, and in many cases if the vagus nerve issue is not addressed soon enough it can result in serious diseases or even death. Research has shown that women who have complete spinal cord injury can experience orgasms through the vagus nerve, which can go from the uterus, cervix, and probably the vagina to the brain.

Blocking the vagus nerve may also help people who suffer from extreme obesity. Vagus nerve blocking therapy is similar to vagus nerve stimulation but is only used during the day. A report issued by the Mayo Clinic says that "in a six month open-label trial involving three medical centers in Australia, Mexico, and Norway, vagus nerve blocking has helped 31 obese participants lose an average of nearly 15 percent of their excess weight."*

There are myriad people around the world who suffer from epilepsy, including more than 2.5 million in the United States. Western allopathic medicine, which generally focuses on treating symptoms rather than treating the true causes, has been befuddled by its cause and possible cure. Presently, thanks to a team of U.S. electromedicine researchers, a successful treatment may be just around the corner, and it doesn't use drugs. Scientists have discovered (as the Chinese doctors did some two thousand years ago) that stimulation of the vagus nerve at certain points can drastically reduce seizures and in some cases totally prevent them from occurring. The electronic stimulator now approved by the FDA sends microcurrent electrical impulses into the cranial vagus nerve. Some devices can actually be planted under the skin, while other vagus nerve stimulators go above the skin on the back of the neck, such as Dr. Bob Beck's brain-tuner device. This and other devices are perceived to work by stimulating the vagus nerve, which directly increases the production of chemicals and neurotransmitters. When the vagus nerve is thus stimulated, it can trigger the secretion of the neurotransmitter acetylcholine, which plays a key role in the body's electrical system. If levels of acetylcholine become abnormally low, diseases of the nervous system have been known to develop. This device is the first nonpharmacological treatment approved by the FDA for epilepsy and may be the first of a new wave of medicine, known as electrical medicine.

---

*"Device Blocking Stomach Nerve Signals Shows Promise in Obesity," *Science Daily,* June 28, 2008.

BOWENWORK

There are many excellent structural healing techniques available today, from cranial-sacral therapy to osteopathy, but none are more simple, effective, and easy to learn than neurostructural therapy, also known as Bowenwork. The body has an innate ability to heal itself, provided conditions are favorable. Bowenwork, a therapeutic technique developed by an Australian, Tom Bowen (1916–1982), recognizes this principle by helping to reorganize the body's intrinsic systems to facilitate healing.

There is a direct relationship between the structural framework of the body, the nervous system, and the internal organs. Bowen technique, or Bowenwork as it is sometimes called, restores their functional integration through gentle moves that relax the muscles, fascial tissues, and the nervous system. It is a gentle, noninvasive, safe method of manipulating of the muscles, nerves, and connective tissue back into their original positions. Unlike many forms of massage and other structural techniques that attempt to force a change in the structural body, Bowen technique works to reset your body so it can heal itself. Because of the safety and ease of application of the Bowen technique, it can be applied to anyone, from highly trained athletes to the elderly, newborns, and pregnant women.

Tom Bowen, a self-studied "manipulative therapist," worked on hundreds of thousands of patients during his life, forever changing the nature of soft-tissue work. It was not uncommon in Bowen's Queensland, Australia, home for people to be lined up on the street outside for treatment. Bowen was neither a doctor nor a physical therapist at the time he discovered his original technique, so it is not derived from or substantially similar to any other physical manipulative modality. Unlike in chiropractic, Bowenwork involves no manipulation of the joints, but it does encourage misalignments to correct themselves, which is a more passive, gentle way of manipulating the muscular-skeletal system. There is no deep tissue penetration or lengthy contact with muscle tissues as in most forms of deep-tissue massage such as Rolfing, yet muscles do relax and lymphatic circulation is improved. As Tom Bowen did not have extensive knowledge of the meridian system, he relied on his own intuition when he created the original sequence, whose effectiveness is evident by the fact that meridians show strong and immediate changes after a Bowenwork session. There are also improvements in scar tissue and stretch marks.

Unlike Reiki and other energetic therapies that are regarded as spiritual or emotional, Bowenwork does not intentionally use channeling or any other form of connection with higher guides. It is more of a system of stimulating body reflexes involving simple movements that are done across muscles fibers, nerves, and connective tissue. This gentle cross-fiber technique is done using your thumbs or index fingers across muscle fibers or nerve sheaths, causing traction, therefore fully stretching the skin in the opposing direction. This simple technique in turn causes the neuromuscular system to reset all related tension levels, promoting natural healing. The relief can be profound and lasting, usually after only two or three treatments, because it treats the causes of structural problems rather than just its symptoms. Because Bowen technique acknowledges asymmetrical muscle tension, tense and dehydrated fascia tissues, and imbalances in the cranial system, especially in the temporomandibular joint, it has beneficial effects on the muscular, digestive, respiratory, glandular, and energetic systems. Moreover, emotional and spiritual changes have been known to be common after Bowenwork treatment.

SEXUAL KUNG FU AND INTERNAL EXERCISES

In *The Tao of Sexology* Taoist master Dr. Stephen Chang says, "When the average male ejaculates, he loses about one tablespoon of semen. According to scientific research, the nutritional value of this amount of semen is equal to that of two pieces of New York steak, ten eggs, six oranges, and two lemons combined. That includes proteins, vitamins, minerals, amino acids, everything. . . . Ejaculation is often called 'coming.' The precise word for it should be 'going,' because everything—the erection, vital energy, millions of live sperm, hormones, nutrients, even a little of the man's personality goes away.

It is a great sacrifice for the man, spirituality, mentally, and physically." For a man, sexual orgasm and ejaculation go hand in hand (pun intended), and excessive ejaculation has become one of the biggest causes of premature aging, depression, and health problems. Taoist teachings state that as soon as a man ejaculates and throws off his seminal emissions he is committing a form of blatant chi loss. This vital form of chi that is depleted from the male kidney energy is what the Taoists called Ching Chi or essential essence and is the foundation of a man's primal physical and spiritual nourishment. Women differ from men and do not lose Ching Chi through orgasm; rather, they lose their essential essence from heavy menses and from having too many babies, especially if they have their children too close together without cultivating their Ching Chi between pregnancies.

Women do not lose their Ching Chi during orgasm even if they ejaculate, yet as soon as a man ejaculates he loses his. For a man to have longevity without health problems and a strong libido well into his old age, it is of vital importance that he learn to master sexual Kung Fu, thus perfecting the art of orgasm without ejaculation. Hair loss, back and knee pain, prostate problems, kidney disease, weak adrenal glands, low digestive strength, poor memory or concentration, tinnitus, low energy, poor motivation, and lack of creative drive are all signs of a depleted Ching Chi from too much ejaculation.

The average normal ejaculation contains approximately two to five cubic centimeters of semen and approximately 200 to 500 million sperm, rich in nuclear proteins, testosterone and other hormones, and many other essential elements. Each individual sperm of those 200 to 500 million carry 23 chromosomes, prostaglandins, genes and essential vitamins, enzymes, and minerals for the creation of another human being when joined with the female's ovum. There are also striking similarities in the analysis of brain cells and semen, as both are rich in phosphorus, sodium, magnesium, and chlorine. From this we could conclude that our sex glands and brain cells are intimately connected yet are also competing for the same nutritional elements drawn from the essence of our blood.

According to the Taoists, of all the treasures that a man seeks, the most precious of them is *ching*. For a man cannot enjoy any other treasure he discovers or creates without this vital essence of Ching Chi and its essential cultivation. In Chinese medicine, ching is known as one of the "Three Treasures" and is the most valuable of the three, with the other two of them being chi (vital energy, life force) and *shen* (spirit, the spiritual self). Ching is the most concentrated and vital substance known to the Taoist Internal Alchemists. It is said to form bone, brain, and nervous tissue and also nourish the other two treasures. In the yogic tradition of ayurveda, the Three Treasures are also explained with ching being equivalent to the substances known as *soma, shukra dhatu,* and *ojas,* chi being known as *prana,* and shen as *atman.**

We inherit a large part of our ching from our parents through genetics (DNA), and the rest is cultivated during life from proper food and good digestive practices such as slow eating, breathing exercises, and Chi Kung, but we must also guard this sacred treasure by learning sexual Kung Fu. From a modern scientific viewpoint we can liken our storage and cultivation of ching to the length and protection of our telomeres, which are the end parts of our DNA and which determine the aging process according to modern science.

The Taoists say that for the formation of one drop of blood, one needs to digest about twenty times more food, but to form one drop of ching approximately forty to fifty drops of blood is required. That being said we must also understand that the energy that is required for this alchemical process to form ching, which comes from good chi and a strong shen, is incidentally also nourished by ching. Taoists state that the prime energetic ingredient of semen is ching, so it is imperative that a man learn the art of orgasm while retaining his semen for optimal physical and mental health. Of all the Taoist internal exercises the art of sexual Kung Fu is primary for Immortal health.†

---

*For more information on the Three Treasures parallels between TCM and ayurveda see http://wailuahealingarts.com/blog/2016/6/9/the-three-treasures-of-traditional-chinese-medicine-an-ayurvedic-perspective.
†For more information on seminal conservation see http://www.ecologyofthespirit.com/_infoexchange/articles/The%20New%20Science%20of%20Seminal%20Conservation.htm.

There are Chinese herbal formulas that can be prescribed by your Chinese medicine practitioner that can help support Ching Chi formation. That being said, it is also important that a man cultivate Ching Chi with internal exercises such as Chi Kung and yoga as well as with a healthy diet and lifestyle. And most important, for the conservation of ching a man should learn the sexual Kung Fu practices outlined in Mantak Chia's books *The Multi-Orgasmic Man, Sexual Reflexology,* and *Chi Kung for Prostate Health and Sexual Vigor.*

Seventh Immortal Healer—Chuan Chung-Li

Your Body Is Electric

If you want to understand the secrets of the universe, think in terms of energy, frequency, and vibration.

NIKOLA TESLA

When we discuss a construct of energy working together, we call it a matrix. The atom in which the proton operates is a matrix. Your entire body is a matrix.

DAVID A. ELLIOTT, FROM THE BOOK
THE ELECTRIC UNIVERSE

Electric healing is symbolized by Chung-Li Chuan, considered the leader or the most ancient of the Immortals. He is said to have been born in the third century CE. During the Han Dynasty he was a well-respected army general, but after meeting an old man who instructed him in the Tao he left government service and went to the mountains, becoming a wanderer and a beggar. Once while he was meditating the stone wall of his mountain dwelling crumbled, exposing a jade box. The box contained secret meditation instructions on how to become an Immortal. He followed the instructions, and one day his chamber

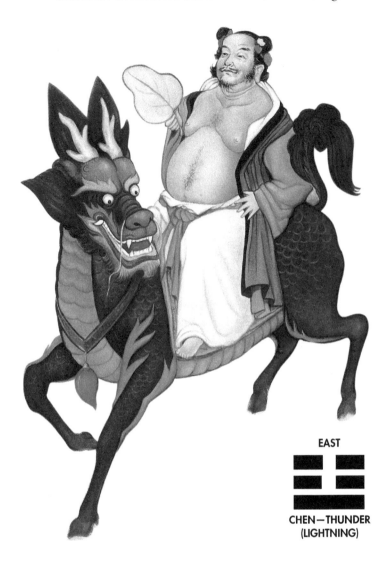

EAST

CHEN—THUNDER
(LIGHTNING)

Fig. 7.1. Chuan Chung-Li (Quan Zong Li)

was filled with rainbow clouds and celestial music. A crane arrived and carried him on its back into the regions of immortality.

Chuan Chung-Li is often represented as a corpulent, bearded, bare-bellied old man of pleasant disposition, often depicted bearing a feathered fan (thought to confer power over the seas or over the forces of life and death) or a peach of immortality. He is a master alchemist and thought to be the teacher of his fellow Immortal Lu Tung-Pin. He represents the element of thunder and lightning, the natural electricity of the cosmos. From this energy the planet recharges its batteries and electrical potentials, cleansing itself and renewing its meridian lines with vital chi. Similarly, our own bodies and cells are electrical in nature, controlled by a supercomputer that is run by a cosmic force the Taoists call *chi*.

UNDERSTANDING THE ELECTRICAL BODY

Our body is described as being electromagnetic because the energy fields within and around it contain both electrical and magnetic qualities. The "electromagnetic spectrum" is the name given to the list of different energy frequencies, which vary from a few cycles per second to several million cycles per second. The official measurement is measured in hertz (abbreviated Hz), where one cycle per second is called 1 hertz. When an atom vibrates at a few hundred cycles per second, this is called a *sound frequency;* a few thousand cycles per second is called a *radio wave,* and several million cycles per second is called *light,* with color being a specific light frequency. The cells of your body vibrate at approximately 1.5 million hertz, and your DNA vibrates at approximately 50 billion hertz.

The scientific study of these frequencies and their relation to healing the body is called *electrical medicine* or *electrical nutrition,* and more recently it has been called *photobiotic nutrition.* Many inventors who have ventured from the norms and limitations of conventional drug medicine have discovered and personally documented the amazing healing abilities that different electromagnetic frequencies and sounds have on the body. Probably the first documented records in the West of using electricity to cure disease came in 46 CE from the Roman physician Scribonius Largus, court physician to Roman emperor Claudius. Scribonius cured health ailments such as headaches and gout by having patients stand on a wet electric torpedo fish. It is believed that electrical fish were actually used for a variety of different illnesses until the invention of electricity in the eighteenth century. Then around that time, drugs became the main treatment option, and the thought of using electrical fish was considered barbaric and foolish. It seems that the move toward treating the chemical body rather than the electrical body has been given priority in medicine ever since. However, over the last hundred years has come a stream of scientists, such as Nikola Tesla, Georges Lakhovsky, Albert Abrams, Royal Rife, and more recently Ed Skilling, Bob Beck, and Hulda Clark, all of whom have played important roles in the development of some of the latest electrical healing devices in the field of electromedicine.

Georges Lakhovsky was one of the first pioneers of electromedicine to theorize that each human cell operates like a tiny battery and when fully charged is able to experience cell balance, creating a feeling of well-being and health. Albert Abrams theorized that a disease condition sends out a radio frequency that is incompatible with normal cells. He believed that if you could alter the polarity of the sick cells and restore their electrical balance, you could accelerate the healing process. Royal Rife believed that germs and other microorganisms are responsible for creating most diseases within the body by attacking the immune system, in turn disabling it. He later went on to discover specific frequencies for healing specific diseases and eliminating specific pathogens. Dr. Rife comprehensively documented what frequencies result in the death of certain pathogens, yet received little recognition for his amazing discoveries until recently, as electrical medicine has become more accepted in natural medicine circles today. He was the first person in history to comprehensively research the unique frequency of specific diseases, and then list the specific frequency that destroys or disenables its ability to function. More recently, it has been discovered that our own white blood cells destroy bacteria and foreign microorganisms when an electrical current is used against them, as concluded by French scientists who summarized in one study that "white cells (leukocytes) kill bacteria and pathogenic fungus by electrocuting them."[*]

The electrical activity that occurs inside the body and especially within the cells is primarily responsible for the manufacture of all body chemicals and their interactions. Medical professionals in the allopathic

---

[*]"Médicine," *Science et Vie* 972 (1998): 44; translated from French.

field to this day primarily focus on the chemical aspect of the body because it is what they are taught in medical school. However, if you limit yourself solely to the observation and treatment of the chemical body, an array of other complications will obviously occur in the form of side effects. Only when a proper electrical balance occurs in the body can there be a corresponding chemical balance. This is exactly how acupuncture is believed to work. The stimulation of acupuncture points on the body's meridians in turn creates electrical signals to the chemical body, thereby increasing the production of certain hormones and neurochemicals. At the same time it delivers messages to the chemical body, acupuncture can also unblock the physical tissues, increasing the circulation of vital nutrients within the blood, especially to deficient areas. The Chinese have documented since the time before Christ the effects of the electrical body and the results of stimulating certain points, but it has only been quite recently that modern medicine with its advancements in electrical measuring devices recognized the existence of the body electric. And even though it has only been researched and studied in the West in the last hundred years, electrical medicine has advanced very quickly. For example, scientists have discovered that the cell membrane is made of fat, which is only one-millionth of an inch thick. Despite this, it has the same electrical potential as a two-thousand-volt power line and far better electrical insulation ability than any other known man-made material.

Our bodies are able to create their own electromagnetic fields by absorbing photons from sources such as the sun, the environment, and the food we eat. While the sun is our primary source of light, food also represents an important sustaining form; hence the term *photobiotic nutrition,* which refers to a high-energy diet. At the same time our bodies are able to use photons of light to create its electrical fields; these electrical fields also produce their own form of light. This storehouse of the body's electrical currents and frequencies is no other than our own DNA, which also acts as the body's electrical transformer. From this information alone one can begin to imagine the complexities and intricacies of the electrical body and its strong effect on the chemical body.

And just as our own bodies depend on electricity for health, so does planet Earth. Our own bodies would perish without the nourishment of electromagnetic fields in the form of light and sound. This fact became evident during Michael Faraday's experiments involving the Faraday cages, which were sealed cages that block all forms of electromagnetic fields. Dr. Faraday discovered that any living organism placed in these cages died as a result of the absence of vital electromagnetic fields. Earth, like us, also depends on environmental phenomena to allow it to sustain other life-forms like us. Planet Earth could be likened to a giant battery or crystal that absorbs both the sun's energy and the electrical energy from lightning. Yes, Earth uses the electromagnetic energy from lightning to fix nitrogen into her soil, which balances the soil's electromagnetic properties and also nourishes vegetation.

HEALING ELECTRICAL CURRENTS

If you or someone you know is suffering from arthritis, diabetes, cancer, AIDS, or any immune-deficiency condition as a result of viral or bacterial infections, the use of electricity may be of prime help. In her book *The Cure for All Diseases,* Dr. Hulda Clark says, "Electricity can now be used to kill bacteria, viruses, and parasites in minutes, not days or weeks as antibiotics require."

The most recent discoveries using electricity and frequency to selectively electrocute pathogens without harming healthy tissue may sound futuristic, but it is fast becoming a well-accepted scientific fact. Modern science now acknowledges that every form of life, whether animal, bacterial, or viral, has a specific frequency at which it oscillates (vibrates). Once you know the frequency at which a specific life-form vibrates, you can also find the frequency that destroys it. Many of us are aware that certain electromagnetic frequencies are disastrous to human health and can even result in death. This includes various forms of radiation and microwaves that can kill human beings while leaving many forms of bacteria and insects completely unharmed. Every virus, bacteria, and parasite also has a unique frequency at which it vibrates and a frequency that destroys it. Since viruses and bacteria are at the root of so many of today's health ailments, the use of electricity instead of drugs to neutralize these pathogens is a step in the right direction.

When we think about it, all life is simply vibrating energy. An atom, for example, is an energy system consisting of electrons, neutrons, and protons whose elements oscillate at a specific frequency, therefore providing electrical homeostasis. Electromedicine researchers such as Dr. Hulda Clark state that any positively offset (DC) frequency can destroy bacteria, viruses, and parasites when given sufficient voltage (5 to 10 volts) and a frequency ranging from 10 to 500,000 Hz. Although "zapping" in this way can get into most parts of the body, it may not reach certain parts of the digestive canal, meaning that herbal medicines for parasites and immunity need to be combined with electromedicine to obtain optimal results.

With the development of such frequency devices as the F-Scan 2, it is possible to scan the body with a wide range of frequencies in order to detect pollutants, pathogens, and parasites, along with their resonating frequencies within the body. These specific disease frequencies come from an internal "library" of frequencies that have been discovered over the decades by electromedicine researchers like Royal Rife. These frequencies are fed into a microprocessor and then sent into the body via a simple wristband or handheld electrodes. Sending out biofeedback messages that return, frequency generators can then indicate if a specific disease pathogen is inside your body. If the feedback information from the body indicates the presence of identical pathogenic frequencies (through the principle of resonance), then the device can administer these frequencies into the body in a corrective dosage in order to neutralize the negative effects of the disease-causing pathogens. One can easily see that if and when these devices are ever accepted by the FDA and become legal for medical doctors to use, this could mean an end to many pharmaceutical drugs, especially all antibiotic medicines and perhaps even vaccines. Using electricity and frequencies to eliminate and destroy disease-causing pathogens while simultaneously stimulating the immune system just seems like a more sensible way to assist the body to heal itself. If this is so, why then does modern medicine fail to spend any of our hard-earned tax dollars on research into the use of electricity for health?

Unfortunately, these devices are just too cheap to be profitable to the medical industry. A simple zapper, for example, can be purchased for as little as a hundred dollars. On top of this, if you have knowledge of electrical circuits and can read basic electrical circuit diagrams you can easily make one yourself from parts from your local electrical store. So in addition to not being profitable, electrical medicine puts too much control back into the hands of the people. Electrical medicine has the potential of making people less dependent on Big Pharma every time they are sick. So is it any wonder that pathogen-zapping devices are not approved by the FDA? At present, these devices are available only from manufacturers, who are not allowed to advertise them as being effective for a variety of health conditions.

THE BECK PROTOCOL, A FIRST-AID KIT FOR THE TWENTY-FIRST CENTURY

The late Dr. Robert C. "Bob" Beck was a highly respected physicist and former consultant to Sandia Corporation, a senior staff scientist at the Eyring Research Institute, and a consultant to the U.S. Navy. He was well known for his leading-edge designs in measuring subtle magnetic fields and extra-low-frequency (ELF) fields. His research project in the early 1980s that focused on the brain and altered states of consciousness resulted in the design of a device he called the Brain Tuner, which won him an award from the John Fetzer Foundation. Although at that time he was living in relative ease because of the money he'd made by holding the patent on the automatic camera flash—just one of his many inventions—Dr. Beck's life changed forever when he read about a research project done at the Albert Einstein College of Medicine in New York City. In March 1991, *Science News* gave a brief report that "zapping the HIV virus" with a low-voltage electrical current can eliminate its ability to infect human white blood cells cultured in the laboratory. Doctors William Lyman and Steven Kaali presented this research at a symposium, but it somehow later mysteriously disappeared, deleted from the symposium report. However, the research sparked Bob Beck's interest in electrical medicine, and he set out to track down this research.

In 1993, Lyman and Kaali filed for a patent with the U.S. Patent Office* that would enable their discovery to become public information for the first time. Dr. Beck soon modified their device and developed a safe, simple, noninvasive method of applying this technique, but rather than patenting his idea, he made his information freely available to all as the device known as the blood electrifier referenced in this section. Beck's invention brilliantly combined the discoveries of Lyman and Kaali with other research from Dr. Robert Becker and his team at Syracuse University, who conducted many years of research into the long-known antibacterial properties of silver. He proved that submicroscopic particles of colloidal silver suspended in water destroyed even the most drug-resistant microbes on contact. Imagine the hidden reactions of the pharmaceutical industry when Bob Beck developed a simple electronic device, affordable by almost anyone, that could destroy virtually all known bacteria, viruses, and fungi instantly. By making his invention freely available to all, Beck made it impossible for the medical and pharmaceutical industries to control or suppress his invention.

Four Easy Beck Protocols

At Master Chia's clinic at Tao Garden, in Thailand, we recommend and use the following four protocols from Bob Beck:

Dr. Beck's blood electrifier: Microcurrents are well known in electrical medicine circles for their ability to eliminate viruses, parasites, fungi, bacteria, and other pathogens in the blood. Pioneering work in this field goes back to 1890, but most of these breakthroughs and patents have either been either lost or suppressed. For example, this method was rediscovered in 1990 at Einstein College of Medicine as an AIDS cure and then silenced. Dr. Beck's blood electrification protocol takes approximately one hour daily for about three weeks and has demonstrated remarkable results not only with the HIV virus, but with a variety of other health-related conditions.

---

*Patent no. 5,188,738.

Pulsed kilogauss magnetic fields using the Beck magnetic pulse generator: Externally applied magnetic resonance of the lymph glands, spleen, kidneys, and liver can help neutralize germinating, latent, and incubating parasites that block the reinfection process. Magnetic fields increase lymphatic drainage elimination, restore the immune system, and support detoxification. Permanent magnets, no matter how strong, will not, and cannot, scavenge pathogens with induced magnetic currents. You must have a sharp time-varying magnetic impulse, and not just a magnet, to get the desired effect.

Silver colloids (ionic/colloidal silver) using the Beck silver maker: With colloidal silver costing only a few cents per gallon to make at home, an ionic colloidal silver maker can greatly assist you in eliminating pathogens and guarding against opportunistic infections and viruses. Silver can actually help to create a "second immune system" and is highly complementary with the other three protocols.

Drinking oxygen-rich water using Dr. Beck's water ozonator: This unit provides fast and natural cell oxygenation through oxygen-rich water without causing free-radical damage. Drinking ozonated water aids in the body's detoxification process by oxidizing wastes and anaerobic pathogens and reducing CO_2 without the hassle of physical techniques. Recall from chapter 1 that no harmful pathogens can live in high levels of oxygen for any length of time.

We highly recommend watching the Beck Protocol video at www.bobbeck.com, which gives an in-depth explanation of how to use each of these protocols effectively and safely.

Beck Pulsar and Clark Zapper

The main difference between Dr. Hulda Clark's zapper and Dr. Beck's blood electrifier unit (or pulsar, as it is also called) is that the former works more with frequency and the latter with current. Dr. Clark's research was heavily influenced by Dr. Royal Rife and his work during the 1930s. Combining this knowledge on specific frequencies to destroy parasites, Dr. Clark uses a positive offset square-wave frequency with a direct current, combined with a voltage of 7 to 8 volts, producing frequencies that can range from 2,500 to 30,000 Hz. The lower frequencies are said to penetrate the body more easily. When this voltage is applied in pulses, it produces what is called a "square wave," which is more likely to affect a large range of different parasites. Even Dr. Clark admits that any frequency with a range from 1 to 400,000 Hz will produce a similar result as long as the wave form is of a positive offset. The positive electrical force that pulses up and down destroys disease-causing invaders while also energizing the white blood cells to attack any other foreign invading pathogens. The Clark zapper is applied using wristbands or hand-held copper pipes applied on both wrists.

The Beck blood electrifier uses a higher voltage of 27 volts that supplies alternating microcurrents of electricity. This voltage is similar to a tense muscle stimulator, but the Beck device uses lower microcurrents applied onto the surface of the radial arteries on only one wrist at a time. The current that enters the blood can be as low as 50 micro amps operating at a frequency of 4 Hz, which is half that of Earth's frequency (which is approximately 8 Hz). Dr. Beck's device uses harmless microcurrents of electricity to literally electrocute pathogens, as opposed to a specific frequency like Dr. Clark's device, destroying them in the bloodstream.

We have seen many cases where clients get more benefit from one particular device over another, and in our experience it all depends on the person and the illness involved. Using both devices and seeing which one feels better is the best way to find out. Both devices use ultrasafe levels of current and frequency to eliminate pathogens from the body and stimulate the immune system. The Clark zapper can be useful especially in children's ailments and for quick zaps to eliminate the onset of cold or flu. Dr. Beck's blood electrifier appears to be more efficient for cleaning the blood of disease pathogens and viruses. Neither device actually enters into the lymph glands or the organs themselves. Because of this, Dr. Beck developed another device, a magnetic pulse generator that penetrates the lymphatic system and other deep tissue areas that the blood electrifier device was unable to reach. Integrating both techniques into a health protocol, in combination with other protocols outlined in this book, is a sure way to benefit your health and reverse disease.

ACUPUNCTURE BALANCES YOUR ELECTRICAL BODY

Acupuncture, although relatively unchanged for thousands of years, is only recently beginning to gain massive worldwide popularity in the complementary health field. One reason for this is that quite simply acupuncture helps to balance the electrical body. Acupuncture stimulates points on twelve major meridians and the eight extra meridians, which are connected to the complex network of thousands of nadis (internal meridian networks) that make up our entire electrical body. Even though acupuncture has only been recognized by allopathy for treating a few conditions such as pain, inflammation, and stress, in reality it has immense potential for a wide range of conditions; inasmuch as stress is probably an underlying cause of many diseases, you can read between the lines to see that acupuncture works wonders for many different ailments. In fact, back in 1972, Dr. Kenneth Riland, an osteopathic physician who attended President Nixon, said, "I am convinced that acupuncture is going to be one of the greatest contributions that any group of people has made to the future of all medicine, if it is handled correctly by the people of the Western world."

As acupuncture is a complex field of study, you may need to search around a bit to find a suitable, appropriately trained practitioner of this healing art. Not all treatments are the same, and many acupuncturists, especially Western medical doctors, have a very limited understanding of the complexity of the meridian networks and subtle protocols of balancing or moving blocked chi. Some allopathic doctors sign up for acupuncture training that is limited to several weekend workshops, whereas a licensed acupuncturist or, better yet, a doctor of traditional Chinese medicine has been educated for a minimum of three years, receiving a full-time education in both classical and modern acupuncture treatment strategies as well as related interventions, such as Asian herbal medicine.

One style of acupuncture that is gaining worldwide popularity in North America, Australia, and recently in Europe, is traditional Japanese acupuncture. This painless style of acupuncture is the one that I use in my clinic and have been using for almost two decades now, with great success. The acupuncture needles are half the thickness of normal acupuncture needles and are extremely tapered, unlike traditional Chinese needles—meaning they can be inserted without causing any discomfort. Japanese-style acupuncture is just as effective as the Chinese style but without any pain. Thanks to teachers such as Shudo Denmei Sensei, Masakazu Ikeda Sensei, Edward Obaidey Sensei, and Alan Jansson Sensei, this gentle yet extremely effective treatment protocol is becoming known worldwide. For more information on the benefits of acupuncture, visit www.cureplanet.com or visit us at www.tao-garden .com, and come and stay with us and enjoy all the benefits of this amazing healing art while also learning all the Universal Healing Tao teachings in beautiful tranquil surrounds with both Master Chia and me.

COSMIC (CHI KUNG) HEALING

According to ayurveda, the subtle body is made of prana, or chi, as it is known to the Taoists and traditional Chinese medicine. The body also contains a light body or aura, which is also made of this substance and is called Wei Chi by the Taoists. Both Hindu and Taoist philosophies believe that we have vortices of energy within our body that are connected to the cosmos. These vortices are the energy centers (chakras), which are essentially spinning wheels of light. The major chakras are on the central axis, which parallels the spine; the minor chakras are around the organs and glands, and in addition there are the mini-chakras, which are referred to as *marma* in ayurveda or as acupuncture points by the Taoists. It is said that all these chakras and acupuncture points have a strong effect on our physical, mental, and emotional bodies; when any of these forces are out of balance or alignment, it can affect the functioning of our chakras and light bodies and thus our nervous system, which is the controlling force in Western medicine. This is the body, mind, and spirit connection, which understands them as all one and not separate entities. Within every cell exists mind, body, and spirit chi, even though many people mistakenly think that mind exists only in the head, modern science is now proving that this misconception is incorrect.

According to ancient Taoist and Chinese medical texts there are five levels of healing skill. In the first level, the healer uses foods and herbs to heal the patient. In the second level, the healer uses his or her hands to massage or apply acupressure. The third level involves the use of acupuncture needles and moxibustion (burning herbs on acupuncture points) to bring about a cure, both of which involve great skill. In the fourth level, the healer is by now so progressed in acupuncture and moxibustion techniques that he or she no longer requires needles or moxibustion and uses only the projection of his or her own chi through the fingers, creating the same effect by touching the acupuncture or marma points. The fifth level of healing requires the highest of all skills; for this the healer must be extremely pure in heart, mind, and intention and have cultivated his or her internal chi to a high level with Taoist Inner Alchemy practices. On this level, physical touch is no longer needed; instead, the healer is able to access chi from the cosmos and project this cosmic chi for the purpose of healing, either at close range or over great distances, with great effect.

Cosmic healing, like the Indian form called Pranic Healing, involves a healing intention to direct chi (prana) toward the patient that comes through the practitioner from the cosmos. The healing energy does not originate with the healer. In cosmic healing the healer is simply a conduit for cosmic energy. The practice uses movements of the hands to clean and regulate the energy fields of the spiritual body and is safe, with no side effects. It is unlike hands-on healing or Reiki; you do not physically touch the body in most cases but rather move the hands slightly above the body. Cosmic healing is not intended to replace allopathic medicine, nor does it diagnose disease; rather, it works on the subtle energy fields in and around the body that are not recognized by modern medicine because they cannot be seen by most of us. Both Master Chia and I have been working with this process for some time, as have numerous other practitioners who practice the Universal Healing Tao. To experience the benefits of cosmic healing please look at the Universal Healing Tao website for registered practitioners in this art.

PHOTON SOUND BEAM:
LIGHT FOR BODY HEALING

Healing both the light body and the physical body with different universal healing frequencies sounds like medicine of the future, almost like science fiction, but it is in fact available today for those who want it. This form of medicine is neither taught nor highly researched in modern allopathic medicine, so don't expect your doctor to provide you with an educated opinion on this form of therapy. Only through educating yourself can you discover the groundbreaking technologies that electrical medicine has to offer.

There are many debates over the incredible work of Dr. Royal Rife and his use of a specific frequency for each disease. One of Dr. Rife's final discoveries was that four universal frequencies could be used interchangeably to treat all diseases. These findings were in fact discovered earlier by Georges Lakhovsky (1869–1942), a Russian engineer, scientist, author, and inventor whose Multiple Wave Oscillator is described as having been used by him in the treatment of cancer. In 1930, Lakhovsky concluded that the frequency carrying the largest amount of harmonics also has the greatest healing potential (with the one in the 727-Hz range said to be more flexible than any other).

The purpose of using different spectrums of high frequencies (in the light and sound ranges) for the purpose of eliminating pathogens and disease must also include the nourishment of cells, in turn making the body stronger for self-healing, as using harmonic-rich frequencies solely for the purpose of eliminating pathogens is just not enough. The electrical body also needs to be stimulated to allow complete healing to occur. All matter, living or not, has its own unique vibrational frequency that forms the "language" that it speaks. This matter is made up of atoms, which are in turn made up of condensed light, or photons, which carry their own form of information that we call *intelligence*. This form of nonphysical intelligence, called chi or prana in Eastern medicine, is a form of information that directs all matter, including your body cells, through the medium of DNA.

The medical terms photobiotic nutrition and electrical nutrition are becoming more common in nutritional circles for several reasons. Nutritional scientists are finally beginning to realize that synthetic vitamins work quite differently inside the body compared to organic (light-containing) sources from whole foods. The main difference between an organic nutrient and a synthetically made one is the amount of light it contains and omits; therefore, the amount of information it can actually provide for your cells and DNA. Once we understand nutrients, especially vitamins, to be living substances and not just dead matter, this opens a new gateway into the field of nutritional and natural medicine.

Since Edgar Cayce's readings in the 1930s and his mention of the violet ray machine developed by Nikola Tesla and presented at the Columbian Exhibition in Chicago in 1893, research into the use of noble gases in light tubes has progressed greatly. Using high frequencies of light and sound through the medium of noble gases such as argon, xenon, and krypton, the photon sound beam delivers a pure dose of bioelectrical energy that provides electrical nutrition to your cells. It also can be used for stimulating the eliminatory organs such as the lymphatic system, thereby increasing detoxification. Today, delivering a full spectrum of bioavailable harmonic frequencies with machines such as the photon sound beam has been found to open and unblock energy channels and meridians with ease, complementing other energetic therapies such as acupuncture and homeopathy. It combines the technologies of Rife, Lakhovsky, Tesla, and others, and it can be performed in the comfort of your own home without having to undergo expensive intravenous medicine procedures such as intravenous ozone or blood electrification.

When noble gases contained within glass tubes are ionized with electricity and magnetic fields, they in turn create millions of harmonic-rich frequencies that can then be directed into the tissues. This photobiotic nutrition is then coupled with the additional healing effects of the gases themselves. As these microcurrents emitted from the noble tubes are the same as the body's, they are able to travel within the physical tissues and along subtle electrical and meridian systems. The noble gases helium, argon, neon, xenon, and krypton not only provide an excellent medium for the transfer of electrical fields, they also have unique healing qualities themselves. The most unique of all the elements in the universe, these gases are called "inert" because their numbers of electrons, protons, and neutrons are completely balanced, making them the perfect medium for electromagnetic transference. The universal frequencies produced can be likened to what Eastern traditions call Sacred Sounds, which have been used in many forms of yoga. These powerful charges have a direct effect on lymphatic drainage, which is just as important, if not more than, blood circulation.

CRANIAL ELECTROTHERAPY STIMULATION

For almost a quarter of a century, cranial electrotherapy stimulation (CES) has effectively treated many forms of anxiety, depression, stress, addiction, insomnia, and learning difficulties. More and more we are being told of the importance of brain waves and the role they play in governing our moods and health. We are told that techniques such as meditation lower brain-wave frequencies, resulting in a sense of well-being. Science has more recently discovered that when we alter these brain waves we can direct our thoughts to positive ones more easily. This is exactly how hypnotists are able to change people's beliefs by taking them into a hypnotic alpha state. Unfortunately, many of us do not take the time to meditate and properly relax, leading to high levels of stress and poor health—which is why a CES device can be vital.

Low-intensity electrical stimulation is believed to have originated in the studies of galvanic currents in humans and animals as conducted by Italian physicists Giovanni Aldini, Alessandro Volta, and others in the eighteenth century. Cranial electrotherapy stimulation was pioneered in the Soviet Union during the late 1940s and has been used effectively and safely by millions of people around the world since then. In 1972, a specific form of CES was developed by Dr. Margaret Patterson. The treatment used small pulses of electric current across the head for acute and chronic withdrawal from addictive substances and was named NeuroElectric Therapy (NET). A prescription cranial electrotherapy stimulation device that was intended as therapy for insomnia became available in the United States in 1963. It was known as an "electrosleep" machine because of its effect on improving sleeping patterns. The device was registered as a Class III device under the Medical Device Amendments Act of 1976, when the name was changed to Cranial Electrotherapy Stimulation. The CES device is a small, hand-size apparatus with a cord that forms a stethoscope-like headpiece. When placed beneath the ears, it delivers a mild stimulation to the hypothalamic area of the brain, resulting in the increased production of endorphins and other mood-enhancing chemicals while also harmonizing neurotransmitter activities. This results in improved relaxation, better sleep, increased vitality, and better health. The alpha state that is produced by the brain when using a CES device also creates a natural high, sometimes called a "runner's high," resulting in improved concentration and moods. Charles McCusker, Ph.D., a researcher in the field of CES, claims that it has "major implications in a number of areas. In the war on drugs, it is a formidable new weapon in the treatment of the symptoms accompanying detoxification and withdrawal. For those suffering from depression and anxiety, it means relief with none of the unpleasant side effects of prescription drugs. For those seeking nothing more than a good night's sleep, it is an alternative to habit-forming tranquilizers."*

CES shows no known side effects, dangers, or serious contraindications. The devices are extremely simple in design and inexpensive to purchase online. It is now estimated that approximately 80 percent of ailments are stress related, so the effectiveness of CES in treating a variety of conditions for which pharmaceutical drugs are otherwise prescribed means these units offer a safe, healthy alternative. And as CES promotes improved brain functioning, it seems logical to also feed the body optimal levels of nutrition when using such devices. Making sure the body is receiving optimal levels of amino acids in organic forms is

---

*Charles McCusker, "Better Living through Chemistry?" http://altered-states.net /barry/newsletter127.

highly recommended, as these are the brain's primary fuels for making neurotransmitters.

MAGNETIC MEDICINE

The Taoist sages have long been aware of the power of magnetic currents in the cosmos and within their bodies, and like nature and all living organisms, the human body is also affected by magnetic fields. Observations as to how magnetic fields affect human health have been recorded as far back as the ancient Egyptian era. It was said that Cleopatra wore a magnetic headband to relieve her migraine headaches and to elevate her mood. NASA and space scientists have also been aware of the effects of magnetic fields on the health of astronauts, so we must be aware of turning off Wi-Fi when not in use and also turning off our phones when we are sleeping.

We all know that advising you to "get enough sleep" is one of the best pieces of medical advice your health practitioner can give you. Now recent research is saying that lying with the top of your head facing in certain directions can affect your sleep patterns due to magnetic fields. Many people have found that simply by switching the orientation of their beds they sleep better due to the body's innate compass. Just like our planet, which has a positive pole in the north and a negative pole in the south, our bodies have a positive pole in the head and a negative pole in the feet. Positive poles repel each other, so aligning our head with the positive North Pole can set up a struggle between the two poles. Taoists have said to avoid sleeping with the head pointing north or west, and even the Sanskrit text the Mahabharata says that man becomes wise by sleeping with the head to east and south.*

Paracelsus, in 1528, was the first to record his success in treating a variety of diseases by using magnets, and shortly after that, around 1600, Sir William Gilbert, the personal physician to Queen Elizabeth I

---

*See www.sanskritimagazine.com/vedic_science/myth-of-sleeping-in-the-right-direction and http://wildalchemist.blogspot.com.au/2011/05/which-direction-should-you -sleep.html.

of England, wrote his pioneering work *De magnete, magneticisque corporibus, et de magno magnete tellure* (*On the Magnet and Magnetic Bodies, and on That Great Magnet the Earth*), regarding the use of magnets in medicine. Forty years after that, Swedish astronomer and mathematician Anders Celsius published his theories on Earth's magnetic fields. By the 1800s English scientist Michael Faraday established the basis for the concept of the electromagnetic field in physics, which became the basis for the modern understanding of magnetic-field therapy today. It was after studies done on electromagnetism in the 1950s by Nikola Tesla and Albert Einstein that Linus Pauling described the biomagnetic property of blood in 1965.

Most of the research on the use of magnets in medicine has occurred in Japan and Russia, where it is an accepted part of complementary medicine, and only relatively recently has interest in the pain-relieving and other health benefits of magnetic medicine sparked interest among doctors and laypeople in the West. William H. Philpott, M.D. (1919–2009), a proponent of magnetic-field therapy and orthomolecular medicine (he won the 2000 American Academy of Environmental Medicine Jonathan Forman Award and the 1997 Linus Pauling Award from the Orthomolecular Health Society, of which he was a founding member), said that "magnetic field therapy will be the most effectual antibiotic treatment for infections (bacteria, viruses, fungi, and parasites) because none of these organisms can tolerate a negative magnetic field." A Hopi prophecy says that after the third tribulation, a new source of energy will be discovered that taps Earth's magnetic field.

It is believed that magnetic fields act on the cells of the body because they can penetrate all organic matter. Because the human body is composed of atoms and molecules that carry electrical charges, magnetic fields actually affect the ion exchange within the cells' nuclei, playing a vital role as the medium of information transference between the cells and their DNA. It has been observed that diseased cells have a reduced electrical potential compared to that of healthy cells. When any area of your body begins to suffer poor circulation, your level of oxygen, which is carried by the blood, also becomes deficient. As oxygen is a fuel for the operation of the electrical ion pump in and around every cell, the electrical potential decreases. On the same note, using magnetic fields on a particular area of the body can lead to improved utilization of oxygen in the cells, thus improving circulation. Remember that diseased cells are sick primarily because they are not receiving enough blood-carrying nutrients and oxygen, which fuel the electrical pumps of the body.

Magnetic Treatment Benefits

Using the therapeutic properties of magnetic fields increases circulation, nutrition, oxygen, and electrical potential to the cells of your body, allowing them to operate at optimal levels. The healing magnetic fields in the form of pulsed fields or attached magnets are one way of reenergizing the affected electrical body and balancing the meridian system. Magnet therapy has the potential to become a common treatment for a wide variety of degenerative health conditions in the near future. Dr. Michael Schachter, founder and director of the Schachter Center for Complementary Medicine in Suffern, New York, says, "I have seen dramatic results when the north magnetic pole is directly applied to a cancer or an area of inflammation." Magnet therapy is economical and easy to apply and has no side effects, making it an excellent adjunct to other complementary therapies. As magnets do not introduce any foreign substance into the body, they are completely safe even when used long term.

Magnetic treatment has a host of health benefits:

- Supports wound healing and bone regeneration
- Improves circulation and nutrients to the tissues
- Treats pain in the nervous system
- Reduces muscle spasms and tension
- Promotes relaxation, reducing stress-related ailments
- Eases migraine headaches, nausea, and vomiting
- Treats metabolic and hormonal disorders
- Treats depression and emotional imbalances

Most body magnets available today work by emitting a concentrated magnetic flux to a single point, whether that is tissue or an acupuncture or trigger point. This concentrated stimulation, which in many types of body magnets is combined with a small nodule in the magnet for added acupressure benefits, induces an electromotive force that directly stimulates blood circulation in the local area, while also stimulating acupuncture reflex points.

Magnetic plasters come in all different shapes, sizes, and gauss strengths so they can be flexibly applied to different areas of the body for different purposes. Many people use them for alleviating pain in the muscles and joints by way of direct stimulation. Most plasters begin at a strength of 800 gauss and go considerably higher. Using one is as simple as locating the tender, stiff, or damaged area of muscle on the neck, shoulders, torso, or legs and directly applying it to the affected area. You can learn about common acupuncture points such as those for stimulating the immune system or relaxing the nervous system from a layperson's acupuncture book or from your natural health practitioner, and you can then apply one of these plasters yourself in the comfort of your home. And if you have doubts about the effectiveness of magnetic fields on a variety of ills, take a look at Bob Beck's magnetic pulse generator,* described earlier in this chapter, which uses pulsed kilogauss magnetic fields that are thousands of times stronger than standard dermal magnets.

NEGATIVE IONS AND THERAPEUTIC IONIZERS

The production of negative ions is nature's way of cleaning its environment. And just like their effect on the environment, they also keep the body youthful by preventing free-radical damage. They react with positively charged pollutants to naturally clean the air we breathe. If you have ever wondered why the air is so much fresher in the forest or mountains and why it gives you more energy, it's because both trees

---

*www.cancertutor.com/bobbeck-mp.

and running water produce large amounts of negative ions naturally, while the concrete buildings, cars, and industrial pollution of the cities all produce positive ions, decreasing the production and survival of negative ions. As bad as our external environment has become today, it is actually our indoor environment that affects us even more, because most people today spend 80 percent of their time indoors, which is where positive ions take hold. As most of us don't have enough indoor plants in our homes to generate negative ions, using a negative ion generator to purify the air at home can assist in reducing allergies and respiratory problems as well as improving overall health and well-being. The negative ions that are released into the air via a negative ion generator act like a magnet, attaching to positively charged pollutants such as dust and pollens, creating a larger particle. Then the natural forces of gravity result in the new larger particle falling to the ground, which can then easily be vacuumed up.

Unlike common air cleaners, which use a filter approximately 0.3 microns in size to clean the air, a negative ionizer filters pollutants as small as 0.01 microns in size. Standard air-cleaning units, with long-term use, can also become breeding grounds for bacteria. Negative ionizers, on the other hand, use a more ingenious system of creating and releasing millions of negative ions that can attach to the smallest airborne particles, removing them from the air. Units such as the XJ-2000 can produce a negative ion density ten times higher than the negative ion level found at Niagara Falls.

Most ionizers use a method called "needlepoint ionization," producing large amounts of microscopic negative ions and safe levels of ozone. Effective units will have at least eight needle points made of corrosion-resistant stainless steel, which can emit trillions of negative ions into the air in seconds. Needlepoint ionization is still the most effective way of producing high levels of negative ions compared to photo-ionization or corona-discharge technology, which produce lower concentrations of negative ions and higher levels of unstable ozone. A good negative ionizer will produce a clean-smelling and sweet odor reminiscent of the fresh smell in the air after a thunderstorm. While most units produce large amounts of negative ions that clean the air, they may not be small enough to be actually breathed in or used by the body, limiting their therapeutic effect. However, a new breed of ionizers called "therapeutic ionizers"—the Elanra unit is an example—claims to produce therapeutic ions small enough to be absorbed into the lungs, thereby having medicinal benefits.

SOLAR (SUNBATHING) TREATMENT

It is not only a boost of vitamin D that we get from exposing our body to the sun, we also get vital electrical energy. For millennia many different cultures have worshiped the sun; poets and sages have written about it, not only because our crops would not grow and animals would not live without it, but also because we humans would not survive without sunlight. The sun sustains our chi, our vital energy that is so important for good health.

Today, most of us spend too much time indoors, on computers and in offices; therefore, we are deficient in vitamin D as well as in the beneficial rays the sun provides. The best times to enjoy the sun are from early morning till 11 a.m., then from 3 p.m. to sunset. Between 11 a.m. and 3 p.m. the sun's damaging UV rays are stronger, so during these times it's best to sit under an umbrella or under the shade of a tree. It is important to expose your legs and arms, or better still your whole body, to the sun regularly. In traditional naturopathic spas in Europe, sunbathing is considered one of the necessary cures along with diet, exercise, and relaxation. The sun feeds the heart in traditional Chinese medicine and nourishes the emotion of joy as well as brightening the *shen* (spirit).

THE DANGERS OF EMFS

Our body contains its own electromagnetic field (EMF) that is constantly reacting with and being affected by other magnetic fields it comes in contact with. It is just plain ignorant to think that with the thousands of magnetic fields we are surrounded by each day, including cell phones and cell phone towers, radio waves, wireless technology, and power lines, none of these affect our own magnetic field. Government regulations concerning these health concerns seem to be lax, especially in light of the well-known dangers of EMFs and other forms of electromagnetic pollution; certainly the companies that sell cell phones, computers, and the like don't want the public to know about the dangers of EMFs. Just try typing in the keywords *electromagnetic radiation dangers* into any search engine and it will bring up hundreds of different devices that claim to protect you from these harmful frequencies. Some of these units attach directly to your cell phone, some you wear around your neck. Others are designed for your PC, and some plug into electrical wall sockets and claim to protect the whole room from EMFs. Unfortunately, most that claim to be effective show questionable studies to substantiate this.

Through my own clinical experience and that of many other health practitioners, I have found that the negative effects of EMFs on human health are obvious. The nervous system is electrical in nature and maintained in a body of water that has a governing effect on the hormonal and immune systems. Something you can do immediately when using a cell phone is to always use earbuds that have a hollow ear tube that keeps it away from your head instead of a wire cord. I highly recommend using protection devices on your cell phone, computer, or any other device to reduce EMF exposure.

Radiation from wireless devices such as cell phones and tablets are more and more linked to cancer, Alzheimer's, Parkinson's, headaches, and more. Scientists claim radiation initiates a damaging process in the body thought to be closely linked to oxidative stress. A 2016 study published in the journal *Electromagnetic Biology and Medicine* examined the effects of radio-frequency radiation in living cells and how cell phones may damage a person's DNA. The researchers claim that oxidative stress due to radio-frequency radiation exposure could explain the link between wireless devices and cancer and other diseases. This theory centers on chemically reactive molecules containing oxygen, known as reactive oxygen species (ROS), which play an important role in cell signaling and the control of internal conditions such as temperature. When ROS levels increase dramatically, this causes significant damage to cell structures and increases the aging process. ROS are generally produced in cells because of aggressive environments, but this study found that they can also be provoked by wireless radiation commonly found in homes, schools, and offices.*

The risks posed by wireless exposure are greatly underestimated because this type of radiation is invisible, yet it is easily measured and understood with an EMF meter. These devices are designed to measure ambient radiation exposures from WiFi, cell phone towers, and cell phones. You can obtain readings in minutes by walking slowly through your home, office, or school environment with an EMF meter. Once you have obtained a reading, you then compare it with safety guidelines and take corrective action as necessary. Unfortunately, there is much controversy about what are safe levels of radiation. The best resource for understanding safe exposure levels is the BioInitiative Report found at www.bioinitiative.org. This is a comprehensive review of thousands of studies compiled by an independent team of researchers; it gives clear guidelines on precautionary levels of EMF radiation.

THE DANGERS OF MICROWAVE OVENS

In the early 1990s, Swiss scientist Hans Hertel performed one of the greatest food studies done in the past century. In the small town of Wattenwil, near Basel, in Switzerland, Dr. Hertel conducted an investigation of the effects of microwaved food on human health that involve the study of a control group of only eight healthy people selected from the Macrobiotic Institute in Kientel, Switzerland. All participants were housed in the same hotel environment for eight weeks; there was no smoking, alcohol, or sex allowed. These strict regulations were designed because the researchers initially believed it might be difficult to clearly see the subtle changes in human blood from the effects of eating microwaved food if these other activities were also involved. The results of this study were published in

---

*I. Yakymenko, O. Tsybulin, E. Sidorik, D. Henshel, O. Kyrylenko, and S. Kyrylenko, "Oxidative mechanisms of biological activity of low-intensity radiofrequency radiation," *Electromagnetic Biology and Medicine* 35, no. 2 (2016): 186–202.

American journalist Tom Valentine's magazine *Search for Health* in the fall of 1992, with follow-up information available in a later issue. Unlike the groundbreaking study done with animals by Dr. Francis Pottenger on the damage to nutritional elements when milk is pasteurized, this study was done with human subjects. In intervals of two to five days, the volunteers in the Swiss microwave-oven study received one of the following food variants on an empty stomach:

- Raw milk from an organic farm
- The same milk conventionally cooked
- Pasteurized milk from a commercial factory
- The same raw milk cooked in a microwave oven
- Raw vegetables from an organic farm
- The same vegetables cooked conventionally
- The same vegetables frozen and defrosted in a microwave oven
- The same vegetables cooked in the microwave oven

Blood samples were taken from every subject immediately before eating. The results of microwaved food showed:

- Decreases in all hemoglobin values and cholesterol values, especially the ratio between HDL (good cholesterol) and LDL (bad cholesterol), which was altered in an unhealthy way
- Lymphocytes (white blood cells) displaying a more distinct short-term decrease following an intake of microwaved food than after the intake of the other food variants
- A highly significant association between the amount of microwave energy in the test foods and the luminous power of luminescent bacteria exposed to serum from test persons who ate that food.*

The results of this study led to the conclusion that when food is microwaved it not only alters nutritional elements, it also causes

---

*Tom Valentine, *Search for Health* (September–October 1992), 2–13.

them to be extremely dangerous in the body and may lead to a variety of disorders due to negative effects on intestinal flora. During microwave cooking, atoms and molecules within your food are hit by strong forms of electromagnetic radiation, forcing them to reverse polarity 1 to 100 billion times a second. Of all the natural substances within food, none react more sensitively to this process than water, which is the main component of most foods. This is actually how microwave cooking works: the friction violence to the water molecules brings about this "heat."

Immediately after Dr. Hertel announced the results of his study, a powerful trade organization called the Swiss Association of Dealers for Electro-Apparatuses for Households and Industry, known as the FEA, forced the court to issue a gag order against Hertel, banning him from publishing his studies or declaring that microwaved food is dangerous. The decision was reversed only in a judgment delivered in Strasbourg, Austria, on August 25, 1998. The European Court of Human Rights stated that there was a violation of Hertel's rights in that decision and ruled that the gag order issued by the Swiss court was contrary to his freedom of expression.

How Do Microwaves Work?

Similarly to light waves and radio waves, microwaves occupy a part of the electromagnetic spectrum, delivering very short waves of electromagnetic energy that travel at the speed of light. Microwaves come from the sun's rays in that the sun's heat is pulsed with direct current (DC), which does not create frictional heat, while microwave ovens use an artificial alternating current (AC), which creates frictional heat. This produces a spiked wavelength of energy with a narrow frequency, unlike the sun, which operates in a wide-frequency spectrum. Basically, the same microwaves being used to relay long-distance telephone signals, television programs, and satellite signals from space are being used to cook your food. If this information is still not enough to make you stop using a microwave oven, then read on.

Microwave Sickness

The Nazi scientists were the first to invent microwave cooking in 1942, using it to heat food for troops during the invasion of the Soviet Union in World War II. After the war the Russians got hold of the information and began experimenting with its biological effects on humans. During their experiments they witnessed a surge in ailments that occurred from people eating too much microwaved food, and in 1976 the government issued a health warning on both the biological and environmental health hazards of microwave ovens and similar electronic devices, as did several other Eastern European states, which reported on the harmful effects of microwave radiation and set up strict environmental limits for their use. At this time microwave ovens were in the process of getting approval in the United States. Despite the warnings issued in Russia and other countries, which were supported by many studies proving the dangers of microwaved food, the United States, United Kingdom, and other Western countries rejected these reports, and microwave ovens became legal in 1978. In response to great marketing campaigns consumers began buying them to the point where presently microwave ovens are now found in 83 percent of American homes, compared to 8 percent in 1978. For some unknown reason, perhaps due to financial gains, the Russian government legalized microwave ovens in the mid-1980s after seeing their successful sales in Western countries. At first the Russian studies described what they called "microwave sickness," with initial symptoms such as low blood pressure combined with a slow pulse. The later and most common manifestations are chronic excitation of the sympathetic nervous system (stress and anxiety), which then sends the body into high blood pressure. This phase includes headache, dizziness, eye pain, sleeplessness, irritability, anxiety, stomach pain, nervous tension, inability to concentrate, and hair loss, plus an increased incidence of appendicitis, cataracts, reproductive problems, and cancer. The chronic symptoms are eventually superseded by a crisis of adrenal exhaustion and ischemic heart disease (blocking of the coronary arteries), leading to heart attacks and death. These symptoms are common ailments in many people today, yet none of this is ever connected to eating microwaved food. The Taoists have always stated that the way food is heated affects the chi and recommend steaming food naturally with water for best results or boiling it when eating soups. And we feel it is not difficult to imagine how the ancient Taoist sages would have felt about using radiation to heat food.

Researcher Lita Lee commented on a 1989 study that appeared in the medical journal the *Lancet,* titled "Microwave heating of milk":

> Microwaving baby formulas converted certain trans-amino acids into their synthetic cis-isomers. Synthetic isomers, whether they are cis-amino acids or trans-fatty acids, are not biologically active. Further, one of the amino acids, L-proline, was converted to its d-isomer, which is known to be a neurotoxin (poisonous to the nervous system) and a nephrotoxic (poisonous to the kidneys). It's bad enough that many babies are not nursed, but now they are given fake milk (baby formula) made even more toxic from microwaving.*

Microwave Ovens Affect the Chi in Our Food

Using photon photography one can clearly see the amount of photons (light) that a substance emits. If you study the mineral analysis of microwaved food compared to that of naturally cooked food using this method, they are identical. The difference is only clear when using devices that measure different forms of light. The basic difference between natural heating and radiation heating lies in their effects on photons (known as prana or chi in traditional Eastern medicine). The universal element that makes up all atoms and molecules of the physical and chemical human body is actually light. Yes, light is the governing functional element that modern science is just beginning to learn about. What traditional medicine has said for so long about the invisible force called prana or chi is slowly "coming to light" in modern

---

*www.litalee.com/documents/Microwaves%20And%20Microwave%20Ovens.pdf.

science. Substances like enzymes are actually the sparks that set off the chemical process that allows the nutrients in food to be combusted and utilized by the body. Without enzymes, nutrients in food simply pass through the body mostly undigested. The effects of using radio waves (microwaves) on food are unquestionable: quite simply, they are damaging to human health. I have seen many positive changes in clients' health solely by eliminating their use of microwave ovens.

Since cigarettes and hard liquor (both known to kill you) are legal, it's easy to understand why multibillion-dollar corporations that manufacture appliances encourage politicians to keep the sale of microwave ovens legal. Even when leading scientists present clear statistics on the dangers of microwave ovens and the effects of microwaved food on health, money and power are the trump cards when scientific evidence is not going your way. The money to be made from selling such a quick and revolutionary cooking device as the microwave oven is not to be downplayed. This brings us the final question: just because it's legal, does that make it safe? Rather than wait for a ban on microwaves, which may not happen in the near future, stop using them altogether and begin using natural cooking methods such as steaming or stir-frying, or add more raw food to your diet, and in this way you'll take a big step toward improving your health.

Eighth Immortal Healer—Lan Tsai-Ho

Emotional Pollution and Spiritual Hygiene

If you want to heal the body you must first heal the mind.

PLATO

Disease will never be cured or eradicated by present materialistic methods, for the simple reason that disease in its origin is not material.

DR. EDWARD BACH

The healing known as spiritual hygiene is symbolized by Lan Tsai-Ho. This may be the least well known of the Eight Immortals. He or she—it appears that the gender of this legendary figure is not clear—was born during the Tang Dynasty and at the age of sixteen became the youngest Immortal. Lan Tsai-Ho is "sometimes regarded as a woman or even a hermaphrodite,"* and typically is seen attired in women's clothes.

---

*Julian F. Pas, with Man Kam Leung, "Lan Ts'ai-ho/Lan Caihe," *Historical Dictionary of Taoism* (Lanham, Md.: Scarecrow Press, 1998).

Considered eccentric, even crazy, much like the Fool of the tarot, he/she is famous for "wearing only shorts and thin shirts in winter, and a thick jacket and long pants in summer. Symbolizing this willfully incongruous conduct, Lan is often depicted walking about with one foot bare and the other shod."* One evening, after singing and entertaining, Lan left a tavern and mounted a crane that had descended amid the sounds of a celestial chorus. The crane gracefully carried this "Holy Fool" off into the sky before an astounded crowd.

This Taoist Immortal is quite the character; we all need to find that character within ourselves to discover our hearts and true spiritual, heavenly selves. Lan Tsai-Ho represents the element of the heavens, or sky, which provides us with the cosmic energy of love, spiritual hygiene, and rejuvenation. This Immortal also represents the "White Tiger" of Chinese Taoist mythology, whom it is said will return to Earth when the emperor (i.e., the heart) rules with absolute virtue. Taoist Immortals teach us that we must become an empty vessel, free from repressed emotional and mental baggage, so we can embrace the mystery that we call God or the Tao.

Of all the spiritual or energy practices, psychic hygiene is the most misunderstood and poorly practiced art of cleansing our energy body, yet it is crucial, for as Bashar, a multidimensional being channeled for over thirty years by Darryl Anka, says, "Everything is energy and that's all there is to it." It helps us to stay in the heart of feeling rather than the egoistic mind, which is the difference between being emotion based and heart/love based. Psychic hygiene allows us to stay "in feeling" and feel the mystery of God and one another. Cleansing the energetic or psychic body is of absolute importance on a daily and several-times-daily basis. Egoistic mind, with its associations of fear, anger, and sorrow, are energetic attachments that get stuck in our energy body and block the flow of love that comes from the heart's true essence. Just as we shower once or twice a day to clean the dirt or sweat from our body, so must we also cleanse our energy body so that it does not become "dirty" with egoistic tendencies.

---

*"Lan Caihe," *New World Encyclopedia*.

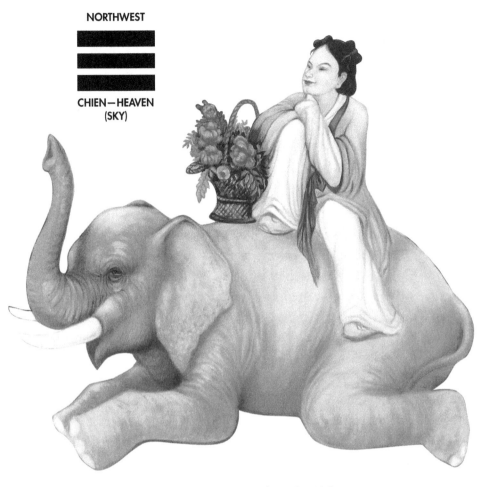

NORTHWEST

CHIEN—HEAVEN
(SKY)

Fig. 8.1. Lan Tsai-Ho (Lan Cai He)

Tai Chi and Chi Kung or yoga practices, walking in the forest, and using crystals, sage, essential oils, incense, bells and chimes, prayer visualizations, water prayer rituals, and other energetic tools are among many that can be used for this purpose. Yes, showering and bathing do help to cleanse the energy body, especially when you swim in the sea or soak in running mountain streams, but often this is not enough. We need to put more attention on cleansing the egoistic mind of the energy of thoughts that are based on fear, sorrow, and anger, which build up as a result of our day-to-day interaction with the ego-based materialistic world.

EMOTIONAL POLLUTION

Those who do not express their emotions and bottle them up, stuffing the resentment, guilt, and other destructive emotions and sweeping them under the rug, get hit with some of the most destructive terminal illnesses around. Many of these people did not smoke or lead an unhealthy lifestyle that would warrant such an attack of a killer disease. Many health professionals scratch their heads, wondering why it happened to such a "nice" person instead of another person who smokes and drinks yet seems unchallenged in comparison.

Suppressing our emotions leads to blocked energy, which then leads to further emotional and ultimately physical problems. On the other hand, experiencing the healthy expression of our emotions provides a free flow of energy and better mental and physical health. It's been proven that bottled-up, repressed, or trapped emotions, all of which can be called *emotional pollution,* have a significant effect on our stress levels. It is widely taught in allopathic medicine that stress shuts down the immune system, the body's main defense system for fighting cancer. Many cancer experts declare that stress is always a factor in the patients they treat. Dr. Linus Pauling said that stress uses up the body's vitamin C supply, which is needed for the immune system to operate. Richard Earle, Ph.D., director of the Canadian Institute of Stress (which was founded by pioneering endrocrinologist Hans Selye), says, "Medical science searches high and low for the causes of cancer, multiple sclerosis, rheumatoid arthritis, chronic fatigue syndrome, and a host of other conditions. Yet it often ignores one of the most pervasive factors leading to illness: the hidden stresses embedded in our daily lives."

Remember that it is primarily the immune system that heals most diseases, and emotional stress is devastating to the immune system. This may be the most difficult area of managing our lives in order to get well. We can be loyal to our relationships at the expense of our health—I have seen it over and over again. Many clients with whom I have consulted just cannot seem to see that certain drastic changes in their emotional state are necessary for them to successfully recover from their ailments. They simply do not see the link between their emotions (or their repressed emotions) and their illness. As leadership mentor, therapist, minister, and author Wayne Muller says, "The last place we tend to look for healing is within ourselves."

There is clear evidence from numerous studies that stress slowly wounds the self-healing process in otherwise healthy people. One such 1998 study revealed that academic exam stress in dental students delayed their wound-healing times by 40 percent compared to healing during summer vacation, when the students weren't stressed. The study also demonstrated a reduction in levels of interleukin-1, a powerful wound-healing chemical produced by the body in around 75 percent of the stressed students.*

The most effective way I have found to balance the emotions is through meditation, yoga, and massage, combined with correct exercise and the dietary principles laid out in this book. With these combined practices, emotional blockages are unlikely to occur. When we repress our feelings, this leads to blocked energies, which then lead to emotional and physical problems. On the other hand, acknowledging and expressing your feelings provides you with a free-flowing energy that is essential for emotional and physical well-being.

FORGIVENESS, THE HIGHEST OF VIRTUES

As Gandhi famously said, "An eye for an eye will only result in us all being blind." On the other hand, negative emotions can be transformed through the energy of forgiveness. The more energy we put into forgiveness, the less time it takes and the less pain you feel. As fear is the basis of all negative emotional states, when we start dealing with our fears, forgiveness becomes easier. It has now been scientifically proven that sustained anger and hostility are risk factors for heart disease, and that forgiveness can be the antidote to hostility. When we become forgiving we begin accumulating health benefits. A 2012 study on the cardiovascular benefits of forgiving found that "forgiveness seems to lower

---

*P. T. Marucha, J. K. Kiecolt-Glaser, and M. Favagehi, "Mucosal wound healing is impaired by examination stress," *Psychosomatic Medicine* 60, no. 3 (1998): 362–65.

reactivity both during the initial cognitive process and, more importantly, during mental recreations of an offense soon thereafter, potentially offering sustained protection."*

There are many techniques that can assist you in forgiving and wiping the slate clean. Sometimes it only comes in time, but even then it
takes work and commitment. One must first have understanding for
forgiveness to occur, because it is through understanding that forgiveness eventuates. "The Work" as taught by author and speaker Byron
Katie is a "a simple yet powerful process of inquiry that teaches you to
identify and question the thoughts that cause all the suffering in the
world. It's a way to understand what's hurting you, and to address the
cause of your problems with clarity."† This practical, simple, four-step
forgiveness process allows you to embrace reality. Remember, forgiving
yourself is just as important as forgiving others. Katie's nonprofit organization offers pages of information detailing the step-by-step work of
this remarkable process. I have been using The Work personally and
in my clinic for several years now and have found it truly remarkable;
I highly recommend it.

AFFIRMATIONS

We all have certain unconscious thoughts and mental programming
that has likely begun at a very early age and that influences our beliefs
about ourselves and our subsequent behavior. These deep-seated beliefs
in many cases do not represent our full potential and may in fact run
counter to who and what we are as authentic human beings. This idea is
not new. Goethe said, "When we treat man as he is, we make him worse
than he is; when we treat him as if he already were what he potentially
could be, we make him what he should be."

In their book *Rebirthing in the New Age,* Leonard Orr and Sondra

---

*B. A. Larsen, R. S. Darby, C. R. Harris, D. K. Nelkin, P. E. Milam, and N. J. Christenfeld,
"The immediate and delayed cardiovascular benefits of forgiving," *Psychosomatic
Medicine* 74, no. 7 (2012): 745–50.
†www.thework.com.

Ray say, "An affirmation is a positive thought that you choose to immerse in your consciousness to produce a desired result." Affirmations are practical tools for reprogramming the unconscious beliefs and attitudes we have about ourselves; they consist of positive statements that you repeat to yourself either verbally or in writing to manifest a specific outcome. Over time, they affect the unconscious by reprogramming it with the thought patterns you consciously select to influence your behavior. In the process, they can unleash and stimulate healing energies in all areas of your life.

As many who have used affirmations have found, the greatest challenge in working with them is to suspend judgment long enough to allow the new, positive messages to produce the results you desire. In addition, it helps to emotionally connect with your affirmations as you recite or write them, since this brings more energy to the experience. The idea is to make the process as vivid and real as possible. Here are some other suggestions for using affirmations:

- Always state your affirmation in the present tense and keep it positive.
- Keep your affirmations short and simple, no longer than two brief sentences.
- Verbalize and preferably write down each affirmation ten to twenty times each day.
- Whenever you find yourself thinking or hearing a habitual negative message, counteract it by focusing on your affirmation.
- Schedule a regular time each day to do your affirmations to add momentum to what you are trying to achieve until it becomes a positive, effortless habit.
- Repeat your affirmations in the first, second, and third person, using your name in each variation. First-person affirmations address any mental conditioning you have given yourself, while affirmations in the second and third person help to release the conditioning you may have accepted from others. In each case, write out or repeat the affirmation ten times.
- Make a commitment to practice your affirmations for at least

sixty days or well beyond the time you begin experiencing the results you desire.

- Visualize your affirmations by closing your eyes and imagining what the affirmation looks and feels like as you say or write it. Try to engage as many of your senses as possible.

Keeping a journal or diary for your personal life and health is just as important as keeping a business diary. Many of us use a journal for business meetings and financial events only and forget to journal our daily feelings, thoughts, and health issues. Napoleon Hill (1883–1970) was an American New Thought author who was well known for his book *Think and Grow Rich*. He stressed the importance of putting your affirmations in writing: "Reduce your plan to writing. . . . The moment you complete this, you will have definitely given concrete form to the intangible desire." When changing your diet or lifestyle it is important to record your progress *daily,* as this allows you to see that things have changed and how you feel from day to day. Remember to record your thoughts and feelings, because getting it on paper allows the mind to rationalize and sort through your thoughts, making them clearer. Writing things down helps your thoughts to become more physical and less mental. Get all your stresses out onto paper and out of your mind, and you can begin to feel and think clearer.

SETTING GOALS

Motivational speaker Denis Waitely, author of such books as *Seeds of Greatness* and *The Winner's Edge,* says, "Happy people don't plan results, they plan actions." Our goals are dreams with deadlines, you could say, the things that we want to achieve and experience in our lifetime, events we want to experience or accomplish. If you do not have goals, you don't move forward, and you will not have what you want because you don't know what you want. Therefore, you probably will end up getting something you don't want. Every person needs direction and a sense of purpose, a reason for living, and it is our passion that fuels this desire. Some spiritual traditions claim that having desires is wrong, that one should not desire things or material possessions, but even spiritually inclined people desire some form of enlightenment or peace of mind, which are both forms of desire. To desire is not wrong; quite to the contrary, it is human, it is what's needed to evolve. But to become obsessed or ruled by one's desires or abuse the gift of creation for the purpose of dominating and controlling others is not what we are talking about here.

Having goals symbolizes that you are taking control of your life. No goal is complete until it's written down, because if it's just in your head, it's still only a dream. When our dreamed-about goals are written down, only then do they become tangible as words. In addition, it's important that you review your goals as much as possible and make "stepping stone" goals that get you to your end goals. For example, if your major career goal is to compete at the next Olympics, then you need to also write down the daily training goals that will prepare you for your end goal. If we don't set goals and discipline ourselves to achieve those goals, then the rest of the world will shape us around *its* ideals, which usually have nothing to do with our own sense of purpose or fulfillment—or as internationally known business leader Jack Welch succinctly puts it, "Control your destiny or somebody else will."

Begin by writing down your goals today. Start with simple goals, whether they are emotional, health, financial, or relationship goals. If you spend all of your energy focusing and achieving your financial and career goals, don't be too amazed if you end up very rich but miserable. Only by carefully managing your goals into categories can you have complete fulfillment. Start with personal goals, such as good health, good attitude, and being an honest, caring person. Then you can begin looking at relationship and career goals. Getting your priorities in order when setting goals is very important. Goal setting is fun, and your attitude toward writing them down, fine-tuning them daily, and achieving them is a fulfilling and rewarding process. God gave us the ability to create, and creating a happy, fulfilling, abundant life is one of the many gifts of life. It is your choice as to whether you want to be in control and create the life you want, or to be a victim and blame others for not having or getting what you want.

Setting goals also increases one's discipline. Look at a simple definition of *discipline:* it's the ability to delay gratification to honor a higher value. This emphasizes the necessity to sometimes postpone what we want in the short term for a greater long-term benefit. On the other hand, it also outlines the importance of performing small, daily actions to eventually reach our long-term goals. Sometimes we're not willing to make the small, daily sacrifices because the end result is not so clear if we haven't set and reviewed our goals. Similarly, undisciplined people usually follow a whirlwind of daily demands, remaining out of control and constantly reacting to the energy of others' demands, so by setting goals we increase our awareness of our own needs and desires and program those into our daily lives as we go about steadily working toward them.

The Five Laws of Health Goals

1. "The first step to becoming is to will it," said Mother Teresa. Sometimes the things we want the most are also the things we fear the most, and sometimes the fear of success is greater than the fear of failure. If this is so, then we will always feel a constant struggle in getting what we want or need in life. Getting what you want and wanting what you have seems to be a closely held secret among those who have both. Like all things in the cosmos, there are universal laws that pertain to both of these. The next four steps outline the laws you can use to manifest your goals. Using this simple outline has helped many people tap into the immense powers that the universe bestows on us human beings. That said, it is very important that you only use this method for good and not to manipulate. If you try to use it to control others it will eventually come back and bite you in the behind.

2. You Deserve It. You must prove to yourself and no one else that you deserve to be healthy, healed, and happy. If you are religious, it is not God to whom you have to prove anything; God does not judge, only humans do. God loves you unconditionally and wants you to have all that you need to be well: "Beloved, I wish above all things that you may prosper and be in health, as thy soul prospers" (John 3:2). You need to be rooting for yourself and on your own side. I like to use affirmations and positive statements about myself to begin to program a sense of self-love and respect. Using these affirmations comes from a sense of worth that is physical, mental, and spiritual in nature.

3. Visualize It and Write It Down. Dr. Carl O. Simonton, founder of the Simonton Cancer Center, a pioneer in the field of psycho-oncology and author of *Getting Well Again,* describes dramatic remissions of cancer in patients to whom he taught a simple visualization technique in which the person sees the white cells of their immune system as an army attacking their cancer cells and destroying them. Dr. Simonton says, "You are more in charge of your life and even the development and progress of a disease such as cancer than you may realize. You may actually, through a power within you, be able to decide whether you live or die." First you see what you want happening, then you visualize it constantly every time you think about it. Whatever you want in terms of full healing, you must visualize it as if it is real. When I first began using creative visualization to imagine my goals I found it difficult. I could not see anything when I closed my eyes except the backs of my eyelids, but with a little persistence and practice I gradually became good at it. Try this: sit quietly and begin to see the outcome of your goal; see it happen and the people involved playing their parts to make it so. Repeat this visualization several times a day for a minute or so each time. Make sure that after each time you do this, you then detach from the outcome. By this I mean let it go and trust that all that happens is for the greater good. Now that you have a clear picture of your goal, bring it into physical form by writing it down on paper or drawing a picture of it, visualizing the words and the picture daily. There is much power in the written word, for words can be brought from the mental plane into the physical plane instantly given there is enough passion. Words become more powerful when written down and also when repeated aloud.

4. The Power of the Spoken Word. Affirm your goal with the spoken word daily; for example, "Every day in every way I am getting better. I am at peace. Thank you for my healing." Do not just think it in your head; say it daily and as often as you can. Refer to the previous pages on affirmations and apply those techniques. Believe it. As Napoleon Hill says, "What the mind can conceive and believe, it can achieve." Belief is a key ingredient for successful healing; sometimes you have to brainwash yourself into believing. Believe in yourself and what you are doing while also acting and believing that your creations are already in motion, that the wheels are turning, and that your creations are in the process of manifesting, as indeed they are. Take daily actions to create positive steps toward attaining your goal, doing something practical each day that helps get you closer to healing yourself in the long term.

5. Give Thanks in Advance. Give thanks to the universe and all sentient beings for what you have now and what is soon about to come. Foster an attitude of gratitude and appreciation for everything you have. Focusing on what you do have rather than on what you don't have gives you a sense of appreciation and humbleness. The ego can sabotage our dreams, but by having an attitude of gratitude, the ego is humbled. Begin now. Declare "I am grateful for my life." "Thank you for my beautiful body." "Thank you for my friends and family." Everything you have in your life, both physically and spiritually, and everything you experience is somehow due to others in some way or form. Think about it, and then "thank about it." As the seventeenth-century French literary figure Francois de La Rochefoucauld put it, "Gratitude is merely the secret hope of further favors."

DEVELOPING DISCIPLINE

The Bhagavad Gita extols the virtues of self-discipline: "He who shirks action does not attain freedom; no one can gain perfection by abstaining from work. Indeed, there is no one who rests for even an instant; every creature is driven to action by his own nature." One great way to get some discipline is to make a list of the benefits you will gain from all the hard work that's involved in the task you need to perform to bring about an outcome such as curing yourself of some illness. This helps you to see your target goal. Imagine what it will be like when you achieve your goal. How will you feel? Sense the enjoyment. Don't be afraid to imagine using your senses to feel what it will be like. It's like dangling a carrot to a donkey. The commitment to delay immediate gratification and instead choose to honor the end result is a simple definition of discipline.

Begin with the end in mind. What this means simply is delaying the quick fix for a long-term cure. Does this sound familiar? In modern medicine we tend to focus on treating only the symptoms of the physical body rather than looking at the big picture, the body-mind-emotion-spirit connection. The discipline needed for life is also the discipline you will need to heal yourself of a serious illness. Rather than succumbing to junk food and a junk lifestyle, see the end in your mind's eye. What is it you are attempting to achieve? Better health and peace of mind? Then be willing to work on it daily. Instead of seeing the work that you need to do each day as a drag, see it as an exciting challenge along the way to success.

REBUILDING YOUR PERSONAL POWER

Personal power is another way of describing the ancient belief regarding living life as a warrior of light, love, and compassion. Long, long ago, in the times of our hunter-gatherer ancestors, warriors roamed and ruled societies and only the strongest survived. So what was it that caused certain humans to survive, and what made them stronger? Why did certain people rule over others, such as Moses, who rose up and led his people out of slavery from Egypt? What made all the great leaders in history actually become great leaders? It was personal power. Today, taking back your personal power does not mean being a warrior in the sense of being a barbarian wielding a weapon; instead it means standing up for your rights and cultivating a solid, persistent motivational belief in yourself to successfully achieve your full potential. It means being your own leader rather than looking to an external authority, and helping others do likewise because you care. As the Bible says, "He that walketh with wise men shall be wise . . ." (Proverbs 13:20).

Taking back your personal power is about choosing not to consort with people who encourage you to feel uneasy within yourself. It's about being willing to learn from those who are more learned than you. It's about understanding that you don't know it all but are willing to learn. It's also about your ability to feel okay about saying no and knowing when you have had enough. Developing self-esteem is fundamental to taking back your personal power. As the old saying goes, "Fake it till you make it," or as American historian and social critic Christopher Lasch says, "Nothing succeeds like the appearance of success." The process of *acting* like you have confidence helps you to gain more self-esteem until you genuinely *do* have that confidence. Dressing confidently, speaking confidently, and acting confident all help you to feel more confident. It's not about being full of yourself—it's a humble power, not an egoistic, narcissistic power.

So what are some more simple things you can do to help build your confidence?

- Look other people in the eyes and gently smile with your eyes when communicating.
- Try using people's names when addressing them.
- Show gratitude to others when they assist you.
- Avoid bragging, as it is commonly known that people who brag suffer from low self-confidence beneath their overconfident exterior.
- Compliment others for their good habits rather than criticize them for their bad ones. Truly confident people always attempt to boost the confidence of others.

The human potential astounds all of us, especially now with the development of advanced technologies for use in instant global communication and space travel. Just when you think humans can go no further, someone comes out with an even smaller computer or more advanced cell phone. While we are all amazed at those nerdy science geniuses who keep coming out with better and better technology, doctors are telling us that we are currently only using 5 percent of our full brain capacity. What will happen when we learn to tap in to all those missing areas of the brain that we currently are not using, the other 95 percent? With processes such as remote viewing becoming more available to more people, we are beginning to get a small taste of the human potential, whether it be physical or psychic. There are certain common denominators that suggest why some people achieve more of their potential than others, and it is mostly because they stop doing things that hold them back.

Common Things That Limit Your Personal Power

- Not feeling good enough about yourself and seeing the world in just black and white
- Being unable to say no because it may mean confrontation or entering into a debate
- Choosing to blame everyone else for your own problems while being caught up in "victim consciousness," instead of taking responsibility for your own situation
- Those who lack personal power also lack a strong sense of boundaries and are not attuned to their surroundings. They are too involved in their own private "I" complex rather than the needs of others. They attempt to control situations and people, only creating unhappiness for themselves and others around them.

Taking back your power is also about learning to make decisions on your own. Sure, consulting a professional is a must in areas you don't know anything about—say, computer technology—but in the end you're the one making the decision on the information you have accumulated, so if anything goes wrong, you're the one who's responsible for sorting it out.

OUR QUESTIONS PROVIDE
THE ANSWERS

Motivational speaker Tony Robbins says, "The questions we ask ourselves affect what we focus on, what we focus on affects the way we feel, and the way we feel affects the way we act. And it is those actions that we make each day that are creating our future." If the questions we ask ourselves direct our focus, then those questions provide the answers. Questions we need to ask ourselves when we are feeling emotional should lead us in a positive direction. Ask yourself, "What can I learn from this?"; "How can I grow from this and become a better person?"; "What do I need to do to turn this situation around?" When we only ask "why," we usually get answers like, "Because I'm not good enough," or "Because I did something wrong." So don't ask why; instead ask, "What can I learn from this?" or "How can I grow from this experience?" Asking "why?" always digs up unconscious negative answers from your ego that interfere with your emotional healing. Begin to ask proactive questions that lead you to the solution to your concerns.

When things happen, they do so for a reason: so we can learn something. A famous quote from William Connor Magee (1821–1891), an Irish clergyman of the Anglican Church, goes, "The man who makes no mistakes does not usually make anything." Often we find ourselves saying, "Why is this happening to me?" and "Why did I do that?" or "Why do I feel like this?" In such cases we feel totally without our personal power. When tragic things happen in life, it's difficult to fathom that they are happening for a higher reason, and it is we who have the choice to learn and move forward. Or we can ask "why?" and become stagnant and emotionally blocked. Tragic events affect us all—the death of a loved one, the breakup of a relationship, the loss of a job and finances. Many times it is our own actions that are involved in most of these sufferings, but many times it can also be totally out of our control. Becoming a better person through right actions and working toward your goals and passions and achieving a better sense of well-being is aided by learning from your mistakes. While it is true we are here to learn, we are also here to love and accept others as they are, and events as they happen. Applying Taoist philosophy means that we follow the water-course way, which means the path of least resistance. It's about giving up the fight with what reality brings us, with what has happened or is happening, and surrendering to the direction in which the universe is guiding us. We cannot change what has happened or what we have done, and in most cases we cannot change others. Yet we can change ourselves and create out of what we are doing now, and what we are doing now contributes with other beings to create the future through the principle of interrelatedness.

During times of crisis or loss we need to talk to someone and be counseled. We need someone to listen to us and support our healing. They can support us to realize that when things happen, they happen for a reason: to learn something. We make mistakes so we can grow, learn, and become a better person. Our attitude toward this kind of suffering and how we embrace it, and how we envision a greater outcome, determines our ability to become a more humble, grateful, and fulfilled person in the long term. Practicing the Eight Immortal Healers in times of trauma and crisis can help with healing and letting go.

LAUGHING CHI KUNG

Facial feedback is premised on the fact that changing the structural parts of our face dramatically affects our thoughts, emotions, and feelings. In this way we can increase the production of endorphins and other chemicals associated with pain or mood, making happiness a conscious choice. This is evident in internal alchemy exercises such as the Inner Smile and the Six Healing Sounds, as described in chapter 6. One of the greatest yogas, the act of laughing, whether naturally or artificially induced, causes the production and release of literally hundreds of different chemicals that assist in healing the body and releasing stress. Studies have shown that laughing seems to reduce stress by releasing excess adrenaline in the blood, as well as the obvious physical effects of opening and releasing tension in the diaphragm and heart muscles, which are both associated with stress, which in turn is commonly known to cause disease. To think that some diseases could be improved or sometimes eradicated through laughter seems almost ridiculously simple, but as researchers begin to understand the complex chemistry of the human brain and body, it seems to make perfect sense.

An old saying from Kahlil Gibran goes, "The deeper that sadness carves its way into your being, the more joy it can contain." That you cannot know happiness until you've known suffering is true for most of us, as we most often grow through suffering, which melts our ego. This new century brought us much bloodshed, with so many terror attacks all over the world on innocent people. What then do we have to laugh about? As strange as it may sound, the times when we feel least likely to laugh are the times when we need to laugh the most. Many people today associate laughing with something that is done only when something is humorous, but like exercise, laughing sometimes needs to be induced. Just like exercise, you force yourself to get out in the park or hit the pool or gym and do some exercise, so if your emotional body is feeling down, you need to get out there and start laughing. Force yourself if need be! Even in some of the most severe states of depression and anxiety, forced laughter brings about a temporary influx of beneficial hormones and other neurotransmitters, which in turn will change your emotional state immediately.

Instructions for Laughing Chi Kung

While this exercise is excellent to practice in groups, in yoga class, or in any classroom situation, to break up excess seriousness and to relax the overall energy within a group, it can also be done when you're by yourself.

1. Lie down in a comfortable, relaxed position on your back or, if you wish, sit in a comfortable chair.
2. Begin laughing out loud; you may need to force yourself, as most do not feel like laughing initially. Start by giggling, and then allow it to take you into full belly laughs (fig. 8.2). After a few minutes of fake laughing (for some it may be longer or shorter), you will

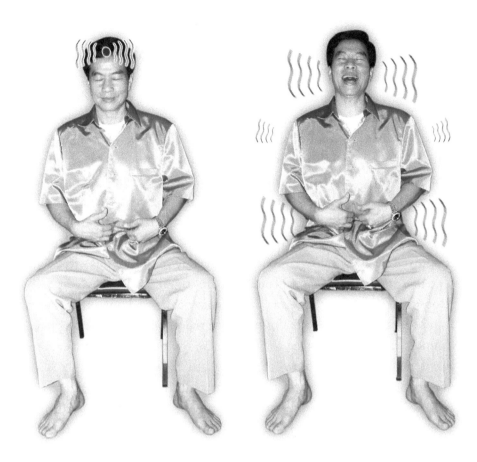

Fig. 8.2. Smile and think of something funny,
then start giggling, eventually allowing it to take you
to full belly laughs.

suddenly feel yourself laughing at yourself or, if you are in a class, at
other people's silly laughter. You can then begin to forget that you
initially started laughing by forcing it and begin to start laughing
naturally as you hear yourself laughing or at things that are funny
(or troubling you) in your own life.

3. Enjoy laughing for as long as your diaphragm allows.

Practice daily for at least five minutes.

MUSIC AS A MEDICINE

Eighteenth-century English playwright and poet William Congreve's most famous line is, "Music hath charms to soothe the savage beast." Congreve was not the first to write about the healing powers that music provides. Plato, Pythagoras, and Aristotle all noted the importance of music in creating emotional and spiritual well-being. The poetic tradition may be one thing, but science is another, and now scientists are discovering a wealth of information about the healing frequencies contained within music. There have been many recent scientific studies on the benefits of listening to music, particularly before and during surgery; these studies demonstrate remarkable results as reflected in improved healing and recovery time. Relaxing music contains frequencies that stimulate the same glands that are stimulated when we eat delicious food or have sex. Anyone with teenage children knows that music can be irritating as well as calming. With that in mind, researchers have found that the right music for the person's individual tastes seems to have the best effect in terms of healing and relaxation, although there are certain sounds that seem to resonate with the majority of people.

Recent university studies in the United States have revealed that sound tones can trigger certain nerve responses in the brain of the listener. It seems apparent that our brains are "tuned" very much the same way that a piano is. What this means is that when certain sounds are heard, it sets off a reaction of responses when the right notes are struck. Many of us are aware of the sense of well-being we get when we listen to our favorite songs or our favorite sounds in nature. Using music to heal illness is not a new idea, but taking it further and studying in detail certain frequencies that create universal healing among us is a relatively new field of inquiry. Organizations such as the Monroe Institute, dedicated to the exploration of consciousness, are gaining much attention by creating music for just this purpose. Harmonic sounds can be tailored with the use of computers to generate specific sacred sounds to achieve specific results. The study of music and sound is becoming a healing science, as music once was considered by the ancient philosophers and sages so long ago.

Singing

The benefits of using the human voice in song were lauded by the ancients, going all the way back to the Bible's admonition to "make a joyful noise to the Lord, all the earth! Serve the Lord with gladness! Come into his presence with singing" (Psalms 100:1–2). The therapeutic benefits of singing for neurological and psychological disorders have been studied for decades. Both singing and playing an instrument can help with our mental and emotional well-being and assist in healing. In traditional Chinese medicine singing is said to help heal the spleen and stomach, which is associated with the earth element. This is the element that is associated with worries and anxieties and digestive problems that are all linked to the enteric nervous system, which has been called the "second brain." Singing literally changes the brain and changes the neuroplasticity of the brain, promoting healing by elevating endorphins and reducing stress dramatically, as well as depression, anxiety, and loneliness. Singing is something intimate because it's a sound that begins inside you. Get out your favorites and start singing, or join your local singing group or choir, and heal your heart and your brain.

DANCE THERAPY

Gabrielle Roth (1941–2012) was a pioneer in the modern dance-therapy movement technique known as 5Rhythms, which is now taught in all major cities. Roth eloquently described the power and purpose of dance:

> To sweat is to pray, to make an offering of your innermost self. Sweat is holy water, prayer beads, pearls of liquid that release your past. Sweat is an ancient and universal form of self-healing, whether done in the gym, the sauna, or the sweat lodge. I do it on the dance floor. The more you dance, the more you sweat. The more you sweat, the more you pray. The more you pray, the closer you come to ecstasy. Disease is inertia. Healing is movement. If you put the body in motion, you will change. You are meant to move: from flowing to

staccato, through chaos into lyrical, and back into the stillness from which all movement comes.

Roth's technique of dance therapy involves five body rhythms: flowing, staccato, chaos, lyrical, and stillness; these dance rhythms facilitate consciousness. Marian Chace (1896–1970), an even earlier pioneer, inaugurated dance therapy in the 1960s and was respected in Western medicine circles for her results in helping people heal their emotional problems. She was influenced by Carl Jung and believed in the strong relationship between the body and mind. Today, dance therapy has become increasingly relevant as a treatment for PTSD and other trauma-related conditions.

E-MOTION YOGA

E-motion Yoga is a revolutionary synthesis of yoga, Chi Kung, kriya yoga (dynamic breath work), tantra, neurogenic tremoring (organic body shaking), and dance that is designed to release trapped and blocked emotions from our past that are stored in the electrical systems of the body, causing physical and emotional health problems, thus preventing us from feeling our deepest form of love. Have you ever held a yoga pose for some time and begun to shake? This is not a sign of weakness or a time to change the pose—it's the beginning of something special, when the nervous system is beginning to heal itself. It was called *shaking medicine* by our ancestors, who used it in a religious setting to heal emotional trauma. Usually the mind tries to stop this shaking process and tighten the core, but when we guide it in an organic way and let it do what it wants to do, something amazing begins to happen: some call it *kundalini rising;* a shaman may call it *spirits leaving the body;* but whatever you call it, science is now proving the effectiveness of the therapeutic process of neurogenic tremoring to heal the mind and body, especially in those who have suffered from some traumatic event. This form of therapy

- Releases trapped/suppressed emotions safely
- Heals trauma and releases the past

- Reduces emotional stress and anxiety
- Gets you out of your head and into your heart
- Frees you from disease (dis-ease) caused by storing stressful emotions

Emotional trauma and subsequent suppressed emotions occur in all human beings after an overwhelming experience. Trapped or suppressed emotions (i.e., trauma) get stored in the nervous system, fascia, and muscles of the body and can be an underlying cause of physical and psychological diseases, according to a number of scientific studies. There are the obvious "hard traumas" such as war, natural disasters, serious accidents, and life-threatening situations, which are usually diagnosed as PTSD; but the forms of trauma that often go undiagnosed and untreated yet are epidemic are the "soft traumas." These are less identifiable and often caused by childhood or relationship emotional abuse, social violence, or a series of stressful events that occur close together, such as loss of a spouse or child; divorce; loss of finances, job, or home; or serious health problems and medical complications.

E-motion Yoga does not claim to fix problems; rather, it aims to support our body to do the organic healing that it is designed to do once we allow it. Your body is a supercomputer with an organic, built-in antivirus program for cleaning itself, and that is shaking and trembling. The organic mechanism that heals emotional trauma has been suppressed because of social programming, usually coming from certain religions that label therapeutic shaking as the "devil's work." In the Taoist viewpoint this movement is called *spontaneous Chi Kung;* it happens naturally when our body releases tension and emotions. The Taoists have always viewed unexpressed or suppressed emotions as a major cause of disease, so they were very interested in working out ways to remedy this, first by studying animals and how they deal with trauma.

You do not need to have emotional trauma to get great benefits from E-motion Yoga, because it also helps a person release chronic stress, which is a form of repressed emotions. Chronic stress is now acknowledged by modern medicine as a major cause of many diseases, so it only makes common sense that we develop natural ways to discharge safely and effectively, using what's natural for the body and mind.

The repetitive recycling of overexcitement/anxiety in the brain (amygdala) and nervous system of a past event that was not discharged at the time and continues long after the event is what is referred to as *trauma,* and for most of us it lies hidden in our body, recreating life events that trigger the original traumas because they are wanting to be released. This recycling can be subtle and unnoticed, or it can be gross and obvious and can often lead to compulsive behaviors, which is when we seek to replay in some way a trauma scenario later in life that mimics a suppressed emotional feeling that was generated during childhood, such as abandonment, unhealthy relationships, and emotional or physical abuse.

It has been suggested that within trauma the original events become trapped in our body, but it is now recognized that it is rather the emotions that do. Because the traumatic experience generated such an overwhelming biological response, the body stores those emotions to then be released at a later date when it is safe, such as hours or days after the event. But due to our ego-focused society we become stuck in the mind, so this natural bodily process has become forgotten, and in most cases the body literally becomes stuck in the past. This then causes an excessive emotional charge to remain in the body; undischarged, it creates a biochemical loop that makes our brain believe this event is continually happening, bringing up emotions such as fear, anger, and sadness to continue in daily life without resolution. The conscious mind is mature and understands the concept of time and realizes that the stressful event happened some time ago and that we are now safe and have survived. Yet the subconscious mind is like an infant: it does not understand the concept of time and believes the event has recently happened or is still happening. It is my understanding that during the process of shaking and tremoring, the body somehow communicates through a universal frequency with the subconscious mind via the nervous system and begins the healing process of bringing it into the present safely.

Only by surrendering on a deep energetic level can we really accept and let go and unlock ourselves from the past and experience the gift that is the present, which great spiritual teachers have taught. The illusive present moment can never be lost or found, nor come when called at will; rather, it only comes fully embodied when one is free on a deep emotional and spiritual level, by being fully in the body and feeling it. The mind, as I understand it, can never really be in the present, only the heart can. The mind is designed to be in the past or future, whereas the heart only beats in the now and can never be anywhere else. When we release the past and our emotional baggage, only then can we fully evolve and fully embrace life's incredible gift of feeling connected; this is called *yog* in Sanskrit, commonly known as *yoga,* which literally means "union with the Divine" and coming into the heart. Johnathon Dao has developed E-motion Yoga using principles of the Universal Healing Tao, yoga and breathwork, neurogenic tremors, and indigenous shamanic cultural practices for a complete release of toxic emotional pollution.*

EMOTIONAL FREEDOM TECHNIQUE

Emotional Freedom Technique (EFT) is a simple meridian technique whereby we tap some basic acupuncture points on the body while simultaneously stating an accepting and loving affirmation. "Even though I am feeling [state how you are feeling], I love and accept myself." It is simple and powerful and has immense benefit in the treatment of depression, pain, emotional worries, and more. It has no side effects, is free, and can help reduce dependence on medications for many. First developed as Thought Field Therapy (TFT) by Dr. Roger Callahan in 1991, it was streamlined by TFT student Gary Craig, who renamed it EFT.

SELF-HYPNOSIS

Your brain is constantly going in and out of alpha states throughout the day and during sleep. In meditation you deliberately take your

---

*For more information visit www.cureplanet.com/e-motion-yoga.

mind into an alpha state, which is when you have a vast learning capacity and your mind can be influenced. A hypnotist, for example, takes you into an alpha state first before he convinces you of certain things. If you don't feel comfortable going to a clinical hypnotist or simply don't have the money to do so, you can do it at home yourself without a hypnotist.

Our reality is formed by our mental state. The English epic poet John Milton said, "The mind is its own place, and in itself can make a heaven of hell, and a hell of heaven." If this is so, then you already possess the ability to change your thoughts and in turn change your life situations dramatically in a relatively short amount of time. You can do this relatively easily with self-made alpha audios. Recording your own alpha-state audio tape is very effective and a simple way to take control of your mental state and reprogram your subconscious mind with new thought patterns. You will need a smartphone with a built-in microphone. Find a quiet place to record your audio, and begin as described below. Use a gentle yet firm voice when you record and remember that your subconscious mind trusts your own voice completely, so even if you do not believe the new affirmations that you are recording at first, your subconscious mind does. This will become evident over the coming days; after listening to your alpha tape regularly, you will begin to act, feel, and think differently. Since your mind goes in and out of hypnotic alpha states during the day and especially during rest, bedtime, when you drift off to sleep, is a great time to use your audios with headphones. Even if you fall asleep, your subconscious mind is still operating and hearing the recorded program.

Recording a Self-Hypnosis Exercise Using Your Own Voice

When you are ready to record your audio, get yourself into a comfortable position with your spine very straight. Then you are ready to begin recording the audio file. Use your own voice on the recording, as your subconscious mind trusts you more than any hypnotist. Unlike affirmations that use "I," subliminal recordings use "you," as if you are being told by someone else, and that someone else is the "new you." Record your audio using a calm, firm voice, speaking slowly but not too slowly, using the following scripts. Once you become more experienced you can change it around. Start with part one, then stop the recorder and rest. Begin recording from the same place as you go on to part two, and then stop the recorder.

◉ Part One:
Autosuggestion Relaxation of the Body

Start the recording here and recite the following script:

Take five long, deep, slow breaths . . . Your body is now relaxing . . . You are becoming totally relaxed . . . With every breath you take, you are becoming more and more relaxed . . . Every muscle in your body is now relaxing . . . Your body is feeling peaceful and relaxed . . . Focus on your breathing . . . particularly the slow, gentle release of your exhalation . . . Your breath is now slow and relaxed . . .

Your scalp is relaxing . . . Your scalp is now relaxed . . . Your eye muscles are relaxing . . . Your eyes are completely relaxed . . . Your jaw is relaxing . . . Your jaw is now completely relaxed . . . Your whole face is now relaxed . . . Relax your neck and shoulders . . . Your neck and shoulders are now relaxed . . . Relax your chest and abdomen . . . Your chest and abdomen are now completely relaxed . . . Relax your arms and hands . . . Your arms and hands are now relaxed . . . Relax your hips . . . Your hips are now totally relaxed . . . Relax your legs and your feet . . . Your legs and feet are now totally relaxed . . . Twitch your toes, and with a deep breath feel all the tension releasing from your body . . . Your whole body is now completely relaxed . . .

Stop recording now.

⚙ Part Two:
Counting Down from 20 to 1, with Suggestions Added

Start recording now as you slowly count down from 20:

20. Your whole body is peaceful and relaxed.
19. Every muscle has now let go.
18. Listen only to my voice.
17. Nothing else disturbs you or worries you.
16. With every breath you relax even deeper.
15. You feel totally content and calm.
14. Your whole body is peaceful and relaxed.
13. Every muscle has now let go.
12. Listen only to my voice.
11. Nothing else disturbs you or worries you.
10. With every breath you relax even deeper.
 9. You feel totally content and calm.
 8. Your whole body is peaceful and relaxed.
 7. Every muscle has now let go.
 6. Listen only to my voice.
 5. Nothing else disturbs you or worries you.
 4. With every breath you relax even deeper.
 3. You feel totally content and calm.
 2. You are too relaxed to move now, focusing now only on my voice.
 1. You are now completely relaxed and listening only to my voice.

Stop recording now.

⚙ Part Three:
Alpha Program of Your Choice

Try not to put too many different messages into one program. Usually it's best to have seven or eight lines and repeat the whole message fifteen to twenty times after the relaxation and countdown. You can keep part one and two of the recording permanently and record part three over again later, when you want to change programs. Start with a basic program for your current personal needs, whether it be confidence, health, making money, or attracting love. Remember to verbalize in a positive manner. Here are some examples:

General Physical and Emotional Health

- Every day in every way you are feeling better and better.
- Your health is improving with each and every day.
- You wake up in the morning feeling totally refreshed and inspired.
- You are relaxed and calm and free from stress.
- Nothing worries you anymore as you know that you can solve any problem that comes your way.
- You are clear in your life's direction, and you exude self-confidence.
- Other people catch colds and flu, but you don't because your body rejects disease and sickness.
- You feel great during the day and sleep soundly at night.

Increasing Your Finances

- Money comes to you easily and effortlessly and in massive abundance.
- You attract financial abundance with everything you touch.
- You now realize that you deserve financial freedom and use it wisely.
- Each day you are coming up with more and more creative ways to increase your finances.
- The decisions you make are based on educated summaries of your genius mind, leading you to sounder investments.
- You feel confident and comfortable having large sums of money and assets.
- You use your money to also assist others and teach them to also accept financial abundance with gratitude.

Quit Smoking

- Whenever you smoke, it makes you nauseous and your breathing is affected.
- You find the taste totally unpleasant and annoy other people when you smoke.
- Your health will be affected if you continue to smoke, and you know that you feel a lot better when you do not smoke and that you can save money when you're not smoking.
- You are now losing the taste for cigarettes, and you're forgetting to light up more and more.
- Your health is improving each day as you no longer need or have the desire to smoke.

Get a Trim, Healthy Body

- Each day your body is becoming thinner and thinner, and your health is improving greatly.
- Your desire for unhealthy snacks is totally nonexistent, as you now only desire healthy foods at mealtimes.
- Exercise and meditation are now a firm part of each and every day, helping you reach your perfect weight.
- You enjoy being trim and fit and realize all the benefits, inside and out, of having a trim, healthy figure.
- Losing weight is easy for you because you know exactly what to eat and how to eat it.
- You know all the secrets of maintaining your ideal healthy weight, using diet, exercise, and mind control.
- Your body is becoming more attractive and your mind clearer each and every day.
- Your friends are astounded at how good you look and want to know your secret to having such a great figure.
- You are now reaching your goal weight of _____ pounds.

Note: You can have fun making up other subliminal alpha recordings. For the most effective results it is best to listen to the recordings every night when going to sleep. Use your headphone as you drift off to sleep each night. Alternatively, you can listen to them anytime while meditating or relaxing.

MEDITATION IS MIND MEDICINE

The Buddha said, "We are formed and molded by our thoughts. Those whose minds are shaped by selfless thoughts give joy when they speak or act. Joy follows them like a shadow that never leaves them." He also said, "Meditation brings wisdom; lack of mediation leaves ignorance. Know well what leads you forward and what holds you back, and choose the path that leads to wisdom."

Meditation is medicine for the mind. There are many forms of meditation, but they all involve slowing the thoughts and getting a clearer impression of our reality or truth. The word for meditation in Sanskrit is *samatha,* meaning "peaceful abiding." With the demanding pace of life in today's world, we need to know how to slow down and meditate to balance our mind and body. Meditation teaches us to observe our emotions rather than becoming a prisoner of them. "I do not have time to meditate" is the classic excuse for not meditating, but in reality this isn't true, as meditation actually provides the clarity and focus that helps you manage your time more efficiently.

There are mountains of medical studies confirming the health benefits of meditation. To date there are over a thousand published research studies that prove it benefits metabolism, blood pressure, brain activation, and immunity and reduces confusion and stress. Meditation is not religious in nature, and anyone of any faith or even an atheist can freely benefit from the practice. Although popularized today by Buddhist teachings that came to the West, the practice of meditation predates Buddhism itself by at least one thousand five hundred years, and the Vedas by five hundred years, having its origins in the ancient Indus Valley (Harappan) civilization, where people practiced it within their culture to attain greater peace of mind. Meditation is not thinking about any particular god, or chanting a mantra, or practicing a concentration "exercise." Meditation simply involves being passively aware of and witnessing in a somewhat detached way your thoughts, emotions, and feelings.

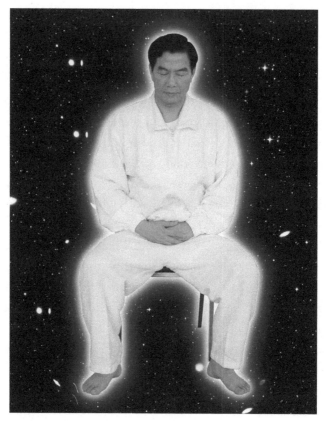

Fig. 8.3. Meditating provides inner clarity and focus that
help you manage your time more efficiently.

It is also a simple reminder that we are here now, living in the present
moment, which is, in itself, impermanent and changing. We spend so
much time regretting the past or worrying about the future, but meditation allows us to live, enjoy, and give thanks for the present moment.

Simple and Effective Breath-Awareness Meditation

Sit comfortably in a chair or on the floor with a cushion or blanket
under the base of your spine or in lotus, a classic yoga meditation posture. What's crucial is only that you have a straight spine and your body
is comfortable.

1. Gently and softly gaze at a single point in front of you, on the floor or wall, with your eyelids completely relaxed.
2. Begin to become aware of your inhalation and exhalation. Focus on observing your breathing, which is slow and full. As you exhale, allow it to be relaxed, and let the breath go completely; don't try to hold on to your breath or force it.
3. As thoughts or feelings enter your mind, keep coming back to feeling and observing your breath, exhaling thoughts and feelings with each breath.
4. As thoughts come and go (as they most certainly will), keep yourself unattached to them; just come back to your awareness of your breath. The thoughts will not stop, but with practice they will slow down dramatically.

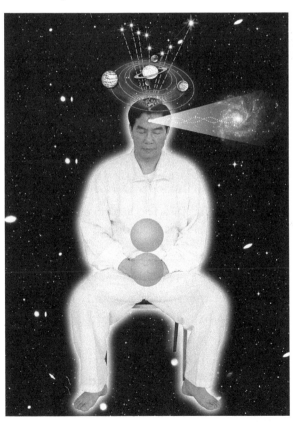

Fig. 8.4. Drawing in healing energy
from the cosmos

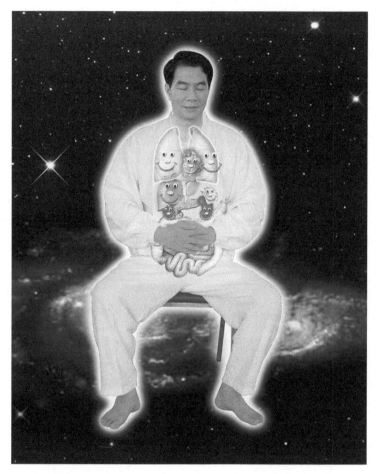

Fig. 8.5. Directing healing energy
to your vital organs

The goal here is to take a break from your thoughts and feelings, not to try to be in denial of them. You are simply having a "miniholiday" from your mind for approximately five to fifteen minutes while being a witness to your breath.

It is highly recommended that you practice meditation daily. Try to find a qualified and experienced meditation teacher with a strong lineage of respected teachers. Your teacher will be able to help you progress much further in understanding the mind, while also being a solid support in your process.

THE HEALING ENERGY OF CHI NEI TSANG (MASSAGE OF THE SECOND BRAIN)

Chi Nei Tsang (CNT) is an ancient Taoist form of detoxifying and energizing abdominal massage that was once a regular practice done in all the Taoist monasteries in China prior to the Cultural Revolution. It blends Chinese and Thai massage and meditation techniques, making it truly different from any other healing modality. The ancient Chinese believed that the mind is concentrated in the abdomen and the internal organs and not in the brain itself. Modern science backs this up by stating that the gut is the "second brain." Chi Nei Tsang works on the organs and viscera directly. As well as detoxing the body, it also has a profound effect on healing the emotions. The Taoists say our emotions are stored in the organs and that each organ has its own spirit. It could be likened to the cellular memory, which is stored over the years during times of stress and traumatic events. Treatment sessions are done regularly over several weeks or more, and their effects are profound for physical ailments as well as for clearing emotional blocks. Today many people in the world suffer from physical disease, but we also suffer from an upsurge in mental and emotional diseases, which is why this treatment is very important. Speaking from personal experience, Chi Nei Tsang has profound benefits for the energetic, emotional, and physical body.

Chi Nei Tsang literally means "the art of moving or transforming the energy of the internal organs." It uses a deep yet gentle and gradual approach, with pressure applied according to what the client can comfortably work with. It is normal for emotional releases to happen during a session, and this is very beneficial. Chi Nei Tsang complements almost any health modality, as it is unlike any other technique. A key to the practice of Chi Nei Tsang is the level of chi and the intention of the practitioner, who works with the client's natural flow of energy within the body. The practitioner does not try to push through resistance but rather allows it to dissolve as emotions are transformed. The intention of this healing art is to allow the free flow of energy in the organ meridians, not to attempt to fix or repair the client's body by working or forcing against it, which would signify that there is something wrong

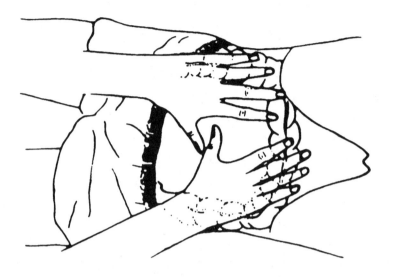

Fig. 8.6. Opening up the small and large intestines

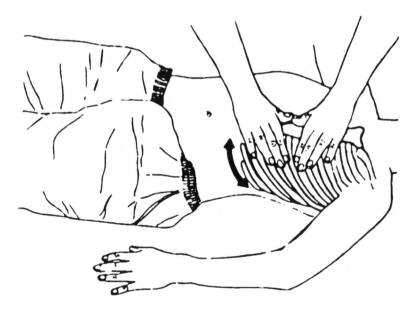

Fig. 8.7. Opening up the lungs

with the body. In this art our intention is to witness the uncomfortable sensations and blockages, which allows these blockages to dissolve, releasing the stagnant blood and chi that has been trapped within them so that the natural flow of energy can return and emotions can be felt and transformed.

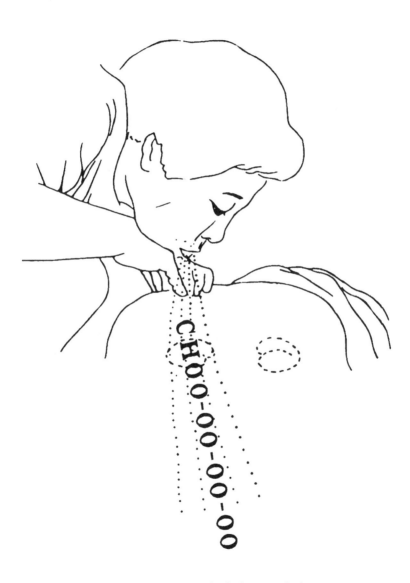

Fig. 8.8. Activating the kidneys with the
kidneys' sound—choo-oo-oo-oo

METTA AND VIPASSANA MEDITATION

"The mind is as restless as a monkey," the Buddha said. It must be trained or it will control you, causing suffering. The Buddha discovered after many years of fasting to the point of starvation and other extreme techniques in an attempt to conquer the elusive mind that the answer was to be found in what is known in Buddhism as the Middle Way and in Taoism as the balance of opposites. If the string of the guitar is too tight it will break, and if it's too loose it will not play; it must be balanced for the tune to come out, which to the Taoists is cosmic love and to the Buddhists metta (lovingkindness). To balance the mind, the Buddha found that the combination of Vipassana (insight meditation) and Metta (lovingkindness practice) are very effective methods for freeing the mind of attachments that cause mental and emotional suffering. Both of these practices help us to explore the root of the mind's suffering and the illusions of fear, anger, sadness, guilt, shame, and so forth, thereby encouraging us to return to our natural state of lovingkindness and compassion. Vipassana is not a religion; it is a technique for taming the mind and, thanks to Burmese-Indian spiritual teacher S. N. Goenka (1924–2013), this art has become more widespread and has popularized the modern Vipassana movement. Mr. Goenka attested to the power of Vipassana meditation when he said, "The only conversion of Vipassana is from misery to happiness, from bondage to liberation."

Vipassana is the art of witnessing and moving into feeling, allowing us to move away from the ego nature of the false self that is termed "I." It encourages us to move away from watching our thoughts, which are not real, toward feeling our body deeply and witnessing the sensations with equanimity. This means not to give any so-called good or bad meaning to the sensations that are felt by the mind, which is a powerful meaning-making machine. Rather our intention in Vipassana is to fully experience all sensations on a deep bodily level, allowing for the memory within the body to be released by the art of witnessing and feeling the body.

Many forms of meditation witness thoughts or imagine beautiful landscapes, whereas in Vipassana we only witness and feel things such as the breath, or witness the gross physical and subtle energetic sensations that make up our cosmic chi body. Once we have begun to witness and feel our body, our true spiritual self, which is the heart intelligence, begins to cultivate *metta,* a Pali language term for the highest form of love, which literally means "benevolent lovingkindness to all sentient beings." By breathing in and out of the heart center we can consciously send good wishes and lovingkindness to those who have harmed us, or to those whom we hold dear, such as our family and friends, and also to all sentient beings. As Vipassana meditation involves sitting for long periods of time, which can damage the chi, we recommend also practicing your Chi Kung and Universal Healing Tao practices, which will provide you with strong chi and healthy kidneys, allowing you to sit for longer periods of time without depleting your chi. This is what we call the middle road between using the benefits of Taoist and Buddhist wisdom for both emotional healing and enlightenment.

THE HEALING POWER OF GRATITUDE

When we focus on what we do not have, the worse off we feel. Conversely, the more we focus on being grateful for what we *do* have, the more peaceful we become. It's a catch-22 type of situation, where you feel you are caught on a spinning wheel like a pet mouse and you just cannot step off. Robert Emmons, a leading figure in the field of gratitude research, says, "Psychology has generally ignored the positive emotions. We tend to study the things that can go wrong in people's minds but not the things that can go right."

The good news is that there is a scientifically proven way to get out of the useless cycle of feeding negative emotions: it's called gratitude, and many of us today have forgotten this virtue's power to catapult us into self-empowerment and spiritual connectedness. All the great philosophers and spiritual teachers over many centuries have commented on the virtues of gratitude and that when extending it into our daily lives through everything we do, it opens closed eyes.

As motivational speaker Tony Robbins puts it, "The purpose of my life is to humbly serve our Lord by being a loving, playful, powerful, and passionate example of the absolute joy that is available to us the moment that we rejoice in God's gifts and sincerely love and serve all his creations."

What you focus on will grow. Is it a coincidence that people who often describe themselves as being grateful for whatever life brings them seem to suffer less stress and have better health? Is this because when we begin to focus on the many things we have to be grateful for, no matter how small they are, we become less materialistic and therefore feel less pressured by society's definition of what brings happiness? Is it any coincidence that highly evolved spiritual persons show tremendous gratitude, no matter how horrendously they may have suffered, and that this is because the act of practicing gratitude took them to the genuine feeling of gratitude in the first place?

The choice is yours; you can either focus on how beautiful the rain is, or on why the sun is not shining. You can focus on people killing one another over religion and money, or you can focus on the privilege of having fast transport, futuristic communications, and decent education—or even on the information in this book. It doesn't matter how silly it sounds—what you focus on grows. If you focus on all the so-called bad things happening in the world, you will feel suffocated by them; instead, if you focus on the achievements of so many amazing people helping others in need, you will experience heartfelt delight. Today we are generally bombarded to say the least with the "bad news" rather than the "real news." Lurid headlines sell by hooking people in; no one's arguing with that. But why are we buying "bad news"? While governments and so-called terrorists are killing innocent persons, humanitarians are feeding the hungry and curing the incurable, but how often do you hear about that? It seems that you're more likely to get a time slot on the world news if you're a murderer than if you save people's lives.

The Buddha said, "Let us rise up and be thankful, for if we didn't learn a lot today, at least we learned a little, and if we didn't learn a little, at least we didn't get sick, and if we got sick, at least we didn't die; so let us all be thankful." If you are alive and reading this book, give thanks. The sheer fact that you have the time and the ability to read this book (or to listen to it) is in itself something to be grateful for. While some people are unable to eat tonight, and others have nowhere to sleep, you have a roof over your head and food on the table and are reading this book. What about the paper this book is written on or the computer it is stored on? How many persons were involved in getting this into that format? Where would we be without them? Every day you walk down the street be thankful for our precious street cleaners. Every time you sit on a public toilet give thanks for the toilet cleaners. Every time you sit down to a meal give thanks for the hands involved in growing that food and bringing it to you, and give thanks for having the money to buy it. American motivational speaker and author of *The Psychology of Winning,* Denis Waitley, puts it succinctly when he says, "I had the blues because I had no shoes until upon the street I met a man who had no feet."

No matter how small, list your grateful thoughts and look for the simple things first. Try this easy experiment: For one whole week keep a gratitude journal with you wherever you go and make a list throughout the week of all the things, large and small, you have to be grateful for. No matter what so-called bad things may be happening in your life at the moment, focus on what you have rather than what you do not have. Regularly review your list several times a day. Gratitude brings us closer to the Creator because it ensures that we focus more on what we have come here to do, which is to return to the natural state of love and happiness.

STAYING CONNECTED TO SOURCE

How many of us actually take a little time out each day to connect with nature? As "hippie" as it may sound, hug a tree. Or probably more fashionable these days, prune your bonsai tree. The fear of loneliness is one of the greatest illusions of humankind and one of the greatest reasons so many people today are unhappy. Many of us stay in or enter into unhappy relationships because the fear of being alone is just too great. Today many relationships end because people see relationships on the material level of what they can get from their partner rather than seeing him or her as a spiritual-growth partner and facilitator. Our inbuilt fear of loneliness is reinforced during our younger years, from experiences such as parental separation, alcoholism, drugs, death of close family members, emotionally unavailable caregivers, and abandonment. The illusion and fear of loneliness is a driving force in the world today, and this is evident in the growing number of suicides and relationship and family breakdowns. Many times it is the fear of something that drives us closer to it. Communication is the key to all relationships—communion with one's true god-self and the other person's.

We must fully realize that we are never alone and that our communication and relationships with one another and with the elements of nature is vital. Mother Teresa said, "The biggest problem facing the world today is not people dying in the streets of Calcutta, and not inflation, but spiritual deprivation . . . this feeling of emptiness associated with feeling separate from God, and from all our sisters and brothers on planet Earth." For religious people, it is God whom they connect to. If you do not like the word *God,* you can substitute *Source, Universal Love, Mother-Father nature, the universal love force, the All That Is,* the *I Am That I Am, Prime Creator,* or any number of sobriquets. It could also be said that GOD refers to the three combined forces of the universe: Generate-Organize-Destroy. Whatever your faith (or nonfaith), it is important that we all feel connected, because in reality all *is* one. His Holiness the Dalai Lama says, "In past centuries, there have been many learned teachers who have laid down various paths to the realization of Truth. Among them, Lord Buddha is one, and my study of Buddhism has led me to form the opinion that despite the differences in the names and forms used by the various religions, the ultimate truth to which they point is the same."

Buddhists get connected by taking refuge in the Three Jewels: the Buddha, the guide who gave the teachings and the lineage of teachers in the first place; the Dharma, the teachings or guidebook that helps to protect the practitioner along the way; and the sangha, all the others who similarly follow the path of love and compassion as taught by the Buddha. Interestingly, the Sanskrit word *sangha* means "inseparable."

A lack of meditative prayer and humanistic compassion for all sentient beings is a core reason behind so much of today's human suffering. In the yogic philosophy of Vedanta, this form of love and relationship with God is called Bhakti yoga, the yoga of devotion, one of the four core yoga paths, the other three being Karma yoga (selfless service), Raja yoga (body and mind control, such as Ashtanga), and Jnana yoga (intellectual development). Bhakti yoga is regarded by many spiritual teachers as one of the most powerful and divine yogas, as it promotes humility and oneness, which leads to what Buddhists call *Sunyata,* or emptiness, and ultimately to nirvana.

It is true that most great saints and sages have been saying the same thing in different ways and languages. I have heard the saying, "There is only one God that we all call by different names." As the translations get changed along the way, the true meaning of the teachings often is misconstrued. Beneath all this, many of the world's great teachings teach us the same things. During my elementary school days, my fifth grade teacher promptly asked our class to make a list of all the people we did not like, as many as we could. After the lists were turned in to the teacher, it was soon shown that the students in the class with the largest lists were also themselves the most disliked. Those who have more understanding and respect for other religions other than their own, and races and ethnicities other than their own, are themselves the most liked. It is sad today that religions are fighting over something that is really all the same. Different religions have different customs and words, but we are all part of the same family that is just listening to different kinds of spiritual tunes. The word *religion* comes from Latin, meaning "to reconnect." The word *yoga* means "to unite or have union with Source." As Gandhi said, "Our ability to reach unity in diversity will be the beauty and test of our civilization."

In January 1987, the British journal *Nature* published a story that shocked the scientific community and challenged many theories of human evolution. Upon studying the mitochondrial genes within the DNA of many people from different races, religions, and parts of the world, scientists realized that all people living today have inherited their DNA from just one woman who lived approximately two hundred thousand years ago in Africa. She is called "Mitochondrial Eve" and is considered the mother of us all. What this really means is not that she was the only woman living at that time or even the very first woman on the planet; rather it means that her genes have been the only ones to survive down through all the bloodlines. When a family has boys only, the female mitochondrial DNA ceases, so therefore this Eve was the only one whose DNA continued. A similar event happened on a small scale on a remote island in Tahiti called Pitcairn Island, which was settled in 1790 by thirteen Tahitian women and six British sailors who had mutinied on the HMS *Bounty*. We know that half the original surnames disappeared in just seven generations, and if the island had remained isolated for a few more generations only one surname would have remained. Whatever way we look at it, the population of the planet has on several occasions been reduced to very small numbers of people because of great floods, ice ages, or perhaps polar shifts. Whatever the scientific explanation, there is a high chance that we are all related in some way down the line. If we can only grasp just a fraction of what this means, perhaps we would try harder to get along with others because we really are all brothers and sisters.

Studies have shown that those who enjoy regular social interaction with good and caring friends enjoy better health and a lower incidence of heart disease. In a 2004 Swedish study that was published in the *European Heart Journal,* 750 males with varying backgrounds were analyzed over a fifteen-year period to see if there was a correlation between social interaction and heart disease. The study showed that those who demonstrated a deep, emotional friendship with their friends during that period had an average of 58 percent less chance of developing heart disease.*

THE HEALTH AND SPIRITUAL BENEFITS OF PRAYER

The fourteenth-century German theologian, philosopher, and mystic Meister Eckhart declared, "If the only prayer you say in your life is 'thank

---

*A. Rosengren, L. Wilhelmsen, and K. Orth-Gomér, "Coronary disease in relation to social support and social class in Swedish men: A 15-year follow-up in the study of men born in 1933," *European Heart Journal* 25, no. 1 (2004): 56–63.

you,' that would suffice." When we make the act of prayer, we are making a special connection of communication. Sometimes there is not always a physiologist to listen to you, so you can use what you always have at your disposal: the power of prayer. It can be likened to getting rid of excess emotional baggage, and also to connecting to a spiritual force that is 100 percent within you and does not judge you. You don't need a church to pray; Jesus did not pray in churches. The universe (oneness/emptiness) listens to your concerns wherever you are, whoever you are, whatever you've done. A 2005 MANTRA (Monitoring and Actualization of Noetic Trainings) II study conducted at Duke University found that patients who received prayer were 50 to 100 percent less likely to suffer from side effects of heart medications. First names only of patients consenting to the study were sent via e-mail to Buddhist groups in Nepal, Hindus in India, Jewish groups in Jerusalem, Catholic nuns, Unity Village Missouri, and a Protestant prayer group in North Carolina.*

Legendary baseball player Satchel Paige said, "Do not pray when it rains if you do not pray when the sun shines." Most of us resort to prayer only in times of crisis or times of sudden danger, but many of the great sages and saints stressed the importance of doing personal prayer regularly and its power in spiritual evolution and in helping one to stay on one's path. For religious people, prayer is when they merge with God or pray to a prophet or messenger or a figure like Jesus. Buddhists pray to the Buddha or to the enlightened ones. God for a Buddhist is rather referred to as emptiness (which is not the same as nothingness). Buddhists interpret this as "within union or oneness lies emptiness." You need to completely empty yourself of ignorance, desire, and attachment to reach nirvana, which is beyond the concepts of the normal mind. Buddhist prayer is not directed to any particular god and is devoid of any self-centeredness or neediness; it is purely about love and compassion for all beings, wishing that all sentient beings may one day end their suffering. Its intention is to open hearts and benefit all beings.

---

*M. W. Krucoff, S. W. Crater, D. Gallup, et al., "Music, imagery, touch, and prayer as adjuncts to interventional cardiac care: The monitoring and actualisation of Noetic trainings (MANTRA) II randomised study," *Lancet* 366, no. 9481 (2005): 211–17.

Buddhist prayer has nothing to do with begging a god for personal, worldly, or heavenly gains. For those with a nonreligious or atheistic outlook, prayer can simply be a way of giving thanks for your body, life, friends, family, and so forth.

Give thanks daily in prayer for what you have and are about to receive. Begin to see the universal force that some call God in everyone and in all things, including yourself. As the ego and emotions can trick us into forgetting these facts, you need to keep your body (your vehicle) and your mind (the driver) clear of emotional pollution and remind yourself that all sentient beings are interdependently connected. Keep your life as simple as possible by handing over material attachments (things) that you no longer use, such as clothes, furniture, magazines, household appliances, etc., to others in need. Use both prayer and meditation daily for healing both physical, mental, and spiritual health complaints. As Swami Sivananda says of prayer, "One ounce of practice is worth a ton of theory."

I remember one particular saying from childhood: "Practice doesn't make perfect; perfect practice makes perfect." Similarly, by creating a daily program of some form of effective and proven spiritual practice, you ensure that you will move toward a place of a greater peace of mind. Whatever your religion or origin, daily practice of prayer, meditation, or spiritual duties of some sort helps you to become increasingly reminded of the awareness of the interdependent nature of all beings and of an omnipotent, omnipresent energy that is always within and around you. Even if you don't follow religion or believe in God, you can give thanks for your life, your family, friends, and everything you have. A Chinese proverb from Confucius goes: "I hear and I forget. I see and I remember. I do and I understand." Listen to your inner wisdom, your higher self, or, as Buddhists call it, your "Buddha mind." By daily practicing seeing yourself as neither above nor below others, you become spiritually equal to all beings. As you become a more aware and less ignorant and more enlightened being, you can share that wisdom with others to help them to suffer less.

You have all the answers inside you, and everywhere around you there are signs to guide you on your path to happiness. People will come in and out of your life for a reason, a season, or a lifetime, but they are never there forever. Use your daily practice of meditation, prayer, lovingkindness, and compassion to access answers within and be guided to the people who can provide help along the way. You are a spiritual sentient being having a human experience. It is easy for us to get caught up in the physical dimension and feel that we are physical beings having an occasional spiritual journey. Reminding yourself of this simple fact through meditation and prayer will help you to avoid getting drawn into the desires of the material world so you can maintain your spiritual evolution. Knowledge can be learned, but true wisdom can only be earned. Every situation is an opportunity to grow and learn; it is called the school of life, and you are enrolled in full-time study for your whole life. There are no mistakes really, only lessons, and these lessons are repeated until they are learned. Learn from your mistakes rather than regret or resent them. As well, learn from the mistakes of others, as chances are you may not live long enough to make all those mistakes yourself. You can learn to transform your fears that overshadow your ability to love by using these emotional healing techniques and incorporating daily spiritual practice into your life.

THE HIGHEST YOGA: HELPING OTHERS

When we are in crisis and stuck in our own suffering, one of the best things we can do is to go out there and help someone else, perhaps someone worse off than you are. It may sound strange, but today most people are less likely to help someone else when their own life is falling apart. Although Karma yoga in the true sense of the word means "doing one's duty," most of us in this fast-paced world have forgotten the importance of the Biblical admonition, "Give without being paid and you will receive without paying" (Matthew 10:8). Being so wrapped up in ourselves has made us forget about one another, and after all, it is by working together that we have progressed this far. An adage attributed to the ancient Chinese philosopher Lao-tzu says, "Being deeply loved by another gives you strength, yet loving someone deeply gives you true courage."

Try forgetting what you want for just a moment, and begin thinking about what others around you may need—friends, family, or even your neighbors. You may realize that most people around you have similar desires and dreams: to be happy, understood, and loved. Helping others also begins to heal one of the most undiagnosed diseases of our time, the loneliness that comes from a sense of separation. A common unspoken affliction in this modern world, it can be cured simply by going out and helping others in need. It is only when we become genuinely interested in others, feeling others and their needs and feeling into them and their hearts, that we truly begin to help ourselves spiritually.

According to all spiritual traditions, death is not the end, for when the physical body gives way the spirit-soul or higher consciousness moves on. While Christians say we go to heaven and Buddhists say we reincarnate, Taoists say we return the five elements to be recycled. Can we really know for sure what happens? What is sure is that consciousness is the essence of the universe and to cultivate the virtues held within are of highest importance. What also seems to hold true is what the Eight Immortal Healers represent in healing the body, which is a temple for the spirit-soul or higher consciousness. That said, no matter how much we cultivate our chi and lengthen our life span and avoid disease using the Taoist arts of Immortality, the physical body will eventually end. Therefore we must understand that Immortality is not the art of making the body live forever; rather, it is the attainment of a deep connection with one's higher nature, which is the consciousness of light. Through this connection we reach spiritual Immortality— setting our spirit-soul free to become one with the energy of the cosmos after our physical body dies. One must be prepared and aware that death can happen at any moment and that we must be grateful for every moment and every breath we take, for there are no ordinary moments. To return to our true self, our spiritual nature, is the reason we are born in the first place: to remember who we really are— spiritual beings having a human experience, not humans having a spiritual experience. In the day-to-day stress of the physical world we can easily forget this and become trapped in the material world and controlled by the sensations of pleasure that are never lasting. The

Eight Immortal Healers serve as a platform for longevity and quality of life so that one may live long enough to realize one's true nature and practice gratitude and happiness daily, self-realizing oneself as a being of love. For as the Tao Te Ching says, "Those who die without being forgotten get longevity."

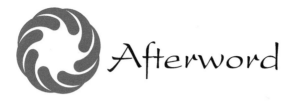 Afterword

"At the center of your being you have the answer; you know who you are and you know what you want."

LAO-TZU

"Mastering others is strength, mastering yourself is true power."

LAO-TZU

Health is becoming more and more a personal responsibility. Educating yourself on the simple laws of the human body, mind, and spirit and on how to keep yourself healthy and free from disease has never been so important. Modern medicine is doing little to educate us on these important facts on preventive medicine, while also outright suppressing many natural, true cures. Remember, true health needs to be cultivated in the same way a flower grows. A healthy flower needs sunlight, water, fertile soil, and clean air; similarly, there is more than one aspect we must address to keep ourselves healthy or to cure an illness. I have found along the way that the Eight Immortal Healers serve as a solid guide in this process. Unfortunately, governments along with the heavy influence of Big Pharma are now trying to implement the Codex Alimentarius, which places bans on natural-food supplements and herbal medicines while simultaneously increasing the production of vaccines, synthetic drugs, antibiotics, and chemicals in our food and in agricultural practices. Please understand that there is large revenue to be earned from the "sickness industry," and that the information in this book is considered a threat to the modern orthodox medical institutions and their governing bodies.

We encourage you to take back your power and your health along with it, living to the fullest, in happiness and health. Remember to help others also along your way who are less fortunate than yourself, with their health and well-being. We challenge you to dream and take action to influence the alignment of both forms of medicine to side by side become effective in easing the suffering of all sentient beings, while simultaneously teaching us how to prevent disease and have a healthier way of life, physically, emotionally, and spiritually. Is this not the job that medicine should be doing? We have relied on scientists to bring us the most advanced computers and communication systems year after year, which they have done. Yet modern medicine has failed to cure or even reduce the incidences of killer diseases like cancer, heart disease, diabetes, and arthritis, which it has promised to do for so long. We can send a man to the moon, build international space stations, connect to the Internet, and speak to one another any place in the world, yet modern allopathic medicine cannot find any real cause or cure for our major chronic diseases. Let the truth be known about the true causes and cures of disease, and may it spread its wings and fly to all the corners of this blue planet!

Remember, love is your gift to the world, not money. Money can buy things to help us survive, and it can even buy people for a while, but it can never buy love. Taoist philosophy tells us that it is love and living in harmony with that love within nature and its laws that is our natural state. In truth, there is only one sickness, and that is homesickness, separation from and longing for our true home—union with God through moving with the Tao and being like water once again.

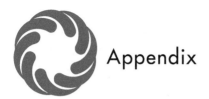 Appendix

The Eight Immortal Healers Nutritional System

This nutritional system is not a diet or fad; it is a balanced Taoist lifetime system based on a predominantly plant-based, whole foods diet that is environmentally friendly and spiritually ethical and should be used along with food-combining guidelines and metabolic typing.

ENJOY EATING THESE FOODS ✦ ENVIRONMENTALLY ETHICAL, ALKALINE-NEUTRAL-FORMING, GLUTEN-FREE, PLANT-BASED, ORGANIC, WHOLE FOODS	AVOID OR LIMIT THESE FOODS ✦✦ NONENVIRONMENTALLY ETHICAL, RAJASIC AND TAMASIC, ACID-FORMING, GLUTINOUS, ANIMAL-BASED OR PROCESSED REFINED FOODS
Foods marked with a diamond (✦) in this "Enjoy" column are high in natural sugars or fat and should always be eaten in moderation—even by those who tolerate them well. For those who have conditions that make them sensitive to sugar or fat, they should only be eaten in small amounts with caution.	Foods marked with a double diamond (✦✦) in this "Avoid" column are best avoided during a detox. They can, however, be eaten in moderation at other times as part of a balanced diet. Always choose organic non-GMO options.
Fresh vegetables (raw salads, lightly cooked/steamed vegetables), herbs and spices, fresh fruits (apples, berries, cherries, etc.), ✦dried fruits	Canned, frozen, microwaved vegetables, canned and processed fruits, ✦✦garlic

ENJOY EATING THESE FOODS◆	AVOID OR LIMIT THESE FOODS◆◆
Legumes (beans, peas, and lentils— soak and sprout for optimal assimilation and digestion), fermented soy products (tempeh, miso, natto, fermented tofu), seaweeds and sea vegetables	Commercially farmed meats & eggs & seafood, ◆◆organic grass-fed meats, ◆◆free-range eggs, ◆◆wild-caught seafood, processed veggie-meats/mock-meats, ◆◆unfermented organic soy (tofu, soy products, etc.)
Raw nuts (almonds, Brazils, walnuts, pecans, macadamias, chestnuts, pistachios), seeds (pumpkin, sunflower, hemp, chia, perilla), sacha inchi, flax, sesame/tahini, carob (activate/ soak/dehydrate all raw nuts to access nutrients and aid digestion)	◆◆Cacao, ◆◆cashews, ◆◆peanuts (avoid all commercial nut butters containing sugar and oil or salted nuts and seeds that are cooked and flavored and contain vegetable oils; instead try almond or Brazil nut butters or tahini)
Gluten-free whole grains (brown/ red/black/wild rice, millet, buckwheat, amaranth, quinoa, sorghum; organic whole grains or stone-ground flours of these grains/seeds), sprouted Essene bread	Gluten grains (wheat, barley, and any products or refined flours and manufactured carbohydrate foods made from these grains), ◆◆rye, ◆◆oats, ◆◆kamut, ◆◆spelt, ◆◆corn
◆Oils and butters (cold-pressed essential oils such as flax, perilla, chia, hemp, black current, coconut) (For high-heat cooking use only coconut and macadamia; for low heat use rice bran and grapeseed; add oils at end of cooking for flavor and nutrition.)	Refined vegetable oils (especially canola), artificial butter spreads (organic raw-mild butters are superior to fake butter that is made with refined vegetable oil containing carcinogenic/ processed trans fats), ◆◆cold-pressed organic olive oil, ◆◆organic raw-mild butter, ◆◆ghee
Plant-based milks (rice, oat, almond, coconut), ◆non-GMO organic whole soy (unfermented soy, even organic, is not recommended during pregnancy, and for babies or those with thyroid/ hormonal issues)	Pasteurized/homogenized dairy products (destroys enzymes and alters fats), ◆◆organic raw-milk dairy products (cow, goat, sheep), ◆◆raw-milk kefir, GM soy milk and soy protein isolate milk, ◆◆organic (non-GMO) whole soy milk (unfermented soy is not recommended for pregnancy, babies, or those with thyroid-hormonal issues or gut problems)
Beverages (pure, fresh water, coconut water), ◆vegetable juices (dilute 50 percent with water) (avoid fruit juices as they are high in sugar; fruits best consumed whole, blended, or add for flavor to vegetable juice; eat some fruit seeds, too), herb teas (roasted dandelion root), ◆raw sugarcane juice	Sodas/soft drinks, energy drinks, yogurt drinks (contain bad sugars), flavored milks, commercial instant coffees and teas, ◆◆organic small-batch coffee, ◆◆water-processed decaf coffee, ◆◆organic teas (chai, green, and oolong, etc.)

ENJOY EATING THESE FOODS*	AVOID OR LIMIT THESE FOODS**
*Organic sweeteners (organic raw honey, *molasses, yakon, maple syrup, stevia, coconut sugar, *rapadura sugar, agave)	White and brown sugar/sucrose, high-fructose corn syrup, artificial sweeteners (saccharin, aspartame, sucralose, asphaltum-K, etc. (all contain neurotoxins that damage the brain and central nervous system), **sugar alcohol sweeteners (**xylitol, **erythritol, **Lakanto), rice malt syrup
Salts (Celtic sea salt, Himalayan pink salt (unprocessed/sun-dried/hand-harvested; both contain trace minerals for nervous system, immunity, blood pressure, hydration)	Salts (common iodized table salt, common refined sea salt (refined salt dehydrates and poisons heart, arteries, kidneys), MSG, maltodextrins
Homemade dressings, sauces, dips (tamari and shoyu; i.e., traditionally fermented soy)	Condiments (commercially made and bottled sauces, dressings, and dips, unfermented soy sauce), refined pasteurized vinegars, commercially pasteurized/fermented foods
Fermented probiotic foods (raw, fermented vegetables such as kimchi, sauerkraut), unpasteurized apple cider vinegar, coconut vinegar	Antibiotics and pharmaceuticals (whenever possible), recreational drugs, tobacco smoking, alcohol
Herbal-mineral antibiotics, antivirals (olive leaf, barberry, andrographis, turmeric, colloidal silver, H_2O_2, Master Mineral Supplement, potassium iodide, grapeseed extract)	Whey protein isolate or concentrate (contains excitotoxins), body-building protein powders and bars with flavorings and artificial sweeteners, **pea protein, **organic cold-filtered whey
Superfoods (organic sprouted/fermented brown rice protein powder, hemp protein powder, super greens and reds powders, superfood formulas, raw superfood bars)	
Note: Eat to 80 percent full, as undereating helps cure illnesses and builds the immune system, while overeating even healthy food causes acid imbalance. Chew slowly. Combine with gentle yoga, Tai Chi, and Chi Kung to help to alkalize and balance the body (too much intense physical exercise can acidify the body).	**Note:** Avoid overeating and eating too fast. Overeating even healthy food causes acid residues and disease. Intense physical exercise can cause acidity and imbalance the body.

METABOLIC TYPE
(FOOD GROUP RATIOS)

There are three types of metabolic constitutions: protein (P), mixed (M), carbohydrate (C). Different metabolic (constitutional) types need different ratios of nutrients as follows:

Protein type (P). Feels better after high-protein/fat meals, but tired after higher carb meals

Mixed type (M). Tolerates both proteins and carbs generally well

Carbohydrate type (C). Feels tired from high protein/fat foods and better after eating higher carb meals

The good old-fashioned food pyramid bases our diet on grains that contain gluten and may have contributed to today's health crisis, so I prefer to use the ratios described in the table below as a guide to a healthy diet for the three metabolic types. The three basic groups of nutrients—proteins, carbohydrates, and fats—can be confusing because no single plant or animal is completely composed of just protein, carbohydrate, or fat alone. For example, nuts are high in protein but also in fat; brown rice is high in protein but also in carbohydrates; avocados are high in fat but also in protein. So where do these mixed foods fit in on our chart? We must put them in the section that corresponds to their dominant nutrient, the nutrient they have the most of.

Note: Animals in nature eat a 100 percent raw diet; only humans cook, and they eat far too much cooked food. Eat at least 50 to 80 percent of your diet as living raw and fermented/cultured foods! Enzymes in raw food are the missing link in healing. Increase gradually, and eat more raw food in summer and less in winter.

METABOLIC-TYPE BASIC GUIDELINES
FOR A BALANCED DIET

NONSTARCHY VEGETABLES AND FRUITS + HERBS AND SPICES (55% P TYPE, 60% M TYPE, 65% C TYPE)

Vegetable to sweet fruit ratio depends on one's metabolic type, sugar tolerance, and climate; start with 80:20 vegetable to fruit ratio and listen to your body. Eat fruits whole and on an empty stomach (avoid juicing fruits except certain low-sweet fruits in combination with vegetables for flavor).

PROTEINS (20% P TYPE, 15% M TYPE, 10% C TYPE)

Sprouted legumes, fermented soy, green beans, peas, lentils, sprouted beans, mushrooms, algae and seaweed, seeds, organic eggs,* organic meat and seafood*

COMPLEX CARBOHYDRATES (10% P TYPE, 15% M TYPE, 20% C TYPE)

Complex, low-glycemic, unrefined, non-GMO, gluten-free whole grains; starchy vegetables (with skins); cooked beans

FATS (15% P TYPE, 10% M TYPE, 5% C TYPE)

Avocados, olives, lychees, nuts and nut butters, seeds, coconut flesh, cold-pressed oils, butter and ghee*

*Not to be taken during detox cleanse.

Digestion begins in your mouth and not your stomach, so chew food well and slowly. Avoid overeating or eating when stressed. Be present with food, and it will be a gift to you. Animal milk is primarily designed for baby animals, not adult humans! Some tolerate dairy in small amounts, especially when fermented, while others don't. If you consume animal milk products (never consume them during a cleanse-detox), choose organic and raw dairy only. Naturally fermented foods aid in digestion and assimilation, while also nourishing the intestinal bacteria and boosting the immune system. Such beneficial foods include raw sauerkraut, kimchi and cultured/fermented vegetables, fermented soy products (macrobiotics), kombucha, and kefir made from coconut milk or raw organic milk.

FOOD-COMBINING LAWS

Eating even healthy food in poor combinations will cause illness. Animals do not combine many different foods in a sitting like humans, and we, unlike animals, also suffer from indigestion, gas, bloating, weight gain, and sluggish digestion when we do.

Proteins and carbohydrates individually combine well with vegetables and fats but do not combine well with each other. Avoid combining animal proteins with high-protein vegetables (beans) in the same meal.

Low-carb vegetables combine well with all food groups except most fruits (certain fruits such as citrus, apple, grapes, and kiwi can be combined with vegetable juices for flavor, usually without any problem).

Fruits combine with nothing else, so eat fruit alone or leave it alone (melons also should be eaten completely alone, even separate from other fruits).

Fats combine well with proteins and low-carb vegetables but poorly with high-carb vegetables.

Milk and dairy products do not generally combine well with any other food group (that said, vegetables are the most tolerable combination). Just as baby animals take them, raw dairy products (the only permitted dairy) are best enjoyed alone, or leave them alone.

DAILY MENU PLAN GUIDE

Break-fast: Choose one of the following (alternate when you feel the need)*

1. Fresh fruits or berries in season
2. Superfood smoothie: use water, coconut water/milk, or grain or nut milk, supergreens powder, fruit (banana, papaya, and/or berries), hemp or rice protein or flaxseeds/sunflowers/almonds, raw carob powder, cinnamon powder, vitamin C or nutritional powder

---

*Try to break your daily fast as late in the day as possible, around noon or midafternoon so you eat your first and second meals as close together as possible to get the maximum results available from daily "cyclic intermittent fasting."

3. Cold-pressed vegetable and fruit juice cocktail (carrots, apple, ginger, beets, grapes, lemon, greens, etc.)
4. Gluten-free organic raw muesli or porridge with grain or nut milk plus supergreens powder
5. Poached eggs or vegetable omelet with steamed greens, green peas/beans, sprouts, and salad
6. Homemade vegetable or unpasteurized miso soup with coriander, mushrooms, and seaweed
7. Raw or lightly cooked vegetable and pea/bean soup with sprouts or cultured/fermented vegetables

Evening main meal: Choose one of the following (alternate when you feel the need)

1. Mixed vegetable salad with sprouts, olives, avocado, or goat cheese, nuts and seeds; use healthy homemade salad dressing (e.g., tahini dressing with hemp or flaxseed oil)
2. Low-fat raw vegetarian meal (raw vegan pasta, lasagne, pizza)
3. Garden salad and vegetable or miso soup and sprouted Essene bread or 100 percent whole-grain bread, rye or brown rice biscuit, or sourdough or gluten-free bread
4. Mixed vegetable and fruit juice cocktail (carrots, apple, ginger, beets, grapes, lemon, greens)
5. Steamed vegetables with tamari and tahini plus garden salad, with brown/red rice or gluten-free grain
6. Baked vegetables (with herbs and coconut oil) plus garden salad, plus brown/red rice or gluten-free grain
7. Vegetable curry or vegetable casserole plus garden salad, plus brown/red rice or gluten-free grain
8. Asian-style spiced vegetable and tempeh soup with coconut milk and mushrooms
9. Raw or lightly cooked vegetable pea/bean soup with sprouts or cultured/fermented vegetables
10. Homemade vegetarian pizza with goat cheese on Essene bread or 100 percent organic whole-grain bread

11. Grilled tempeh, fish, sardines, or organic chicken with steamed greens plus garden salad
12. Mixed vegetable/fruit juice cocktail (carrots, apple, ginger, beets, lemon, grapes, and greens)

Snacks

- Fresh fruit eaten whole or unsweetened organic dried fruit (figs, dates, and apricots)
- Cold-pressed vegetable juice cocktails (add the aforementioned fruits for flavor only)
- Raw, dehydrated, homemade vegetable chips (made from vegetable juice, extracted pulp, and herb seasonings)
- Raw, dehydrated, homemade kale chips
- Raw vegan dessert
- Nuts and seeds
- Whole tender coconut or coconut water
- Herbal teas

If you do intense physical labor you may need three meals per day but still do your best to eat these three meals in a window between noon and 8:00 p.m.; otherwise eat twice daily. We overeat, plain and simple! Eat twice daily, and have those two meals as close together as you can for best "cyclic intermittent fasting," which Taoists have always said promotes longevity, and which is now backed up by modern scientific proof. Place these charts on the refrigerator or pantry door. Then you'll know all this by heart very soon; also take a copy of it when you go shopping to make food selections easier!

About the Authors

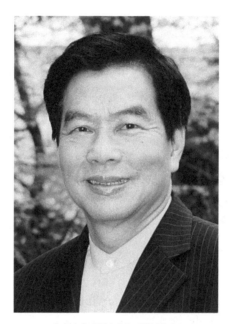

MANTAK CHIA

Mantak Chia has been studying the Taoist approach to life since childhood. His mastery of this ancient knowledge, enhanced by his study of other disciplines, has resulted in the development of the Universal Healing Tao system, which is now being taught throughout the world.

Mantak Chia was born in Thailand to Chinese parents in 1944. When he was six years old, he learned from Buddhist monks how to sit and "still the mind." While in grammar school he learned traditional Thai boxing, and he soon went on to acquire considerable skill in aikido, yoga, and Tai Chi. His studies of the Taoist way of life began in earnest when he was a student in Hong Kong, ultimately leading to his mastery of a wide variety of esoteric disciplines, with the guidance of several masters, including Master I Yun, Master Meugi, Master Cheng Yao Lun, and Master Pan Yu. To better understand the mechanisms behind healing energy, he also studied Western anatomy and medical sciences.

Master Chia has taught his system of healing and energizing practices to tens of thousands of students and trained more than two thousand instructors and practitioners throughout the world. He has established centers for Taoist study and training in many countries around the globe. In 1990 and in 2012, he was honored by the International Congress of Chinese Medicine and Qi Gong (Chi Kung), which named him the Qi Gong Master of the Year.

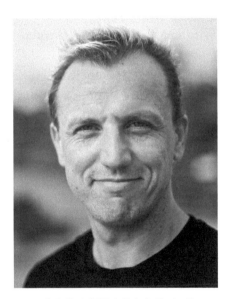

JOHNATHON DAO

Johnathon Dao is a clinical health practitioner and medical researcher of natural medicine with twenty-two years of clinical experience, including a Universal Healing Tao practice. He holds degrees and diplomas in traditional Chinese medicine (TCM), acupuncture, herbal medicine, shiatsu, kinesiology, medical Chi Kung, yoga therapy, and several other natural medicine therapies, including a doctorate M.D.(A.M.) (doctor of medicine in alternative medicines). He is also the founder of E-motion Yoga, which is aimed at healing emotional pollution and recovering from PTSD and associated mental health problems. His studies began at the age of eighteen, when he came across a book by Master Mantak Chia.

In his practice of medicine he endeavors to continue learning and maintain a constant state of humble surrender and being willing to make mistakes and learn from them, turning them into lessons, which is how he came upon the Eight Immortal Healers. He believes that healing is a choice, and that disease is not something that randomly or unfairly affects one "victim" over another, but rather something that is created gradually or in some cases rapidly by dietary choices and lifestyle and through our thoughts and actions.

Johnathon is available to perform consultations for clients worldwide via Skype and offers his services as a public speaker on natural medicine. He currently resides on the Gold Coast, Queensland, Australia, and can be contacted directly through his website:

www.cureplanet.com.

The Universal
Healing Tao
System and
Training Center

THE UNIVERSAL HEALING TAO SYSTEM

The ultimate goal of Taoist practice is to transcend physical boundaries through the development of the soul and the spirit within the human. That is also the guiding principle behind the Universal Healing Tao, a practical system of self-development that enables individuals to complete the harmonious evolution of their physical, mental, and spiritual bodies. Through a series of ancient Chinese meditative and internal energy exercises, the practitioner learns to increase physical energy, release tension, improve health, practice self-defense, and gain the ability to heal him- or herself and others. In the process of creating a solid foundation of health and well-being in the physical body, the practitioner also creates the basis for developing his or her spiritual potential by learning to tap into the natural energies of the sun, moon, earth, stars, and other environmental forces.

The Universal Healing Tao practices are derived from ancient techniques rooted in the processes of nature. They have been gathered and integrated into a coherent, accessible system for well-being that works directly with the life force, or chi, that flows through the meridian system of the body.

Master Chia has spent years developing and perfecting techniques for teaching these traditional practices to students around the world through ongoing classes, workshops, private instruction, and healing sessions, as well as books and video and audio products. Further information can be obtained at www.universal-tao.com.

THE UNIVERSAL HEALING TAO TRAINING CENTER

The Tao Garden Resort and Training Center in northern Thailand is the home of Master Chia and serves as the worldwide headquarters for Universal Healing Tao activities. This integrated wellness, holistic health, and training center is situated on eighty acres surrounded by the beautiful Himalayan foothills near the historic walled city of Chiang Mai. The serene setting includes flower and herb gardens ideal for meditation, open-air pavilions for practicing Chi Kung, and a health and fitness spa.

The center offers classes year-round, as well as summer and winter retreats. It can accommodate two hundred students, and group leasing can be arranged. For information on courses, books, products, and other Universal Healing Tao resources, see below.

RESOURCES

Universal Healing Tao Center
274 Moo 7, Laung Nua, Doi Saket, Chiang Mai, 50220, Thailand
Tel: (66)(53) 921-200
E-mail: universaltao@universal-tao.com
Web site: www.universal-tao.com

For information on retreats and the health spa, contact:
Tao Garden Health Spa & Resort
E-mail: reservations@tao-garden.com
Web site: www.tao-garden.com

Good Chi • Good Heart • Good Intention

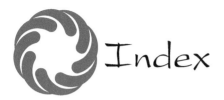

Index

Numbers in *italics* indicate illustrations.

BOOKS OF RELATED INTEREST

EMDR and the Universal Healing Tao
An Energy Psychology Approach to Overcoming Emotional Trauma
by Mantak Chia and Doug Hilton

Chi Self-Massage
The Taoist Way of Rejuvenation
by Mantak Chia

Craniosacral Chi Kung
Integrating Body and Emotion in the Cosmic Flow
by Mantak Chia and Joyce Thom

Iron Shirt Chi Kung
by Mantak Chia

Chi Kung for Prostate Health and Sexual Vigor
A Handbook of Simple Exercises and Techniques
by Mantak Chia and William U. Wei

The Six Healing Sounds
Taoist Techniques for Balancing Chi
by Mantak Chia

Healing Love through the Tao
Cultivating Female Sexual Energy
by Mantak Chia

Healing Light of the Tao
Foundational Practices to Awaken Chi Energy
by Mantak Chia

INNER TRADITIONS • BEAR & COMPANY
P.O. Box 388
Rochester, VT 05767
1-800-246-8648
www.InnerTraditions.com

Or contact your local bookseller